Neuromuscular Problems in Orthopaedics

Neuromuscular Problems in Orthopaedics

EDITED BY

C. S. B. GALASKO

MSc, ChM, FRCS(Eng), FRCS(Edin)

Professor of Orthopaedic Surgery
University of Manchester
Consultant Orthopaedic Surgeon
Royal Manchester Children's Hospital
and Hope Hospital, Salford

BLACKWELL SCIENTIFIC PUBLICATIONS

OXFORD LONDON EDINBURGH

BOSTON PALO ALTO MELBOURNE

© 1987 by
Blackwell Scientific Publications
Editorial offices:
Osney Mead, Oxford, OX2 0EL
8 John Street, London, WC1N 2ES
23 Ainslie Place, Edinburgh, EH3 6AJ
52 Beacon Street, Boston
   Massachusetts 02108, USA
667 Lytton Avenue, Palo Alto
   California 94301, USA
107 Barry Street, Carlton
   Victoria 3053, Australia

First published 1987

Set, printed and bound by Holmes McDougall Ltd.,
Edinburgh.

DISTRIBUTORS

USA
   Year Book Medical Publishers
   35 East Wacker Drive
   Chicago, Illinois 60601

Canada
   The C.V. Mosby Company
   5240 Finch Avenue East
   Scarborough, Ontario

Australia
   Blackwell Scientific Publications
     (Australia) Pty Ltd
   107 Barry Street
   Carlton, Victoria 3053

British Library
Cataloguing in Publication Data
Neuromuscular problems in orthopaedics.
   1. Orthopedia   2. Neurology
   I. Galasko, C.S.B.
   617'.3   RD732
   ISBN 0-632-01347-8

Contents

Contributors

P. AICHROTH MS, FRCS. *Consultant Orthopaedic Surgeon, Westminster Hospital and Westminster Children's Hospital, London, UK.*

N. J. BARTON FRCS. *Consultant Orthopaedic Surgeon, Department of Hand Surgery, University Hospital, Nottingham, UK.*

J. C. DRENNAN MD. *Director of Orthopaedics, Newington Children's Hospital, Newington, Connecticut, USA.*

V. DUBOWITZ BSc, PhD, MD, FRCP, DCH. *Professor of Paediatrics, Department of Paediatrics and Neonatal Medicine, Royal Postgraduate Medical School, London, UK.*

E. N. FEIWELL MD. *Associate Clinical Professor, Department of Orthopaedics, University of Southern California School of Medicine. Attending Orthopaedic Surgeon, Rancho Los Amigos Hospital, Downey, California, USA.*

C. S. B. GALASKO MSc, ChM, FRCS(Eng), FRCS(Edin). *Professor of Orthopaedic Surgery, University of Manchester, UK. Consultant Orthopaedic Surgeon, Royal Manchester Children's Hospital and Hope Hospital, Salford, UK.*

J. Z. HECKMATT MB, BCh, MRCP. *Nattrass Memorial Lecturer in Paediatric Neurology, Department of Paediatrics and Neonatal Medicine, Royal Postgraduate Medical School, London, UK.*

M. M. HOFFER MD. *Chief, Children's Orthopaedic Service, Rancho Los Amigos Hospital, Downey, California. Professor and Chief, Division of Orthopaedic Surgery, University of California, Irvine, Orange, California, USA.*

J. D. HSU MD, CM, FACS. *Clinical Professor, Department of Orthopaedics, University of Southern California School of Medicine. Attending Orthopaedic Surgeon, Rancho Los Amigos Hospital, Downey, California, USA.*

M. KOFFMAN MD. *Assistant Clinical Professor, Department of Orthopaedics, University of Southern California School of Medicine. Attending Orthopaedic Surgeon, Rancho Los Amigos Hospital, Downey, California, USA.*

M. J. McMASTER MD, FRCS. *Consultant Orthopaedic Surgeon, Princess Margaret Rose Orthopaedic Hospital and Royal Infirmary, Edinburgh. Honorary Senior Lecturer, University of Edinburgh, UK.*

A. M. K. RICKWOOD FRCS. *Consultant Paediatric Urologist, Alder Hey Children's Hospital, Liverpool, UK.*

B. A. ROPER MA, FRCS. *Consultant Orthopaedic Surgeon, The London Hospital. Honorary Consultant Hand Surgeon, Hospital for Sick Children, Great Ormond Street, London. Consultant Orthopaedic Surgeon, King Edward VII Hospital for Officers, London, UK.*

W. J. W. SHARRARD MD, ChM, FRCS. *Consultant Orthopaedic Surgeon, Sheffield Children's Hospital. Professor of Orthopaedics, University of Sheffield, UK.*

J. A. YOUNG MB, ChB, FRCP(Glas), MRCP(Lond). *Consultant Paediatric Neurologist, Tayside Health Board. Honorary Senior Lecturer in Child Health and in Neurology, University of Dundee, UK.*

Preface

Neurological problems are responsible for a large part of children's and adult orthopaedic practice. They include injuries to the spinal cord, cauda equina, nerve roots and peripheral nerves; compression of the spinal cord, cauda equina, nerve roots and peripheral nerves by prolapsed disc, tumour and a variety of other lesions; and a variety of conditions that primarily affect some part of the nervous system and which frequently are associated with secondary deformities that affect adversely the patient's quality of life.

It is not possible in a book of this size to deal with every neurological problem that may require orthopaedic intervention. The detailed techniques of repair of nerve injuries have not been included, but methods of tendon transfer to improve function following nerve damage in the upper limb have been mentioned. The management of spinal injuries, quadriplegia and paraplegia has not been included but the treatment of spina bifida has. Although spina bifida is a congenital anomaly of the spine, it is a neurological problem in that the spinal cord, nerve roots or both are often involved. This leads to secondary deformity, and a multitude of orthopaedic procedures have been designed to improve the quality of life of these patients. The treatment is multidisciplinary, orthopaedic surgery only playing a part. Therefore, separate chapters have been devoted to the general management and the orthopaedic management of this condition.

The medical management of cerebral palsy, and the dystrophies, neuropathies and myopathies is ill understood by the average orthopaedic surgeon, whereas the average neurologist and paediatrician may not fully appreciate what modern orthopaedic surgery can offer children with these conditions. Therefore, the medical and orthopaedic management have been described in separate chapters. Poliomyelitis is rarely seen in Europe or North America, although it still frequently occurs in the undeveloped world. It has not been discussed in a separate chapter, but the principles of treatment are mentioned in chapters discussing the orthopaedic management of regional problems.

The orthopaedic management of the effects of neuromuscular disorders in specific areas such as the spine, upper limbs, hips, knees and feet is so important that it has been discussed in separate chapters.

The orthopaedic management of the stroke patient is an often neglected field and, therefore, a chapter has been devoted to this subject.

During the past few years there has been an increasing recognition of the need for orthopaedic surgery in the management of many patients with neurological disorders. The aim of this book is to present the orthopaedic management of patients with neurological disorders, to indicate the place of orthopaedic surgery in the overall care of these patients and particularly in the treatment of secondary deformities.

Although the book is aimed primarily at orthopaedic surgeons, it is hoped that it will also be of interest to neurologists and paediatricians by demonstrating how modern orthopaedic surgery can help their patients.

C.S.B.G.
Manchester, 1986

Acknowledgements

I am most grateful to the contributors to this volume, without whom it would not have been possible to produce the book. I would like to thank the publishers for their help, my secretary, Mrs Margaret Powis, for all her work, the Department of Medical Illustration at the Royal Manchester Children's Hospital for its help and in particular my wife and children for their unstinting support.

This book is dedicated to the staff of the Royal Manchester Children's Hospital, without whose hard work I would not be able to treat patients with orthopaedic problems secondary to neuromuscular disorders.

Chapter 1
Medical Aspects of Cerebral Palsy

J. A. YOUNG

Cerebral palsy is 'a disorder of movement and posture due to a defect or lesion of the immature brain' (Bax 1964). A single definition does not describe adequately the great variety of clinical states encompassed by it. These range from the intelligent, educationally and socially successful child with an awkward gait to the profoundly retarded, immobile, deformed epileptic who is totally dependent on others. The classification used here closely follows that suggested by Ingram (1964), with the addition of the dysequilibrium syndrome (Hagberg *et al.* 1972), and is shown in Table 1.1.

Table 1.1 Classification of cerebral palsy.

Type	Qualification
Hemiplegia	left
	right
Double Hemiplegia	
Diplegia	hypotonic
	dystonic
	rigid
	spastic
Ataxia	
Dysequilibrium	
Dyskinesia	dystonic
	choreoid
	athetoid
	tension
	tremor
Mixed	for example, ataxic diplegia

It is important to note that double hemiplegia is not the simple arithmetic sum of two hemiplegias. The terms tetraplegia and quadriplegia will not be used here. They are usually considered to be synonymous with double hemi-plegia but are sometimes less accurately used to describe any condition in which all four limbs are involved. This is clearly undesirable.

The fact that this descriptive classification reflects the motor disorder should not disguise the fact that many and in some cases most of the cerebral palsied child's difficulties stem from damage to other areas of the nervous system. These difficulties include mental retardation, specific cognitive and perceptual problems that cause social and educational failure, defects of hearing and vision, speech disorders, central sensory defects, vasomotor disturbances in the limbs, convulsions, poor physical growth and disturbed behaviour.

Aetiology

Aetiological factors are usually considered under the headings Prenatal, Intranatal, Postnatal and Unknown. In recent years opinion has swung back to the view that prenatal factors are of considerable importance (Holm 1982). They are the major causes of hemiplegia, double hemi-plegia, the congenital ataxias, the dyse-quilibrium syndrome and also the diplegia of the children born at term described by Hagberg *et al.* (1975): whereas for spastic diplegia of pre-maturity, ataxic diplegia and the dyskinetic cerebral palsies, intranatal and immediately postnatal factors are mainly to blame.

In early pregnancy, damage is caused by various teratogens: chemical, such as foods and drugs; physical, such as X-rays; and intrauterine infection by such organisms as *toxoplasma gondii*, rubella virus or cytomegalovirus. In most cases, however, the cause is not identified. In later pregnancy, placental dysfunction causing fetal undernutrition and asphyxia is mostly involved. During birth, hypoxic–ischaemic damage and intracranial haemorrhage assume major importance.

The ability to carry out serial study of the neonatal and early infantile brain by realtime ultrasound through the anterior fontanelle has enhanced our understanding of the relative importance of haemorrhage and anoxic–ischaemic infarction. Periventricular and intraventricular haemorrhage are common findings in preterm babies, but are of little consequence unless accompanied by persistent dilation of the ventricles or parenchymal extension of the haemorrhage (Stewart *et al.* 1983, Catto-Smith *et al.* 1985). Anoxic–ischaemic induced cystic leucomalacia which occurs in the periventricular region in preterm babies and in the subcortical vascular watershed zones in term babies, is always accompanied by poor neurodevelopmental outcome (De Vries *et al.* 1985, Trounce & Levene 1985). Periventricular leucomalacia is associated with spastic diplegia whereas subcortical leucomalacia results in double hemiparesis and a high incidence of cortical blindness and other defects of higher neurological function. It often seems that devastation of the brain is caused by the summation of a series of individually minor incidents, whereas full recovery is frequently possible after a single major insult to a previously well fetus or neonate. In the postnatal period, haemorrhage, infection, metabolic disturbance and trauma including baby battering become the most frequent causes. The small preterm baby is especially prone to intraventricular haemorrhage as a complication of hypothermia, apnoeic attacks or assisted ventilation. In any population of children with cerebral palsy, low birthweight, multiple pregnancy and the male sex are over-represented. In those cases where the cerebral palsy is symmetrical and a clear aetiology cannot be demonstrated it is probable that the disorder is inherited (Bundey & Griffiths 1977).

Survival of babies of very low birthweight, that is 1500 g or less, is providing an interesting new group. In a recent review Levene and Dubowitz (1982) calculated that roughly 10% of survivors have obvious cerebral palsy and about 15% are mentally retarded. These very low birthweight babies account for most of the diplegia of prematurity that is now seen (Davies & Tizard 1975), although in those surviving mechanical ventilation more severe 'cortical' defects are to be expected (Marriage & Davies 1977).

Pathophysiology

In all but the mild and localized forms of cerebral palsy, the basic defect is a failure of the higher centres to impose their function on the primitive brain stem responses of the neonate. This deprives the child of voluntary control over his own posture and can be recognised by the retention of the repertoire of primitive responses. The most disabling of these is the tonic labyrinthine response which causes extensor hypertonus when the child is supine or the head is extended, and flexor hypertonus when the child is prone or the head is flexed. In the child with the asymmetric tonic neck reflex (Fig. 1.1), turning the head to one side results in extension of the arm on the side to which the face is turned with flexion of the other arm. Similar but less marked changes occur in the legs. In the symmetric tonic neck reflex, extension of the neck muscles results in extension of the arms and flexion of the legs with the reverse on flexion of the neck. Development of the parachute and equilibrium responses is delayed.

There also is inefficiency of postural fixation without which the child cannot counteract the force of gravity and develop voluntary control over the position of his own body (Fig. 1.2).

Spasticity

Spasticity may be defined as an increase in muscle tone, often of clasp knife quality, due to damage to the upper motor neuron and accom-

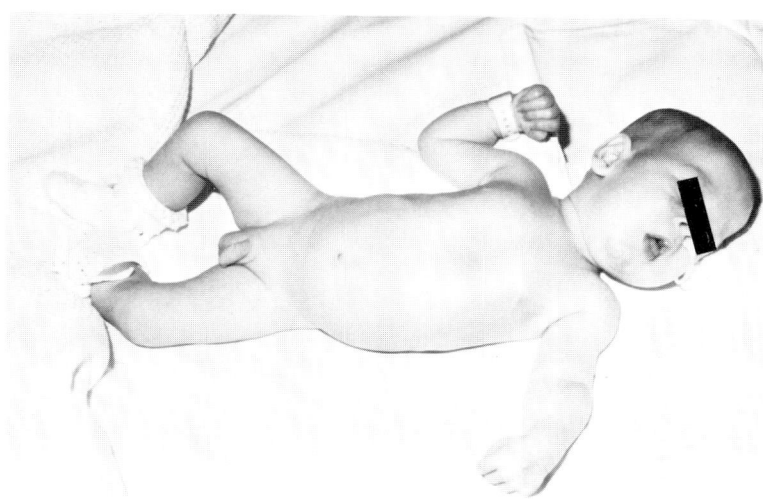

Fig. 1.1. The asymmetric tonic neck reflex.

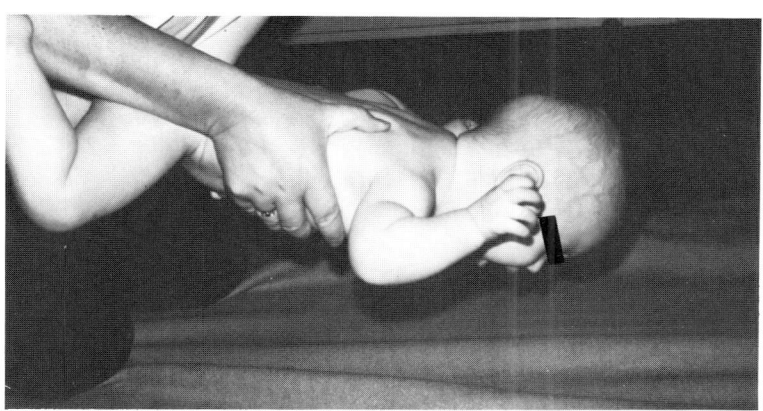

Fig. 1.2. The absence of forward parachute response in a spastic baby.

panied by increased stretch reflexes, clonus and an extensor plantar response. Unfortunately, most of the spastic cerebral palsied patient's difficulty is due not to this simple spasticity but to more complicated neurological dysfunction. The main functional defect resulting from the upper motor neuron lesion is loss of voluntary innervation and of an important inhibitory function that regulates the timing and degree of innervation of muscles within a synergic group. McLellan (1977) and Milner-Brown and Penn (1979) have shown that co-contraction occurs instead of reciprocal inhibition when all but the most mildly spastic patients attempt voluntary movements. It is this and not the increased mus-

cle tone that impairs voluntary activity. The findings of Knutsson and Richards (1979) in a group of adult hemiplegics may well be relevant to the problem in children with spastic cerebral palsy. They identified three patterns of muscle activation. *Type 1* consisted of abnormal early activation of calf muscles and sometimes of adductors induced by stretch. This group had only mild gait impairment. *Type 2* patients had spastic stretch reflexes but they showed reduced EMG activity in peripheral muscle groups. In *type 3* abnormal co-contractions disrupted the normal sequential shift of activity in antagonistic muscle groups. In a few cases they found more complex abnormalities. These findings have relevance to the discussion on the place of anti-spastic drugs and neurosurgical therapy in cerebral palsy.

Weakness is universally found in spastic muscles but sometimes what appears to be weakness is in fact reciprocal inhibition.

Clinical presentation

The very early diagnosis of cerebral palsy is notoriously difficult, but Ellenberg and Nelson (1981) have shown that on clinical examination at age 4 months the finding of excessive muscle tone in neck extensors, arms, legs or trunk is associated with an increased risk of subsequent cerebral palsy as high as 74-fold. A note of caution must be sounded about the early diagnosis of cerebral palsy because a significant proportion of children lose their signs as they grow. The children that are most likely to outgrow their physical signs are those with mild changes, with monoparesis, with one of the ataxic syndromes or with diplegia. Unfortunately these children in later years of childhood show a high incidence of mental retardation, speech defects, seizures, squints and behavioural difficulties (Nelson & Ellenberg 1982).

Causing distress to parents by wrongly diagnosing a disorder of development must be avoided, but it is useful to recognize the early signs.

Hemiplegia

Children with congenital hemiplegia usually present between the ages of 3 and 9 months when inadequate use of the affected hand is noted and there is poor weightbearing on the affected leg. However, careful observation in earlier months will show poverty of movement with hypotonia and a posture of pronation in the forearm and fisting of the thumb. The arm tends to lie alongside the baby's body. There is no difficulty with the diagnosis of the fully developed clinical picture when there is paresis of the limbs of one side, the upper limb usually being more severely affected than the lower. Posture is dominated by flexion, adduction, internal rotation and this determines the nature of the fixed deformities that tend to develop. The limbs may be dwarfed to varying degrees and some show thecutaneous changes of vasomotor instability. Cortical sensory loss tends to be associated with more marked degrees of dwarfing and more severe loss of function in the limb. Some severely affected children show also the choreo-athetoid type of associated movements. There may be visual field defects or convulsions. Intelligence can be normal or low and children of normal intelligence can have specific learning disorders.

Acquired hemiplegia may present as part of an acute illness with seizures if an acute encephalopathy is the cause, or it may be an isolated event of quiet onset if the aetiology is carotid artery obstruction. The flaccid stage lasts days or weeks and is followed by spasticity.

Double hemiplegia (totally involved)

Double hemiplegia is almost always obvious in the neonatal period with either the apathy or the irritability syndrome. There is a high incidence of convulsions and of feeding difficulties associated with pseudobulbar palsy. Spasticity of decorticate or decerebrate pattern quickly replaces hypotonia and motor development is severely impaired. The upper limbs are at least as severely affected as the lower. The development of the windswept posture (Fulford & Brown 1976) is frequent in these children if they are allowed to lie in a posture that is dictated by the asymmetric tonic neck reflex (Fig. 1.3). Almost all of these children are profoundly mentally retarded and epileptic. Other developmental malformations are common.

Diplegia

The earliest stage of diplegia is usually hypotonia but with brisk tendon reflexes. There is poverty

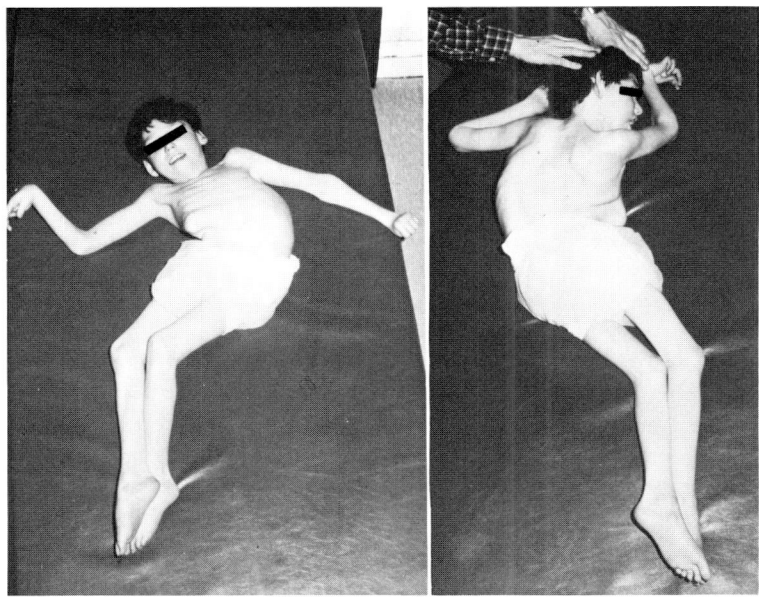

Fig. 1.3. The windswept deformity.

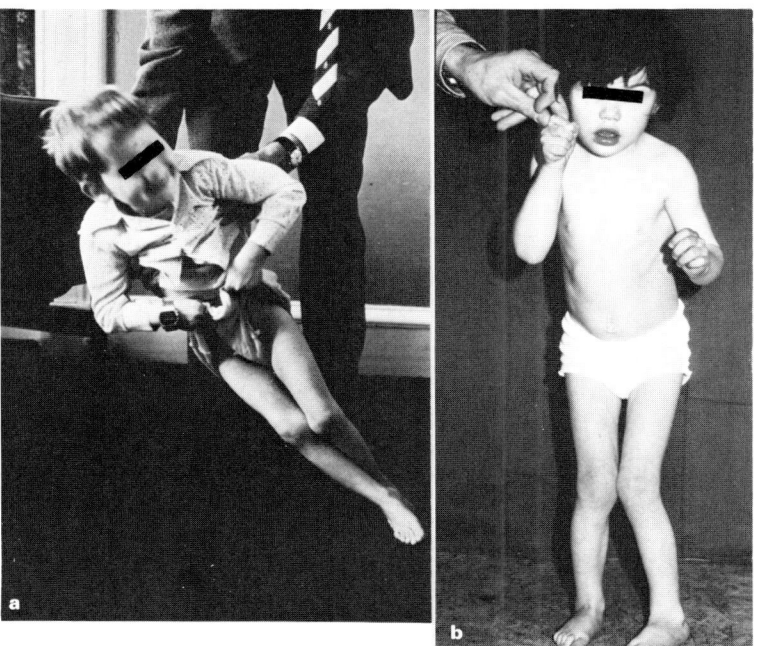

Fig. 1.4. Spastic diplegia.
(a) Dystonic phase, showing the typical posture of the lower limbs with an absence of parachute and equilibrium reactions.
(b) Spastic phase.

of spontaneous movement. Later, as head control develops, tone increases and in vertical suspension the baby assumes a dystonic posture (Fig. 1.4) with extended adducted legs, equinus, flexed pronated arms and fisted thumbs. At this stage there is a tendency to bouts of excessive extensor tone. A phase of rigidity follows when there is generalized extensor hypertonous and this is followed by the spastic phase (Fig. 1.4b), with the characteristic flexed adducted internally rotated posture, most marked in the lower limbs, and a tendency to develop fixed deformities. Diplegic babies are frequently first referred to an orthopaedic surgeon in this phase because of limited hip abduction and suspected dislocation or because of an equinus position of the feet. It is important to distinguish the simple diplegia of prematurity, where the child has suffered damage only to the periventricular white matter and therefore is of normal intelligence and usually free from fits, from the diplegia associated with more widespread brain damage and therefore with the whole range of neurological problems.

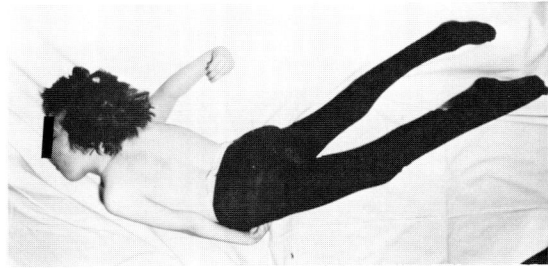

Fig. 1.5. Severe dystonic spasm.

Ataxia

The infant destined to have ataxia is hypotonic with diminished tendon reflexes and general immobility. Motor development is slow and characterized by incoordination and poor balance. As the child's mobility increases, intention tremor and other cerebellar signs become increasingly obvious but nystagmus is rare. Such children are usually of normal intelligence although some are mentally retarded. Epilepsy is rare.

Dysequilibrium syndrome

The baby with dysequilibrium syndrome is profoundly hypotonic to a degree that suggests weakness. Tendon reflexes are diminished and there is virtually no control of posture. Motor development is extremely slow and the child may not walk until the age of 8 or 9 years, if at all. A degree of mental retardation frequently adds to the child's difficulties but convulsions are rare.

Dyskinesia

The dyskinetic cerebral palsies present in the neonatal period with apathy, hypotonia and a tendency to apnoeic spells. This stage is followed by irritability, convulsions and transient hypertonicity which in turn is followed by a latent period in which hypotonia reappears. There is slow motor progress and persistence of the primitive responses. This latent period lasts for months and then the involuntary movements become increasingly obvious. The first sign of this stage is that any attempted activity by the baby results in an uncontrollable mass movement usually of an opisthotonic nature. Severely damaged babies may never grow out of this stage (Fig. 1.5), others progress to more discrete involuntary movements that occur against a background of low resting tone and persistence of the primitive responses. These children have profound motor difficulty and delay. Intelligence is frequently normal, convulsions are rare but difficulties with speech and with feeding are inevitable.

Investigations

The EEG will show a wide range of focal and generalized abnormalities. It may occasionally influence the choice of anticonvulsant but it is the presence or absence of clinical seizures in the child and not the findings on EEG examination that will determine whether anticonvulsants are indicated or not.

Computerized tomography (CT scan) may show ventricular dilation in diplegia, cerebral atrophy in double hemiplegia, porencephalic cyst with or without atrophy and ventricular dilation on one side in hemiplegia, or occasionally congenital defects of the cerebellum in the ataxic syndromes. There is however no one-to-one relationship between appearances on the CT scan and the clinical picture and once again this examination has very little or no bearing on therapy, unless serial examinations show increase in the size of the ventricles or of a porencephalic cyst in association with a deteriorating clinical picture. On the whole, investigations that will explain the aetiology, and therefore help with genetic counselling, or those that will assist in differential diagnosis are more important. These include the search for serological evidence of intrauterine infection, biochemical disturbances and defects of lysosomal enzymes that are associated with the inherited, progressively deteriorating conditions such as metachromatic leucodystrophy. Investigations that have a direct bearing on clinical management are the usual orthopaedic X-rays. Dynamic EMG studies provide a more realiable basis for the planning of orthopaedic surgery (Csongradi *et al.* 1979, *see also* Chapter 2), this technique may usefully be supplemented by the full facilities of a gait analysis laboratory equipped with a television computer gait analysis system which includes force plates to measure ground reaction forces (*see* Chapter 2).

Management

Management of the child with cerebral palsy often must begin before a definitive diagnosis is reached. The central theme must be instruction of the parents on how to cope. The handicapped child does not elicit the responses from his attendants that the normal child does, so the parents must learn how to take the initiative in introducing each new stage of development. The diagnosis of a type of cerebral palsy or the identification of the aetiology is useful as a basis for genetic counselling and for formal medical and surgical treatment, but it is of negligible value in guiding the overall management of the child. For this purpose a functional profile of the child's abilities and disabilities must be constructed and this is best achieved by a multidisciplinary team (Young 1977). In this way an integrated programme of therapy can be devised with the object of helping the child to reach the next stage of his developmental sequence. As each new stage is reached the functional profile changes and the therapy programme is adjusted. It is essential to establish the child's visual and auditory abilities, to correct any correctable defects and compensate for others by appropriate training methods. During brain development there is a sensitive period for the development of each function. We must make sure that the child is not deprived of the opportunity to develop each skill during its sensitive period. Language must be assessed and either the development of speech assisted if necessary, or an appropriate system of nonverbal communication provided. Most handicapped people are of the opinion that communication is more important to them than ambulation.

Physiotherapy and occupational therapy are often best provided together. There has been a tendency in recent years for therapists to concentrate more on posture and function than on work with individual muscle groups. Thus in the first year or so of life, therapy will consist largely of instruction of the parents in such simple techniques as how to lift, carry and feed their infant. Guidance must be provided about such things as resting posture that will avoid windsweeping in inactive children, or about seating arrangements that will facilitate hand function or feeding in children with retention of primitive reflex patterns or in those lacking postural control. There have been few controlled studies of the benefit of physiotherapy. Wright and Nicholson (1973) found it to be of no value in preventing physical deformity but there is a widespread belief that children and their parents who have the benefit of a therapist are improved in a general way.

What is appropriate will vary with the developmental age of the child (Potter & Harryman 1973). For instance, parents of children with extensor hypertonus are encouraged to avoid placing the child supine, when the tonic labyrinthine response will increase the tendency to hyperextension. In side-lying, a forward position of the shoulders is encouraged and the hands come towards the midline. The parents are shown how to carry and feed the child in a flexed position which will facilitate head control and diminish the tendency to tongue thrust. The child's acquisition of head control is assisted by play in the prone position, perhaps with the chest supported on a wedge and by pulling-to-sit with the shoulders held forward; as head control improves, support is provided further and further down the trunk. The hypotonic baby with poor postural control must be provided with seating that gives stability to the trunk and if necessary the head, so that the child does not just lie on his back looking at the ceiling and so that the hands can be free to grasp and explore objects.

As the child passes through the various stages that lead to walking, different techniques of therapy will be appropriate. Some will benefit from orthoses, sometimes to prevent deformity, sometimes to stabilize posture and sometimes to guide movement. Some will progress through the use of standing frames and walking aids to independent walking, some will always be dependent on aids, others will never proceed beyond a wheelchair. Such a chair must be carefully designed to prevent deformity and to allow maximum function. In the design and manufacture of all of these aids, the cooperation of a bioengineer and an orthotist is invaluable.

The occupational therapist must devise ways of providing the child with experiences that promote his perceptual–cognitive development. This involves giving him experience of different positions, for instance on top of and underneath furniture, and of watching brick building and the completion of shape puzzles as a child at that stage of development would attempt them. Effort must be made to increase the child's awareness of his own body. When the child reaches school age education must take priority, but the therapists still have an important part to play in advising about posture and mobility aids that prevent deformity and allow the child to reach his educational potential.

Drug treatment of convulsions

The traditional anticonvulsants Phenobarbitone and Phenytoin cause such a high incidence of unwelcome side-effects, especially those affecting behaviour and educational performance, that they should not be used until other drugs have been tried and have failed. Carbamazepine is the drug of choice for tonic–clonic seizures, both focal and generalized, and for psychomotor attacks. Sodium Valproate is useful for generalized epilepsies both of the tonic–clonic and of the absence types, but is of less use in focal seizures. Important but rare side-effects such as liver damage, pancreatitis and bleeding tendency due to platelet dysfunction limit the use of this drug. The benzodiazepines, Nitrazepam and Clonazepam, are useful in the myoclonic epilepsies.

Drug treatment of spasticity

The hope of uncovering a function that has been obliterated by spasticity has led to the trial of many agents that reduce muscle tone. The three drugs that are used for this purpose at present are Diazepam, Baclofen and Dantrolene (*Drug and Therapeutics Bulletin* 1983). Diazepam acts on polysynaptic reflexes and so reduces tonic activity but it also has prominent central effects. On the whole it is more useful in athetoid than in spastic patients. Sedation, ataxia, disinhibition and drooling are prominent side-effects.

Baclofen has an action that is similar to but does not exactly mimic the actions of gamma-aminobutyric acid. It acts mainly on presynaptic terminals in the spinal cord where it depresses the release of an excitatory transmitter. It seems to be particularly active in the fusimotor system and has been shown in many controlled studies to relieve spinal spasticity, being particularly effective in the treatment of painful flexor spasms. More recently it has also been shown to reduce spasticity due to a cerebral lesion, but the few controlled trials of the drug in cerebral palsy, while confirming the antispastic action, show disappointingly little change in the quality or quantity of unassisted voluntary activity (McKinlay *et al.* 1980). Nausea, sedation, confusion, nocturnal enuresis and loss of posture are prominent side-effects of Baclofen.

Dantrolene acts in the muscle itself; normal depolarization of muscle membrane takes place but Dantrolene causes a decrease in the release of activator calcium from the sarcoplasmic reticulum thus diminishing the force of contraction. Dantrolene too has been shown to reduce muscle tone in all forms of spasticity. It reduces clonus, hyper-reflexia, stiffness and cramps but once again there is not a lot of evidence that this leads to improved function in cerebral palsy (Joynt & Leonard 1980). Prominent side-effects of Dantrolene include drowsiness, dizziness, weakness, general malaise, diarrhoea and liver damage. The serious nature of these side-effects limits the use of this drug.

Neurosurgery

Attempts to reduce tone by neurosurgical means such as chronic cerebellar stimulation have produced similar overall results to drug therapy. In some patients it has been possible to demonstrate reduction of spasticity but double blind studies have not really confirmed functional benefit (Penn 1982). Selective posterior rhizotomy will interrupt the afferent fibres from the muscle spindles and thus decrease the facilitatory effect on the alpha anterior horn cells, so reducing tone in the muscle served by that nervous arc. Peacock and Arens (1982) have reported good results in a group of spastic patients, but one suspects that more extensive study will show that it is only in those patients in whom spasticity is the major cause of the problem that benefit is obtained, and that the procedure will not help the majority whose difficulty lies in co-contraction. Stereotaxic

neurosurgical procedures such as ventrolateral thalamotomy or dentatotomy give mixed results (Gornall *et al.* 1975), but they may have a place in the management of very carefully selected patients.

The intramuscular injection of 50% solution of alcohol in normal saline gives effective but temporary relief from spasticity. The main value of this procedure is that it gives the physiotherapist and orthopaedic surgeon an opportunity to assess the probable success of surgery to that muscle (Carpenter & Seitz 1980).

Drug treatment of dyskinesia

Drug treatment has little to offer this group of patients but in athetosis Diazepam may be tried. Tetrabenazine has been of very doubtful value in this condition (Heggarty & Wright 1974) but it does help patients with chorea (Swash *et al.* 1972). Drowsiness and depression are frequent side-effects that limit its use.

References

BAX M.C.O. (1964) Terminology and classification of cerebral palsy. *Developmental Medicine and Child Neurology*, **6**, 295–7.

BUNDEY S. & GRIFFITHS M.I. (1977) Recurrence risks in families of children with symmetrical spasticity. *Developmental Medicine and Child Neurology*, **19**, 197–91.

CARPENTER E.B. & SEITZ D.G. (1980) Intramuscular alchohol as an aid in management of spastic cerebral palsy. *Developmental Medicine and Child Neurology*, **22**, 497–501.

CATTO-SMITH A.G., YU V.Y.H., BAJUK B., ORGILL A.A. & ASTBURY J. (1985) Effect of neonatal periventricular haemorrhage on neurodevelopmental outcome. *Archives of Disease in Childhood*, **60**, 8–11.

CSONGRADI J., BLECK E. & FORD W.F. (1979) Gait electromyography in normal and spastic children with special reference to quadriceps femoris and hamstring muscles. *Developmental Medicine and Child Neurology*, **21**, 738–48.

DAVIES P.A. & TIZARD J.P.M. (1975) Very low birthweight and subsequent neurological defect (with special reference to spastic diplegia). *Developmental Medicine and Child Neurology*, **17**, 3–17.

DE VRIES L.S., DUBOWITZ L.M.S., DUBOWITZ V., KASER A., LARY S., SILVERMAN M., WHITELAW A., & WIGGLESWORTH J.S. (1985) Predictive value of cranial ultrasound in the newborn baby: A reappraisal. *Lancet*, **II**, 137–140.

Drug and Therapeutics Bulletin (1983) Drugs to relieve spasticity. **21**, 1–3.

ELLENBERG J.H. & NELSON K.B. (1981) Early recognition of infants at high risk for cerebral palsy: examinations at age 4 months. *Developmental Medicine and Child Neurology*, **23**, 705–16.

FULFORD G.E. & BROWN J.K. (1976) Position as cause of deformity in children with cerebral palsy. *Developmental Medicine and Child Neurology*, **18**, 305–14.

GORNALL P., HITCHCOCK E. & KIRKLAND I.S. (1975) Stereotaxic neurosurgery in the management of cerebral palsy. *Developmental Medicine and Child Neurology*, **17**, 279–86.

HAGBERG B., SANNER G. & STEEN M. (1972) The dysequilibrium syndrome in cerebral palsy. Clinical aspects and treatment. *Acta Paediatrica Scandinavica*, **Supplement 226.**

HAGBERG B., HAGBERG G. & OLOW I. (1975) The changing panorama of cerebral palsy in Sweden 1954–1970. II Analysis of various syndromes. *Acta Paediatrica Scandinavica*, **64**, 193–200.

HEGGARTY H. & WRIGHT T. (1974) Tetrabenazine in athetoid cerebral palsy. *Developmental Medicine and Child Neurology*, **16**, 137–42.

HOLM V.A. (1982) The causes of cerebral palsy. A contemporary perspective. *Journal of the American Medical Association*, **247**, 1473–7.

INGRAM T.T.S. (1964) *Paediatric Aspects of Cerebral Palsy.* p. 12 E. & S. Livingstone Ltd., Edinburgh and London.

JOYNT R.L. & LEONARD J.A. (1980) Dantrolene sodium suspension in treatment of spastic cerebral palsy. *Developmental Medicine and Child Neurology*, **22**, 755–67.

KNUTSSON E. & RICHARDS C. (1979) Different types of disturbed motor control in gait of hemiparetic patients. *Brain*, **102**, 405–30.

LEVENE M.I. & DUBOWITZ L.M.S. (1982) Low birthweight babies: long-term follow-up. *British Journal of Hospital Medicine*, **28**, 487–93.

MCKINLAY I., HYDE E. & GORDON N. (1980) Baclofen — a team approach to drug evaluation of spasticity in childhood. *Scottish Medical Journal*, **Supplement 1**, S26–S28.

MCLELLAN D.L. (1977) Co-contraction and stretch reflexes in spasticity during treatment with Baclofen. *Journal of Neurology, Neurosurgery and Psychiatry*, **40**, 30–8.

MARRIAGE K.F. & DAVIES P.A. (1977) Neurological sequelae in children surviving mechanical ventilation in the neonatal period. *Archives of Disease in Childhood*, **52**, 176–82.

MILNER-BROWN H.S. & PENN R.D. (1979) Pathophysiological mechanisms in cerebral palsy. *Journal of Neurology, Neurosurgery and Psychiatry*, **42**, 606–18.

NELSON K.B. & ELLENBERG J.H. (1982) Children who 'outgrew' cerebral palsy. *Paediatrics*, **69**, 529–36.

PEACOCK W.J. & ARENS L.J. (1982) Selective posterior rhizotomy for the relief of spasticity in cerebral palsy. *South African Medical Journal*, **62**, 119–24.

PENN R.D. (1982) Chronic cerebellar stimulation for cerebral palsy: A review. *Neurosurgery*, **10**, 116–21.

POTTER P. & HARRYMAN S. (1973) Physical and occupational therapy for the handicapped child. *The Paediatric Clinics of North America*, **20**, 159–76.

STEWART A.L., THORBURN R.J., HOPE P.L., GOLDSMITH M., LIPSCOMB A.P. & REYNOLDS E.O.R. (1983) Ultrasound appearance of the brain in very preterm infants and neurodevelopmental outcome at 18 months of age. *Archives of Disease in Childhood*, **58**, 598–604.

SWASH M., ROBERTS A.H., ZAKKO H. & HEATHFIELD K.W.G. (1972) Treatment of involuntary movement disorders with tetrabenazine. *Journal of Neurology, Neurosurgery and Psychiatry*, **35**, 186–91.

TROUNCE J.Q. & LEVENE M.I. (1985) Diagnosis and outcome of subcortical cystic leucomalacia. *Archives of Disease in Childhood*, **60**, 1041–1044.

WRIGHT T. & NICHOLSON J. (1973) Physiotherapy for the spastic child: an evaluation. *Developmental Medicine and Child Neurology*, **15**, 146–63.

YOUNG J.A. (1977) The multidisciplinary approach to assessment and treatment. In Drillien C.M. & Drummond M.B. (eds) *Neurodevelopmental Problems in Early Childhood*. pp. 16–21. Blackwell Scientific Publications Ltd, Oxford.

Chapter 2
Principles of the Orthopaedic Management of Cerebral Palsy

M. M. HOFFER

Introduction and classification

A child with cerebral palsy suffers a non-progressive, non-hereditary disease with diffuse neurological manifestations (Chapter 1). There are three descriptive types of cerebral palsy. The *spastic* patient has hyperactive reflexes, clonus and stretch reaction. Most cerebral palsy bracing and surgery have been applied to this group of patients with good results. A second type of cerebral palsy is that of the *motion disorders*. These have been called athetosis, chorea, dyskinesia and ataxia. These motion disorders have slightly different meanings neurologically (*see* Chapter 1), but the differences are inconsequential as far as an orthopaedic surgeon is concerned. This is because we have little to offer these patients with motion disorders. A third type of cerebral palsy is that of *mixed problems*. Here the spasticity co-exists with the motion disorder. It is important to distinguish these patients because the surgical procedures and the bracing that we use for such individuals may not be as effective or predictable as they are for the patient with spasticity alone.

Cerebral palsy patients have involvement either of one side *(hemiplegic)*, both lower extremities *(diplegic)* or all four extremities *(totally involved* or *double hemiplegic)*. The author prefers not to use the terms paraplegic and quadriplegic to identify involvement of the lower extremities, and of all four extremities respectively. The reason not to use these words is that they imply spinal cord problems. Diplegic patients, for example, always have some involvement of their upper extremity and totally involved patients, for example, usually have major problems in communication and cognition.

In making prognostic predictions in these patients, it is important to realize that most hemiplegic patients will ambulate without any surgery. Surgical procedures are designed to help them ambulate better. Diplegic patients with balance reactions by the age of three will ambulate. At the time they develop balance reactions, they will lose the primitive asymmetric and symmetric tonic neck reflexes. The totally involved patient will rarely ambulate and it is extremely important to set realistic goals for patients in this group. Walking requires a great deal of support for them. Braces are cumbersome and crutches difficult to use for many of these children. Ambulation is usually not practical. Patients may require surgery and orthoses to aid in sitting. However, it must be realized that any operative procedure that sacrifices hip and knee flexion helps these patients appear straighter, but can also affect their ability to sit. These patients' basic orthopaedic problems are those of sitting. Scoliosis and painfully dislocated hips are the most common problems that affect sitting in these children. The painful dislocated hip in these patients is distinctly different from the non-spastic dislocated hip associated with congenital dislocations or paralysis (Chapter 8).

Reflex levels are most important in determining balance reaction required for independent sitting and ambulation (Evans 1971, Goldner 1971, Bleck 1975). The most easily determined and probably the most significant are the asymmetric and symmetric tonic neck reflexes (Chapter 1). Patients with obligatory tonic neck reflexes rarely develop balance and are poor candidates for ambulation. The parachute reaction, on the other hand, suggests that balance will be achieved. Patients who do not achieve parachute reactions and have persistent obligatory tonic neck reflexes by the age of three years should not be considered candidates for functional ambulation. If they do not develop these reactions within six years they may have difficulty in independent sitting.

When studying individual limbs, two general factors must be determined:

1   The sensation in the limb and the control of the muscles in the limb. Sensory defects should not be studied by primitive pain tests but by the more sophisticated tests of sensibility *(see below)*. This is especially true in the upper limbs. Sensation is the 'soul' of the upper extremity and no surgical procedure or orthosis can substitute for it.

2   Control refers to the ability of the patient to call on muscles to work singly in a specific manner. If muscle testing is done with joints restrained in disadvantageous postures, some muscles will appear totally paralysed. When allowed facilitation of pattern in their motion, these muscles may show unrestrained strong contractions. For example, testing anterior tibial activity with the hip and knee extended may show weak activity. However, if the testing is done with the hip and knee flexed strong anterior tibial muscle activity may be noted. Flexing these joints adds power to the anterior tibial muscle. Muscle grading alone is insufficient; control is the problem. The muscle may not be weak; it may be a slave to pattern.

Classification of sitting and ambulation

There are three types of sitting. *Propped sitting* is the least sophisticated type. All that is necessary is a straight back and loose hips. In patients with poor balance reactions, a loose cerebral palsy body brace may be used as a propping device,

and various head supports may be required in other cases. Ankle and knee orthoses are not necessary in these patients, nor are surgical procedures on the foot or knee. Surgical spinal stabilization (Chapter 7) and hip procedures (Chapter 8) may be required to keep these patients sitting.

Self-propped sitters need support but can maintain sitting balance momentarily. In these patients all that may be required is a modified wheelchair.

Independent sitters have support reactions and need no orthotic devices for their hip or back. Special attention should be given to their wheelchairs, as these patients have the potential for independent transfer and should have removable arm rests. In addition, patients may require surgical procedures on their knees (Chapter 9) and feet (Chapter 10) to allow them to utilize their lower limbs to transfer to and from a chair.

There are four types of ambulation in disabled individuals (Hoffer *et al.* 1973). In *community ambulation,* patients walk both indoors and outdoors during most activities and may need crutches, braces or both. They use wheelchairs only for long trips out of the community. In *household ambulation,* patients only walk indoors with the support of some type of apparatus. They get in and out of chairs or beds with little, if any, assistance and may need a wheelchair for some indoor activities at home or at school. In *non-functional ambulation,* walking is a therapy session in the home, school or hospital. Patients use a wheelchair for all functional needs. In *non-ambulation,* patients may stand and transfer but they are truly sitters as they cannot maintain the balance necessary for forward progression.

Hemiplegics can achieve functional ambulation; diplegics who develop balance reactions by the age of three years and whose hips are stable and not dislocated will walk functionally, whereas few totally involved patients achieve functional ambulation.

Surgical plans for ambulatory patients

Only the principles will be outlined in this chapter. The details of surgery to the hip, knee and foot are discussed in Chapters 8, 9 and 10 respectively.

Spastic diplegia

These patients' hip problems interfere with ambulation more than the knees and feet. Adduction contracture permitting less than 30° of abduction requires gracilis and adductor longus release and if at the time of surgery there is residual contracture, adductor brevis release. The author advises against obturator neurectomy in these patients because of the risk of hyperabduction. Obturator neurectomy is reserved for the subluxing hip of the totally involved.

For the flexed posture in the spastic diplegic patient, there are two schools of thought; one group advises iliopsoas myotomies whereas the other suggests release of rectus femoris and all the other hip flexors, but sparing iliopsoas. Ambulatory electromyography (Perry *et al.* 1976) may help distinguish the hyperactivity of the iliopsoas from the rectus femoris, and help determine which procedure is required for the individual patient.

In the spastic diplegic patient who has no significant hip contractures, the knee and foot should not interfere with knee walking. If the patient can knee walk independently of hand use, but has fixed contractures of the knee and ankle, appropriate releases of these areas should be carried out. Hamstring lengthening should be done cautiously and only when there is some fixed contracture. The problem here is that over-lengthening results in recurvatum.

The spastic diplegic often has equinovalgus feet. Heel cord lengthening, peroneus brevis lengthening and a Grice procedure (Grice 1952) usually corrects this posture. Tendon transfers for valgus of the hindfoot have not been successful in cerebral palsy. The Grice procedure the author likes to perform utilizes a calcaneal plug taken by the Cloward instrument and a staple over the sinus tarsi.

Hemiplegia

Most of the problems are distal, usually an equinovarus deformity of the foot. Here there is a dilemma as to what is the deforming force. Is it the anterior tibialis, the posterior tibialis or the triceps surae? The gait electromyogram (Perry *et al.* 1974) helps differentiate the possible causes. The author advises that if the orthopaedic surgeon does not have this facility, the heel cord and tibialis posterior are lengthened. If the surgeon is fortunate enough to have these gait studies, and can distinguish between gastrocnemius and soleus hyperactivity, a decision can be made as to whether gastrocnemius slide or heel cord lengthening is indicated. The surgeon can also distinguish a tibialis posterior active in stance and swing and a tibialis anterior active in stance and swing.

The overactive anterior tibial muscle in stance and swing requires a split anterior tibial tendon transfer (Hoffer *et al.* 1974, Chapter 10). The anterior tibial tendon is split longitudinally from its insertion and is transferred subcutaneously to the cuboid. Immediate ambulation in a short leg plaster is permitted, and a brace is applied at four weeks to be worn for at least a year.

The overactive posterior tibial muscle in stance and swing requires lengthening at the musculotendonous junction (Ruda & Frost 1971). In the rare situation when a posterior tibial muscle is active exclusively in the swing phase, an anterior muscle transfer is indicated (Bisla & Louis 1975).

If the varus deformity is fixed, an osteotomy of the calcaneus may be required in addition to the above (Silver *et al.* 1967).

Surgical procedures for the totally involved

Here the basic problems are those of hip motion and spine deformity. It is often difficult to control the hip position unless the spine is well controlled. It has been our experience that for minor curvatures of the spine of less than 20°, body jackets can be used for control. Beyond that point early fusions may be necessary (Chapter 7). Lower limb deformities are amenable to soft tissue releases and obturator neurectomies. However, the totally involved child who had a hip that is subluxed will require a varus osteotomy and even a Chiari acetabuloplasty. If the hip is truly dislocated, and has ascended from the acetabulum, it is too late for these more complex operative procedures. The author's results with shortening these high dislocated hips have been variable, probably because of early degenerative changes. It is suggested that this procedure is not used without a great deal of discussion with the family. Girdlestone head and neck resections, including proximal third femoral resections, have been fraught with problems including heterotopic bone and significant bone loss and we no longer advise these procedures. Total joint replacements have also resulted in problems primarily due to loosening.

Upper extremity surgery *(see also pp. 206–210)*

The key issues in the upper extremity are the cognition of the patient, the sensibility of the extremity, the ability to place the hand, and the control of the muscles in the upper extremity.

Cognition is that complex of processes that indicate intelligence. Perception, abstract reasoning and communication are all part of this complex. Testing for this may be very difficult in these children. Children falling within the first standard deviation of normal are termed normal; between the first and second standard deviation educable (IQ 50–70); and between the second and third standard deviations trainable (IQ 30–50). Children below this level are severely or profoundly retarded. In general, only those individuals with educable or higher cognitive capacity may expect functional results from upper extremity surgery.

Hand placement is dependent on shoulder and elbow control. It consists of range of motion, precision of placement and time requirement for placement (Hoffer 1978). The range of motion is limited by spasticity and contractures. Precision is limited by motion disorders. Time of placement is limited by those motion disorders affecting the pathway of motion. In general, only individuals who can place the affected hand on the head and then the opposite knee within a period of five seconds can expect good functional results from upper extremity surgery (Fig. 2.1, Hoffer 1978).

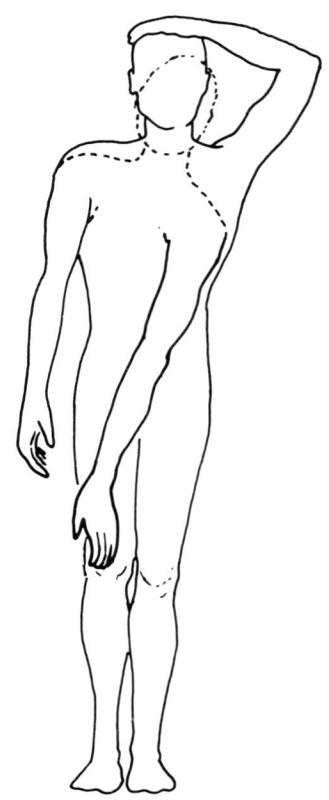

Fig. 2.1. The ability to place the hand. The patient is asked to touch his head and then the opposite knee. He should be able to do this accurately and within 5 seconds if good functional results are to be expected from surgery.

Sensibility is best tested by texture discrimination in the 2–3 year old, object identification in the 4–5 year old, graphesthesia in the 6–9 year old, and two point discrimination in the older child. Only those children with 3 of 5 object discrimination, number perception in the palm, or 2 point discrimination of less than 10 mm can be expected to have functional results after upper extremity surgery.

Individuals with intelligence quotients of less than 50, poor placement and poor sensibility rarely have decent control of muscles in their upper extremities. For these individuals, the goals will be those of hygiene and perhaps cosmesis. Derotation osteotomies of the contracted shoulder, musculocutaneous neurectomies, biceps releases, wrist fusions, lengthening of the flexors of the forearm and the fingers have been used to accomplish these hygiene goals.

Functional goals are appropriate for the patient who has reasonable cognition, sensibility of sophisticated type and the ability to place the hand in space. Releases of contracted muscles either by flexor slide or the fractional lengthening method have been carried out with good results.

Tendon transfers are a more complex issue in these patients and they require knowledge of where is the need of the hand and what is the activity of the donor muscle. The requirement is usually for opening of the hand, and occasionally for grasp. When opening of the hand is needed, the transfer should be to the finger and thumb extensors. When the need is in grasp, the transfer should be to the central wrist extensor. Donor muscles that are working in the phase of the need should be the ones utilized for transfer. Here, the electromyogram helps determine which tendon should be used. The traditional use of the flexor carpi ulnaris has been found most effective, but on occasion the results of the electromyogram suggest that the brachioradialis, extensor carpi ulnaris or pronator teres can be utilized.

Thumb web release by Z-plasty of skin and partial transverse myotomy of the adductor muscle can increase the depth of grasp. Total myotomy of the adductor is advised against because the patient may lose the ability to side pinch. The hyperextendable metacarpo-phalangeal joint of the thumb is treated with a capsulodesis. This is a relatively effective procedure, especially when supported temporarily with a Kirschner wire. Similar capsulodesis of the proximal interphalangeal joints are not as effective and sublimus tenodesis works best for these joints when they are hyperextendable and tend to lock in the recurvatum position.

Summary

The orthopaedic procedures for the cerebral palsy patient are not in and of themselves difficult to perform. The main problems are those of realistic goals and appropriate operative choices.

References

BISLA R.S. & LOUIS H.J. (1975) Transfer of the tibialis posterior tendon in cerebral palsy. *Journal of Bone and Joint Surgery*, **57A**, 137–8.

BLECK E.E. (1975) Locomotor prognosis in cerebral palsy. *Developmental Medicine and Child Neurology*, **17**, 18–25.

EVANS E. (1971) Knee flexion deformity in cerebral palsy. In *The American Academy of Orthopedic Surgeons: Instructional Course Lectures*, Vol. 20. C.V. Mosby Co., St. Louis.

GOLDNER J.L. (1971) General principles in cerebral palsy. In *The American Academy of Orthopedic Surgeons: Instructional Course Lectures*, Vol. 20. C.V. Mosby Co., St. Louis.

GRICE D.S. (1952) Extra-articular arthrodesis of the subastragalar joint for correction of paralytic flat feet in children. *Journal of Bone and Joint Surgery*, **34A**, 927–40, 955–6.

HOFFER M.M. (1978) The upper extremity in cerebral palsy. In Fredericks S. & Brody G.S. (eds.) *Symposium on the Neurological Aspects of Plastic Surgery*, Vol XVII. C.V. Mosby Co., St. Louis.

HOFFER M.M., FEIWELL E., PERRY R., PERRY J. & BONNETT C. (1973) Functional ambulation in patients with myelomengocele. *Journal of Bone and Joint Surgery*, **55A**, 137–48.

HOFFER M.M., REISWIG J.A., GARRETT A.M. & PERRY J. (1974) The split anterior tibial tendon transfer in the treatment of spastic varus hindfoot of childhood. *Orthopedic Clinics of North America*, **5**, 31–8.

PERRY J., HOFFER M.M., GIOVAN P. & GREENBERG R. (1974) Gait analysis of the triceps surae in cerebral palsy. A pre-operative and postoperative clinical and electromyographic study. *Journal of Bone and Joint Surgery*, **56A**, 511–20.

PERRY J., HOFFER M.M., ANTONELLI D., PLUT J. & LEWIS G. (1976) Electromyography before and after surgery for hip deformity in children with cerebral palsy. A comparison of clinical and electromyographic findings. *Journal of Bone and Joint Surgery,* **58A,** 201–8.

RUDA R. & FROST H.M. (1971) Cerebral palsy: spastic varus and forefoot adduction treated by intramuscular posterior tibial tendon lengthening. *Clinical Orthopaedics and Related Research,* **79,** 61–70.

SILVER C.M., SIMON S.D., SPINDELL E., LITCHMAN H.M. & SCALA M. (1967) Calcaneal osteotomy for valgus and varus deformities of the foot in cerebral palsy; a preliminary report on twenty-seven operations. *Journal of Bone and Joint Surgery,* **49A,** 232–46.

Chapter 3
Congenital Lesions of the Spinal Cord — General Considerations

A. M. K. RICKWOOD

Orthopaedic surgeons are naturally mainly interested in spina bifida as it affects their own special interests and other aspects of this condition are, quite properly, usually delegated to different specialists. Nevertheless, patients with spina bifida are frequently admitted to orthopaedic wards, sometimes for prolonged periods, and a recent survey indicated that the majority of adult patients are primarily cared for by orthopaedic surgeons. Therefore it is appropriate to provide those with an interest in the surgery of neurological disease with a broader view of spina bifida, particularly with regard to various practical aspects of management.

Historical review

Myelomeningocele has always been the most common congenital lesion of the spinal cord but, until comparatively recently, few born with this condition survived beyond infancy, the majority succumbing from infection of the central nervous system or from progressive hydrocephalus. The development in the 1950s of shunting devices to control hydrocephalus, plus the realization that prompt neonatal closure of the spinal lesion materially reduced the risk of central nervous system infection, enabled the survival of many infants who previously would have died.

Throughout the 1960s it was widespread practice to treat surgically almost all babies with myelomeningocele in the anticipation that the results would be comparable to those obtained with traumatic paraplegics. Later it became evident that this view was overoptimistic for three major reasons:

1 the adverse effects of hydrocephalus on intelligence plus the technical complications inherent in shunt surgery;

2 the high incidence of major deformities of the spine and legs;

3 the difficulties peculiar to the management of a congenital neuropathic bladder.

These considerations prompted a change to a more selective policy, with active treatment reserved for those with smaller lesions whose handicaps could be expected to be comparatively mild (Lorber 1972). Although the ethics of this policy have been disputed, the practical results appear to be justified (Lorber & Salfield 1981).

The incidence of myelomeningocele in the United Kingdom has declined from a peak of 1 per 350 live births in 1965 to only 1 per 600 live births in 1982. This is partly the result of developments in antenatal screening. Estimation of serum alphafetoprotein levels in the second trimester is now offered routinely in most centres, with estimation of amniotic fluid levels when serum levels are elevated. False negative results are rare and most false positives can be excluded by fetal ultrasound examination. Termination of affected pregnancies is usually advised even where ultrasound demonstrates only a small spinal lesion. More recently the goal of prevention has come nearer with reports that multivitamin supplementation in the first trimester to mothers 'at risk' substantially reduces the incidence of neural tube defects (Smithells et al. 1981).

Covered congenital lesions of the cord are far

less common and affected patients have usually survived childhood. The major factor limiting their life-expectancy has been, and remains, a neuropathic bladder. The incidence of these conditions does not appear to be changing and most cannot be detected by present antenatal screening procedures even if this were thought desirable.

Classification and pathology of congenital lesions of the cord

Congenital lesions of the cord may be divided into 'open' types, where neural tissue lies exposed at the surface (myelomeningocele), and 'closed' varieties where the cord is enclosed by some form of epithelium.

Myelomeningocele

This is employed as a general term for 'open' lesions; others are used to describe variations in the gross anatomy, some of which are of functional significance, others not.

The cause(s) of myelomeningocele is unknown. Although hereditary factors are important, 95% of cases occur sporadically. Females outnumber males by 1.4 to 1.

The essential embryological feature is failure of closure of the posterior neuropore resulting in a variable length of neural tube (the neural plaque) remaining exposed at the surface. Because the posterior neuropore is the last part of the distal neural crest to close, myelomeningocele almost always extends to the tip of the cord. Cases where there is normally formed cord distal to the plaque are exceptional.

The anatomical distribution of myelomeningoceles is set out in Table 3.1.

Because myelomeningocele is almost invariably associated with hydrocephalus there is doubt as to which is the primary embryological disturbance. On balance, the evidence suggests that the spinal lesion is the primary anomaly with hydrocephalus occurring as a secondary phenomenon.

The exposed neural plaque is covered by degenerate ependymal tissue. Within the plaque, grey matter lies dorsally and white matter ventrally. The grey matter is not usually fully organized into separate dorsal and ventral horns, but neuron clusters often lie in relation to ventral nerve roots. In the more extensive lesions white matter is grossly disorganized and ascending and descending long fibres are scarcely recognizable although short interneurons may be found.

Table 3.1. Anatomical distribution of myelomeningoceles (Lonton 1977).

	%
Cervical	0.3
Thoracic	1
Thoracolumbar	45
Lumbar	10
Lumbosacral	30
Sacral	14

The cord is also abnormal above the plaque. The diameter is small because of the reduced population of long fibres running to and from the plaque. The central canal is irregular with alternating segments of obliteration and cystic dilatation. The latter may occasionally result in signs identical to those of syringomyelia. As a result of tethering of the cord below and pressure from hydrocephalus above, the lumbar segments are elongated and the cervical segments compressed.

Several varieties of myelomeningocele are described. In the classical form the neural plaque lies flat like a filleted anchovy (Fig. 3.1) (*myeloschisis*). With *meningomyeloceles* the meninges present as a cystic swelling; the neural plaque, which lies at its apex, is less everted and less obvious (Fig. 3.2). There is no functional distinction between these two types. In some 1% of cases there are *multiple myelomeningoceles*, the most caudal being a typical open lesion while those above tend to be membrane covered. The neurological level usually corresponds to the most cranially disposed lesion. *Hemimyelomeningocele* accounts for 2% of cases. Here

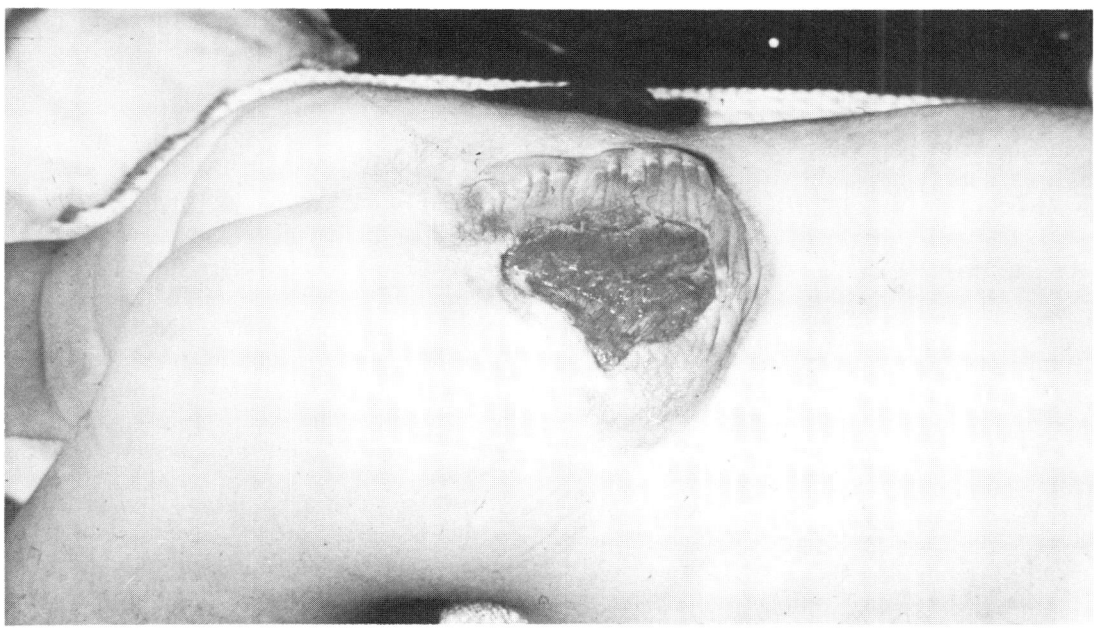

Fig. 3.1. Myeloschisis in a neonate. The lumbar neural plaque lies at the surface and is surrounded by meningeal tissue. The groove along the plaque represents the central canal.

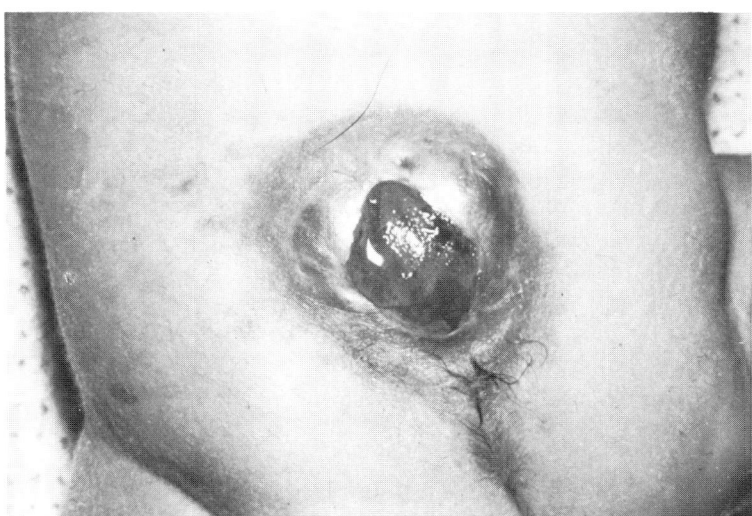

Fig. 3.2. Meningomyelocele in a neonate. There is a cystic bulge of meningeal tissue surmounted by a relatively small neural plaque.

only one half of the cord is malformed resulting in a grossly asymmetrical neurological deficit. Despite its unilateral nature, bladder function is usually abnormal.

The bony defect associated with myelomeningocele will be familiar to orthopaedic surgeons. Neonatal kyphosis due to anterior wedging of the underlying vertebral bodies occurs only in more extensive lesions. Hemivertebrae are common, either at the level of the plaque or more cranially when they are often associated with fusion or absence of ribs.

More remotely, congenital anomalies of other systems (notably cardiovascular and genito-urinary) are more prevalent than in the population at large, but are seldom life-threatening in themselves and rarely influence the decision as to whether to treat the spinal lesion or not.

Closed lesions

Uncomplicated spina bifida occulta

Laminal defects of the 5th lumbar or 1st sacral vertebrae are very common and can be regarded as a variant of normal. Usually discovered during the investigation of backache or functional bladder disorders, this finding can safely be ignored in the absence of any overlying cutaneous abnormality or positive neurological signs.

Meningocele

Textbook meningocele, with a cystic meningeal bulge through a bony and cutaneous defect, but no underlying abnormality of the cord, is rare and usually to be found in the lumbosacral region. Many so-called meningoceles are either examples of myelocele or, at exploration, prove to overly some abnormality of the cord. Genuine examples cause no neurological deficit and are seldom associated with hydrocephalus.

Myelocele

Usually located in the cervical or midthoracic regions, these present as small, midline, membrane-covered structures which extend intrathecally as a stalk of glial tissue and terminate in an area of cystic dilation of the central canal. Cervical lesions may cause a minor neurological deficit in the arms and upper motor neuron signs in the legs. Bladder function is occasionally affected. These are the only 'closed' lesions commonly associated with hydrocephalus, which occurs in some 10% of cases.

Congenital dermal sinus

These generally occur at the lumbosacral junction. The sinus, which is often surrounded by an angiomatous 'blush', penetrates intrathecally with the result that meningitis or intradural abscess may occur as complications. This potentially dangerous condition should be distinguished from the much more common and quite harmless blind-ending pits overlying the tip of the coccyx.

Lipoma of the cauda equina (lumbosacral lipoma)

This is the commonest of the clinically significant 'closed' lesions although occurring in no more than 1 per 10,000 live births. The term is well established but is something of a misnomer in that while there may be fatty tissue surrounding the cauda equina, this is no more than an incidental finding. The lesion presents as a fatty swelling, sometimes in the midline, more often over the upper part of one or other buttock. Deeply it extends intrathecally as a fibrofatty stalk which blends intimately with the tip of the conus medullaris (Fig. 3.3).

Diastematomyelia

Here the cord is split in the midline by a fibrous or bony bar running from the laminal arch to the vertebral body (Fig. 3.4). It occurs most commonly in the lower thoracic region and there is often an overlying hairy patch. Diastematomyelia may also be associated with myelomeningocele and lipoma of the cauda equina.

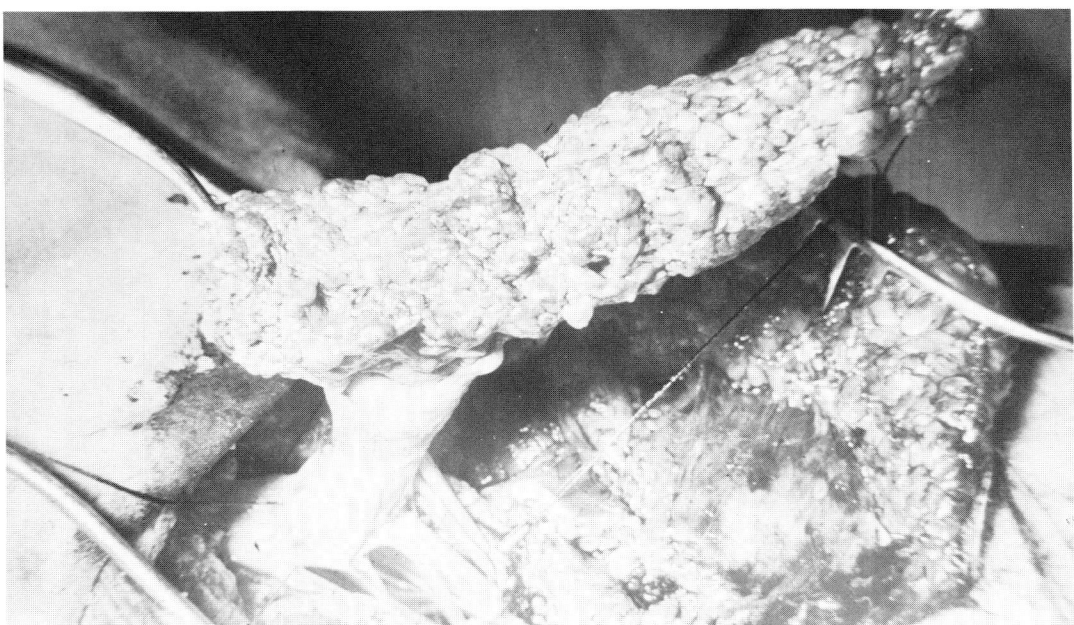

Fig. 3.3. Lipoma of the cauda equina. Operative photograph after freeing the lipoma and laminectomy. The lipoma overlies the stalk which blends imperceptibly with the conus medullaris. Cauda equina roots are seen running from the latter.

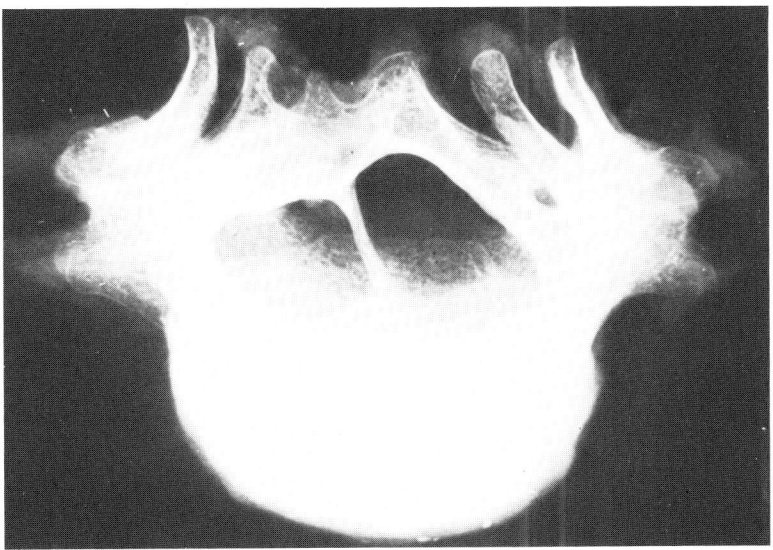

Fig. 3.4. Vertebral body with bony diastematomyelia.

Intraspinal lipomata and dermoid cysts

These can accompany other 'open' or 'closed' lesions, or may occur in isolation. In the latter instance they usually present during childhood or later with some neurological disturbance usually first affecting the bladder.

Sacral agenesis

Pure sacral agenesis is an example of 'caudal regression' syndrome rather than spina bifida. However the neurological manifestations are similar and the two conditions are found together in 8% of cases. At least three sacral segments must be absent before there is any neurological disturbance. In extreme examples even the lower lumbar spine may be deficient (Fig. 3.5). Although flattening of the buttocks is quite characteristic of the condition, minor degrees of sacral agenesis are often overlooked until the child presents with some disturbance of bladder function.

The neurology of congenital lesions of the spinal cord

General

Contrary to widespread belief, there is nothing peculiar in the neurological disturbances produced by congenital lesions of the cord. Myelomeningocele is unusual in that an isolated but intact lower motor neuron innervation of apparently paralysed muscles is often present and can be demonstrated by Faradic stimulation (Sharrard 1976). This phenomenon may have some bearing on the development and treatment of deformities but otherwise is without clinical significance.

Neurological examination should be directed to three basic aspects of cord function:

1   the primary neurological level in terms of motor and sensory function; the former includes assessment of power in non-paralysed muscles and the latter separate testing of dorsal column and spinothalamic tract sensibility;
2   whether the neurological deficit is complete or incomplete and, if incomplete, whether this is manifest in terms of sensory function, motor function or both;
3   the presence or otherwise of reflex activity below the primary neurological level; the conus

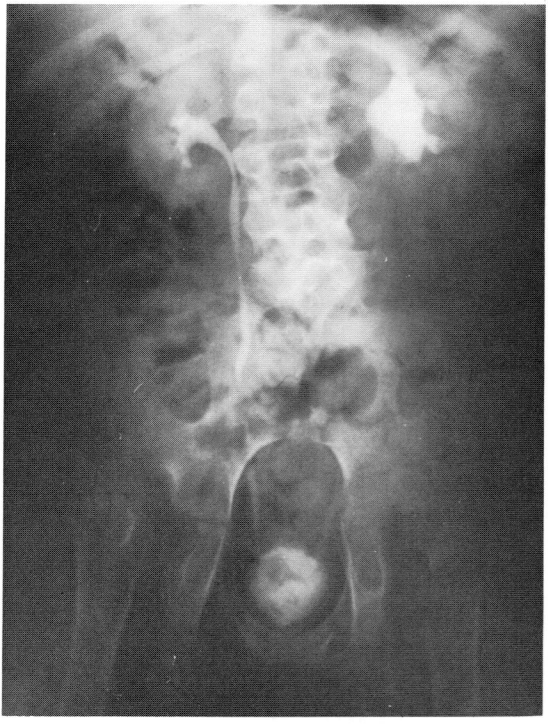

Fig. 3.5. Sacral agenesis with involvement of the 5th lumbar vertebra.

reflexes (anocutaneous and glans-bulbar) are particularly relevant to bladder, bowel and sexual function.

The terms complete and incomplete paraplegia and complete and incomplete cord lesion are frequently, but incorrectly, used interchangeably. The former refers only to whether there is or is not voluntary motor power in the lower limbs. In a complete cord lesion there is no motor or sensory function below a certain neurological level (although sensory and motor levels need not be identical). With an incomplete cord lesion there is sensory or motor sparing (or both) in the lowermost sacral segments; this may coexist with loss of sensory or motor function in more cranially disposed segments. It is thus quite possible to have a complete paraplegia with an incomplete cord lesion, an incomplete paraplegia with a complete cord lesion and so on. The distinction is important in that only patients with incomplete cord lesions have normal bladder and bowel function.

Neurological assessment of older patients poses no problems but there are obvious difficulties in examining infants and younger children in whom accurate definition of dorsal column sensation is virtually impossible as is precise evaluation of muscle power. Nonetheless with patience and experience it is usually possible to define motor and spinothalamic sensory levels with reasonable accuracy and to determine whether the cord lesion is complete or incomplete. A problem in neonates lies in distinguishing reflex from voluntary movement. Should there be any doubt, the dictates of common sense may be applied; movements occurring in association with large spinal lesions are very likely to be reflex and vice versa.

Myelomeningocele

The extent of the neurological deficit is largely dependent on the size of the neural plaque and, as a rule, the primary neurological level corresponds with the upper level of the bony spinal defect. The motor and spinothalamic sensory levels usually coincide while the dorsal column sensory level tends to lie a segment or two below. Except in hemimyelomeningoceles the deficit is generally symmetrical to within a segment or so. The cord lesion in patients with thoracolumbar and lumbar myelomeningoceles is almost always complete. More caudally the proportion with incomplete lesions is appreciable and exceeds 60% in sacral myelomeningoceles. Often this consists only in dorsal column sparing which is of functional importance only in that preservation of postural sense may improve walking. Conus reflexes are present in some 25% of cases and this incidence is fairly evenly distributed regardless of the extent of the neural plaque. A few patients with thoracolumbar myelomeningoceles have spastic paralysis of the lower limbs.

There has been much discussion as to whether the neurological picture changes during the first few months of life. It is the author's experience that it very rarely does regardless of whether the spinal lesion is closed at birth or not.

Closed lesions

Lipoma of the cauda equina

Some 10% of patients have no peripheral neurological deficit and most of these have normal bladder and bowel function. Among the remainder the deficit is usually confined to the sacral segment and incomplete cord lesions are the rule. Conus reflexes are usually absent.

The neurological picture can deteriorate in time but on occasion this is apparent rather than real. Minor degrees of paresis of the muscles acting around the feet and ankles may not be evident in neonates but become quite obvious when the child walks. Increasing deformity should not necessarily be equated with deteriorating neurology.

Diastematomyelia

Characteristically there are long-tract signs in the form of spasticity, exaggerated deep tendon reflexes and upgoing plantar responses. A sensory deficit is unusual. Again it is often difficult to be certain whether these signs represent real neurological deterioration or not.

Sacral agenesis

Even with the most extensive lesions it is unusual to find any sensory deficit, while the motor function is often only patchily affected. Conus reflexes are usually absent.

Management of the spinal lesion

Myelomeningocele

Assessment

Lorber (1972) has defined five adverse criteria, the presence of any one of which contraindicates neonatal surgical closure of the spinal lesion:

1 extreme prematurity or birth trauma (for example, anoxia, cerebral haemorrhage)
2 major associated congenital anomalies
3 gross hydrocephalus
4 spinal deformity
5 complete paraplegia

In the author's view one simple criterion usually suffices, namely whether there is, or is not, good quadriceps function. If there is good function, then the child will almost certainly walk and it is unlikely that any of Lorber's first four criteria will apply. The converse also holds.

The repair

The objective is to obtain good cover over the cord and so prevent bacterial infection of the central nervous system. It is customary to mobilize dural flaps from the lining of the sac and to close these over the cord. In neonates it is almost always possible to close the skin directly without need for flaps.

Timing

The lesion becomes colonized with Gram-negative organisms from the bowel within 48 hours of birth and delayed closure runs the very real risk of precipitating Gram-negative meningitis or ventriculitis. Closure within the first 24 hours is advisable. If this is not possible a case exists for delay for 3–6 months by which time the infant will have become more immunologically competent.

The fate of the untreated infant

Reported survival rates in infants *not* selected for neonatal surgical treatment vary from 0 to 30%. This discrepancy is largely accounted for by the management of these babies in the first few weeks of life and whether developing hydrocephalus is treated or not. If antibiotics are withheld, but the baby is otherwise nursed and fed normally, and if hydrocephalus is treated surgically by the normal criteria, the survival rate is of the order of 15–20%. The survivors probably fare no worse in the long-term than if their spinal lesion had been closed at birth.

Closed lesions

Congenital dermal sinuses clearly require excision to prevent infection while meningoceles and myeloceles are repaired to prevent rupture and for cosmetic reasons. Intraspinal lipomata and dermoid cysts presenting with fresh neurological signs also require surgery.

There is some debate about treatment of a lipoma of the cauda equina or diastematomyelia. With both it is generally assumed that neurological deterioration results from traction of the cord or roots during growth. The greater part of the ascent of the cord is completed by the 25th week of gestation and from birth to full maturity the conus rises by less than one vertebral level (Barson 1970). The role of traction as a cause of neurological deterioration may be less than generally supposed. With lipoma of the cauda equina there is reason to believe that the neurological deficit derives largely from inherent myelodysplasia within the conus.

Of the three possible policies (do nothing, operate prophylactically or intervene only when there is neurological deterioration) the last would seem to be the most sensible with the proviso that it should be certain that it is the neurology, rather than just deformity, which is changing.

Hydrocephalus

Almost all patients with myelomeningocele have hydrocephalus and it is this, more than anything else, which sets them apart from patients with other diseases of the cord, congenital or acquired. The complications of hydrocephalus, or rather of its treatment, are many and frequent while the effects of hydrocephalus on mentation are profound and are at least as important to the patient's rehabilitation as any physical disability.

Pathology

Research continues to uncover new facets of cerebrospinal fluid (CSF) production, circulation and absorption and as yet the precise mechanisms in the generation, evolution and arrest of hydrocephalus remain to be elucidated. In practice hydrocephalus in patients with myelomeningocele can be regarded as obstructive (noncommunicating) and due partly to displacement of the fourth ventricle below the foramen magnum (the Arnold–Chiari malformation) and partly to secondary distortion of the cerebral aqueduct. Arrested hydrocephalus presumably occurs when secondary channels of CSF circulation become established. Continuous monitoring of intracranial pressure in hydrocephalic patients has shown wide diurnal fluctuations which probably reflect varying rates of CSF production. Events such as viral infections may increase CSF production and precipitate intracranial hypertension in patients with long-standing arrested hydrocephalus. Associated with hydrocephalus are numerous gross and microscopic abnormalities of the brain, particularly of the cerebellum and cerebral cortex.

Assessment

Few myelomeningocele patients have a grossly increased head circumference at birth, but, even when head size is well within normal limits, underlying hydrocephalus may be suspected if there is bulging of the fontanelle or separation of the lambdoid sutures. The degree of hydrocephalus may be assessed by air ventriculography, by CT scanning or by ultrasound examination across the anterior fontanelle. The last, which is noninvasive and widely available, is most commonly employed and air ventriculography has largely been abandoned.

Prognosis may be gauged from the thickness of the cerebral mantle; if this is less than 10 mm hydrocephalus is likely to be rapidly progressive, while if it exceeds 25 mm shunt treatment is unlikely to be necessary.

Sophisticated investigations are not usually required to assess these babies during the first few weeks of life, and the necessary tools are no more than a tape measure, a head growth chart and a modicum of clinical sense. Indications for shunting are a rapid increase in head circumference across centile lines and signs of intracranial hypertension in the form of irritability, poor feeding and vomiting. There are no absolute criteria for the timing of shunt insertion and on the whole surgeons now tend to be more conservative than previously.

The severity of hydrocephalus, as judged by the need for shunt procedures, is related to the extent of the spinal lesion (Table 3.2).

Table 3.2. Myelomeningocele and hydrocephalus (Lonton 1977).

Site of lesion	Shunted hydrocephalus (%)
Thoracolumbosacral	100
Thoracolumbar	87
Lumbar	91
Lumbosacral	74
Sacral	30

Treatment

No treatment

Progressive hydrocephalus, left untreated, results, if not in death, then in massive enlargement of the head, profound mental retardation, spasticity, and blindness. Although surgical treatment is not without drawbacks it is clearly better than doing nothing at all.

Non-surgical treatment

From time to time various forms of nonsurgical therapy have been advocated; these include head binding and diuretics (notably Isosorbide). On occasion they can delay the need for a shunt or may result in a more cosmetically satisfactory head size in those whose hydrocephalus was destined to arrest, but it is doubtful if they have ever achieved more than that.

Surgical treatment

Several nonshunting procedures have been devised (e.g. excision of the choroid plexus) but none has proved to be of much value.

Many shunting devices are now marketed, all based upon the same principles, namely of shunting the CSF from one or other lateral ventricle to the vascular tree (via the right atrium), to the peritoneum or, rarely, to the pleural cavity, and of incorporating some stratagem to ensure unidirectional flow and to regulate the minimum intracranial pressure at which CSF flows through the system. The Holter and Pudenz systems have been the most commonly used and more modern devices are based upon one or other of these. Many incorporate a tapping chamber to obtain CSF specimens or to measure intracranial pressure. Some systems can be switched 'on and off' at will while others have an antisyphoning device to prevent overdrainage of peritoneal catheters.

In recent years the trend has been to use shunts with higher 'spill over' pressures in the hope that this will lessen the incidence of overdrainage. Originally the lower catheter was usually placed in the vascular tree. Provided the catheter remained in the right atrium it continued to function for long periods if not indefinitely. Unfortunately during growth it was drawn up into progressively smaller vessels where sooner or later it blocked and required lengthening, often on several occasions. Routine shunting into the peritoneal cavity is now in vogue because long lengths can be left *in situ* to allow for growth while revisionary surgery is generally easy and safe.

Complications of shunts

General

Complications are frequent and on average 3.8 revisionary procedures are required during childhood. In principle, detection of shunt malfunction is straightforward and in practice this is often the case. On other occasions it is not, and shunt malfunction is best regarded as a diagnostic minefield through which only the experienced should tread. It would be no exaggeration to say that, in these patients, even the most unlikely symptoms should arouse suspicion of shunt malfunction until proved otherwise.

Shunt blockage

Most patients remain shunt-dependent during childhood and blockage is life-threatening, sometimes very rapidly so. Even if a delayed diagnosis does not result in death there may be permanent sequelae by way of blindness, spasticity or gross mental retardation.

In the first two years of life blockage of the ventricular catheter by choroid plexus is the most common problem. Thereafter the distal catheter is more often at fault.

The symptoms and signs are typically those of intracranial hypertension, with headaches, drowsiness and vomiting, and bradycardia, hypertension and papilloedema. The last is always a reliable sign of raised intracranial pressure but often is not present in the early stages and may not occur at all. Other indications are a rapidly increasing head circumference and bulging fontanelle (in infants), a fresh or worsening squint, deteriorating mental performance and spasticity. Convulsions are common in hydrocephalic patients but are rarely a presenting symptom of shunt occlusion. Many patients complain of neckache rather than headache.

There may be neck rigidity occasioning an erroneous diagnosis of meningitis. Meningitis is exceedingly rare in these patients and lumbar puncture is contraindicated since it may cause coning if the intracranial pressure is raised.

In theory palpation of the pumping chamber of the shunt provides information as to the site of the blockage; if the chamber is stiff the distal catheter is occluded and if it fails to refill, the ventricular catheter is blocked. Unfortunately, in practice these signs are frequently misleading.

The full-blown clinical picture is the exception rather than the rule and it is not uncommon to find patients with suspicious symptoms but no signs and others with gross papilloedema but no symptoms. The diagnosis may still be equivocal even after a period of observation. Serial CT scans can be helpful in detecting progressive ventricular enlargement. It may be necessary to measure intracranial pressure via a tapping chamber (if the ventricular catheter is patent) or directly from the ventricle via a burr hole. Single measurements of intracranial pressure can be misleading and continuous monitoring over 24 hours is advisable in equivocal cases.

When shunt blockage is life-threatening, aspiration of CSF from the tapping chamber or from the ventricle via a needle passed alongside the ventricular catheter may retrieve the situation until expert help is available.

Shunt infection

Bacterial colonization of the inside of shunt systems follows some 10% of primary and 3% of revisionary procedures. The infecting organism is *S. albus* in more than 90% of cases; being a universal skin commensal, this organism is introduced during surgery and has a unique ability to adhere to silastic. Although occurring at the time of surgery, colonization may not become clinically manifest for months or years afterwards. Secondary colonization is rare if it occurs at all. Internal colonization may be present throughout the shunt system (and may be accompanied by ventriculitis) or may be confined to the more distal parts of the system.

External infection around shunt devices is uncommon and the organism is usually *S. aureus*.

Colonization of vascular shunts leads to septicaemia (often with splenomegaly) and shunt nephritis due to deposition of antigen/antibody complexes within the glomerulus. Haematuria and proteinuria are features of this complication. Colonization of peritoneal shunts only rarely results in frank peritonitis. More often the system blocks as omental and other adhesions form to wall off the infection.

Patients with shunt colonization need not appear to be particularly ill and many of the symptoms resemble those of urinary infection. The two conditions often coexist and certain antibiotics used to treat urinary infections (notably cotrimoxazole) may mask the symptoms of colonization.

Positive blood cultures and rising antibody titres to *S. albus* are features of colonized vascular, but not peritoneal, shunts. The C-reactive protein level is nearly always elevated but this is nonspecific and may occur with almost any infection at any site. Aspiration of CSF from the shunt or the ventricles is often necessary to confirm a diagnosis of colonization.

Only rarely can shunt colonization be treated conservatively with antibiotics. It is generally necessary to remove the whole of the shunt system and to replace it with a new one. An intervening period of external ventricular drainage is required if there is ventriculitis.

Overdrainage

Overdrainage of shunt systems in infants has long been recognized but it is only since the advent of CT scanning that it has been appreciated how common it is for chronic overdrainage to result in ventricular systems of subnormal size (slit ventricles). This may cause three complications:

1 the obvious, and sometimes intractable, difficulties in replacing blocked ventricular catheters;

2 low pressure headaches from intracranial *hypotension;* characteristically these are aggravated by standing and relieved by lying;
3 repeated cycles of overdrainage and blockage of the ventricular catheter; the ventricles shrink down beyond the tip of the catheter, the system blocks, the ventricles enlarge, the system drains again, then over drains and the cycle is repeated.

Disconnection

Disconnection of the shunt system may cause blockage or blockage may cause disconnection. Both clearly require attention. Quite often a disconnected shunt system is discovered at a routine visit or on a radiograph taken for some unrelated purpose. If there are no symptoms or signs of raised intracranial pressure there is usually no indication to reconnect the system.

Sequelae of hydrocephalus

The gross complications of hydrocephalus are largely preventable, but no amount of expert care will secure fully normal intellectual function. This applies even to those with arrested hydrocephalus requiring no shunt surgery. The effects of hydrocephalus on intelligence are set out in Table 3.3 from which it will be observed that, because the severity of hydrocephalus is related to the extent of the spinal lesion, increas-

Table 3.3. Myelomeningocele and intelligence (Lonton 1977).

Site of lesion	Mean IQ*
Thoracolumbosacral	74
Thoracolumbar	84
Lumbar	88
Lumbosacral	88
Sacral	100

* Wechsler intelligence scale for children, full scale performance.

ing physical and intellectual disabilities tend to go hand in hand. These effects of hydrocephalus on mentation are not uniformly distributed; verbal skills are relatively spared, giving the superficial impression of normal, or even superior, intelligence, while performance skills particularly those requiring hand—eye coordination, are more severely impaired. It is this last aspect that results in myelomeningocele patients achieving less by way of self care than others with similar paralysis.

Neuropathic bladder

General

Normal urinary control exists in only some 20% of myelomeningocele patients most of which have low, small, spinal lesions. Neuropathic bladder is present in more than 50% of patients with lipoma of the cauda equina and all those with sacral agenesis. The incidence in other types of 'closed' lesions is comparatively low.

For patients with 'closed' lesions, as well as those with small myelomeningoceles, neuropathic bladder is often the major handicap or even the only one and their quality and expectation of life are largely governed by how well the bladder is managed.

The problems peculiar to the congenital neuropathic bladder are:

1 the high incidence of secondary upper renal tract complications (hydronephrosis, renal parenchymal damage);
2 the difficulties of handling incontinence in a patient population which is predominantly female.

It was once common practice to treat incontinence in girls and upper renal tract complications in patients of both sexes by permanent urinary diversion, usually using refluxing intestinal urinary conduits. It is now clear that the long-term results of such procedures performed in childhood are poor and that they themselves are responsible for fresh or further renal deterioration in more than 50% of cases followed for 15 years or more (Middleton & Hendren 1976). The results with antirefluxing conduits are better but still far from ideal (Altwein *et al.* 1977). In addition fitting stomal appliances may become difficult or impossible in patients who develop major spinal deformities.

As a result urinary diversion has largely been abandoned as a means of treating patients with congenital neuropathic bladder and the conservative approach now practised promises better results. However, effective conservative management requires some knowlege of normal micturition and the ways this can be disturbed by neurological disease.

Normal micturition

The nerve supply to the detrusor is parasympathetic from the 2nd, 3rd and 4th sacral segments and the neurotransmitter is acetylcholine. The same segments somatically innervate the striated external urethral sphincter. There also is an alpha-adrenergic sympathetic innervation of the smooth muscle of the trigone, bladder neck and proximal urethra but the importance of this is debatable (Nordling 1983). The ascending sensory fibres run adjacent to the spinothalamic tracts and the descending motor tracts adjacent to the lateral horns. The events of normal micturition are coordinated at brain stem level.

Much of our knowledge of normal and abnormal micturition derives from urodynamic studies and these are now a routine investigation in patients with a congenital neuropathic bladder. In this study total intravesical pressure is measured during filling and voiding via a catheter. This pressure has 2 components, that due to the activity of the detrusor itself and that due to general intra-abdominal pressure. The latter is measured via a rectal catheter and is subtracted from the total pressure to give the pressure generated by the detrusor. Bladder outflow rate and volume are measured and sometimes the EMG activity in the external urethral sphincter. Addi-

tional information is gained if the study is combined with simultaneous cine-radiographic examination.

The urodynamic features of normal micturition are that during filling the detrusor pressure remains low and no involuntary contractions occur even when the bladder feels full. The bladder neck is closed and remains so despite any rises in intra-abdominal pressure. Voiding occurs by a voluntary detrusor contraction, which can be turned 'on and off' at will, and which is sustained until the bladder is empty.

Pathophysiology of the congenital neuropathic bladder

Classification

The classification of neuropathic bladder was considered formerly in relation to a supposed sacral reflex micturition centre. This could be destroyed in conus lesions to give a flaccid paralysis of the detrusor and external sphincter (the lower motor neuron or autonomous bladder) or left intact but isolated by a lesion higher in the cord resulting in reflex but involuntary micturition (the upper motor neuron, automatic or hyper-reflexic bladder). It is now realized that neuropathic bladder dysfunction cannot be accommodated within so simple a framework but for present descriptive purposes a modification of this classification is adopted:

1 *hyper-reflexic bladder,* voiding only by reflex detrusor contractions;
2 *autonomous bladder,* no detrusor contractions and voiding only by raising intra-abdominal pressure;
3 *intermediate bladder,* voiding by both means.

This classification is of some practical consequence in that patients with autonomous and intermediate bladders can void at will by a deliberate act to raise intra-abdominal pressure whereas those with hyper-reflexic bladders have no such facility.

Hyper-reflexic bladders

During filling detrusor pressure remains low and the bladder neck is competent (Fig. 3.7). At capacity there occurs a reflex detrusor contraction with simultaneous contraction of the external urethral sphincter (*detrusor–sphincter dyssynergia*) (Figs. 3.6 and 3.7). This sphincteric contraction is initially complete and allows no urine to pass. Later, outflow begins but is obstructed since the sphincter does not fully relax. Because of this obstruction detrusor voiding pressures are usually abnormally high but often these strong contractions fade away before the bladder is empty (*nonsustained detrusor contractions*) (Fig. 3.7).

The capacity of these bladders is determined solely by the point at which filling stimulates a reflex detrusor contraction, while their ability to empty is limited partly by detrusor–sphincter dyssynergia and partly by whether the detrusor contraction is sustained or not.

Autonomous bladders

Here it is necessary to introduce the concept of *sphincter weakness incontinence* (SWI), definable as leakage of urine as a result of a rise in intra-abdominal pressure and indicating incompetence of the bladder neck and urethral sphincter. Absent in normal and hyper-reflexic blad-

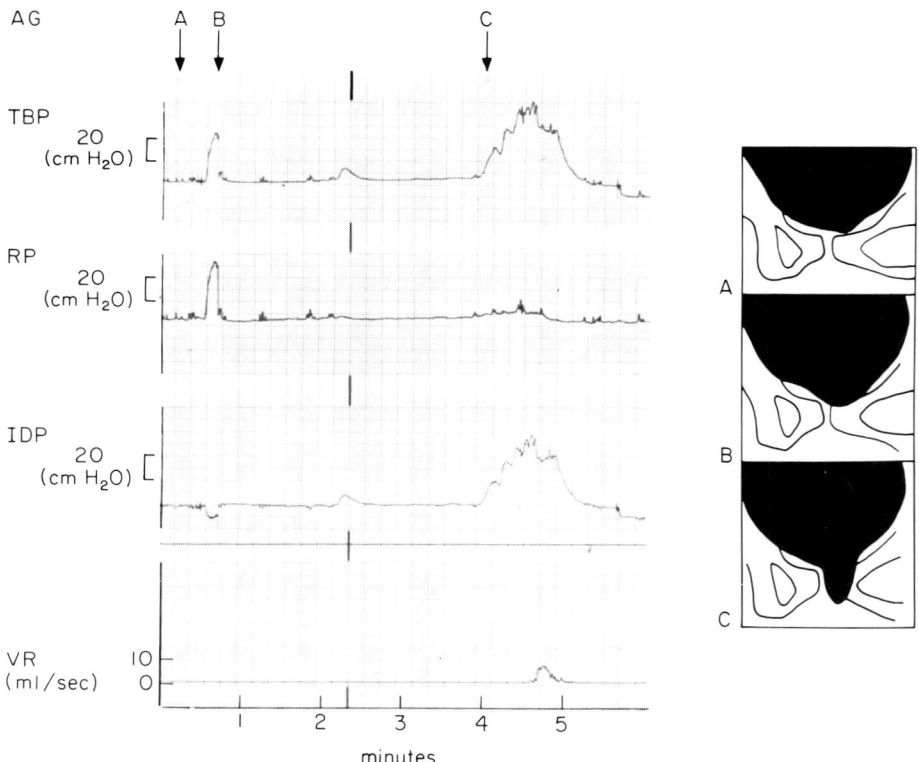

Fig. 3.6. Hyper-reflexic bladder (urodynamic study: TBP = total bladder pressure, RP = rectal pressure, IDP = intrinsic detrusor pressure, VR = void rate). During filling the bladder neck is closed (A) and remains so despite a rise in intra-abdominal pressure (B) produced by straining. A reflex detrusor contraction (C) opens the bladder neck but there is simultaneous contraction of the external urethral sphincter (detrusor–sphincter dyssynergia).

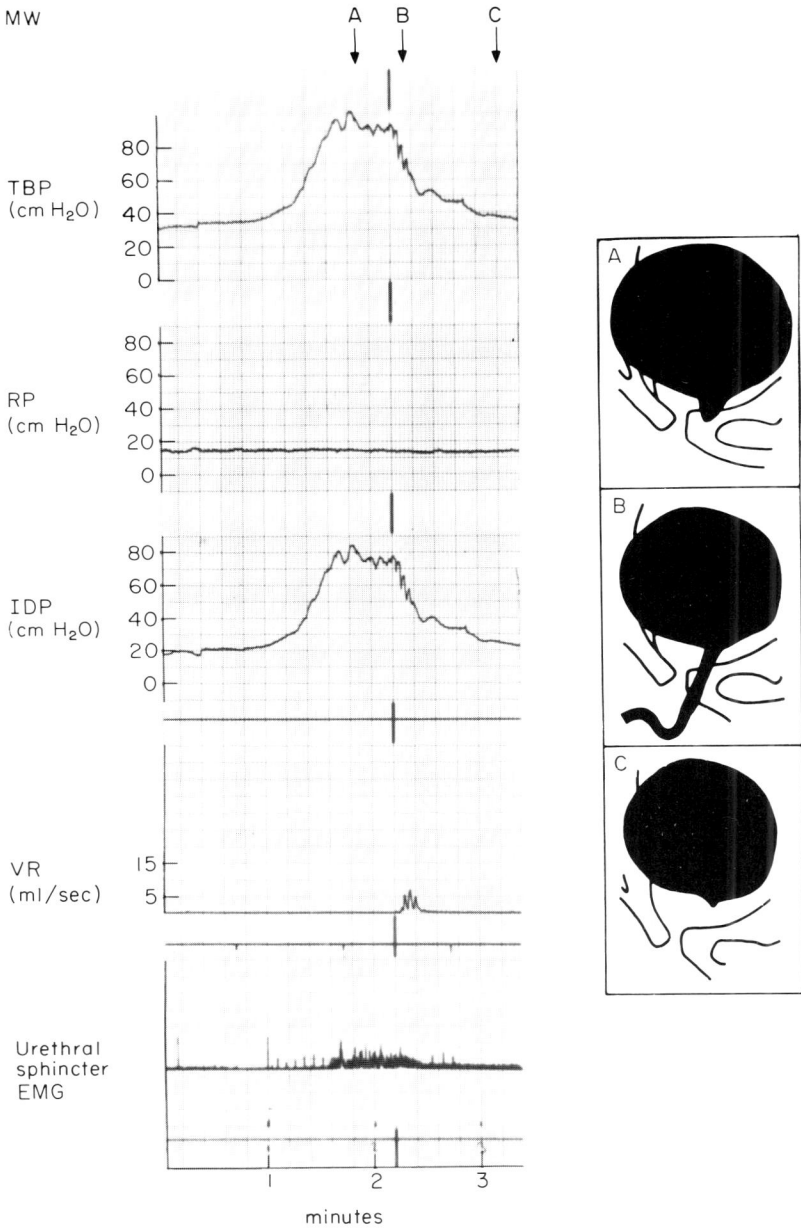

Fig. 3.7. Hyper-reflexic bladder. A reflex detrusor contraction at low capacity (A) is initially associated with complete detrusor–sphincter dyssynergia. Later there is outflow as the sphincter relaxes (B) but the detrusor contraction fades away before the bladder is empty (C). (TBP = total bladder pressure, RP = rectal pressure, IDP = intrinsic detrusor pressure, VR = void rate.) Reproduced with permission from Rickwood (1984).

ders, SWI is present by definition in patients with autonomous and intermediate bladders. Were it not they would be unable to void by raising intra-abdominal pressure. However, the degree of SWI varies enormously from one patient to another. At one extreme are those with gross SWI severely limiting functional bladder capacity (Fig. 3.8), but having a small residual urine in consequence, and at the other those with marginal SWI who have a good functional capacity but usually a large residual urine also.

capacity of the bladder but also results in ureterovesical obstruction because the pressure which ureteric contractions can generate is comparatively low. If there is a large residual urine, the intravesical pressure is permanently elevated and the ureters are constantly obstructed.

Voiding occurs by abdominal compression or straining. If there is outflow obstruction, this is again manifest at the level of the external urethral sphincter (Fig. 3.9). This obstruction is not, by definition, detrusor–sphincter dyssynergia

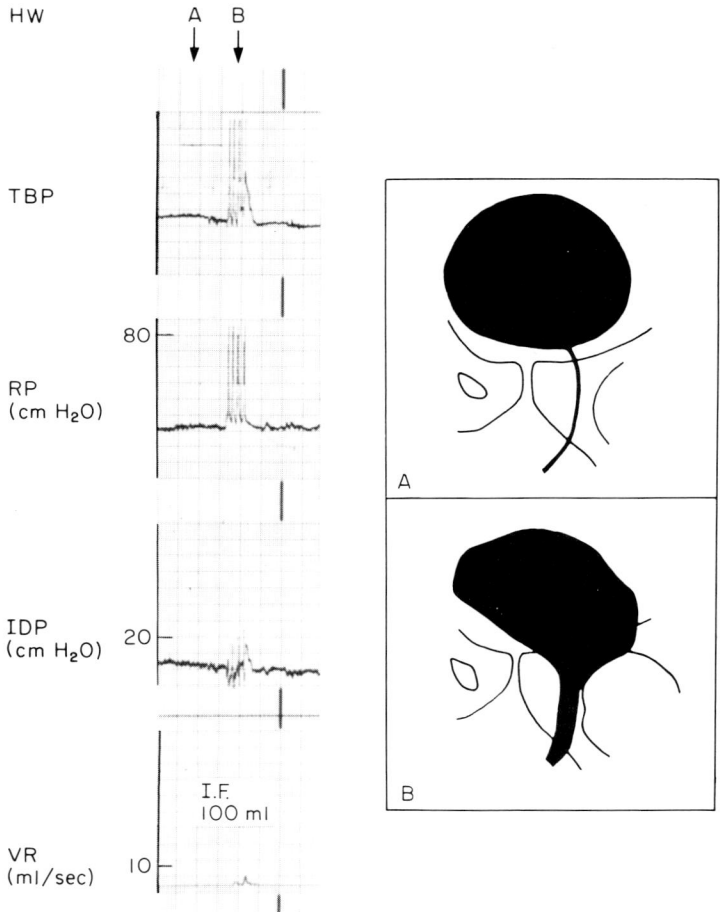

Fig. 3.8. Autonomous bladder (contrast filled urethral catheter *in situ*). The bladder neck is closed at rest (A), but coughing (B) causes leakage of urine past the bladder neck and external urethral sphincter (sphincter weakness incontinence). (TBP = total bladder pressure, RP = rectal pressure, IDP = intrinsic detrusor pressure, VR = void rate.) Reproduced with permission from Rickwood (1984).

During filling the detrusor pressure usually remains low but in some cases there is a steady rise in baseline pressure (*reduced detrusor compliance*). Reduced compliance not only limits the

and is termed *isolated distal sphincter obstruction*. Its cause is unknown but is unlikely to be due to somatically mediated contraction of the striated external sphincter. Some believe it

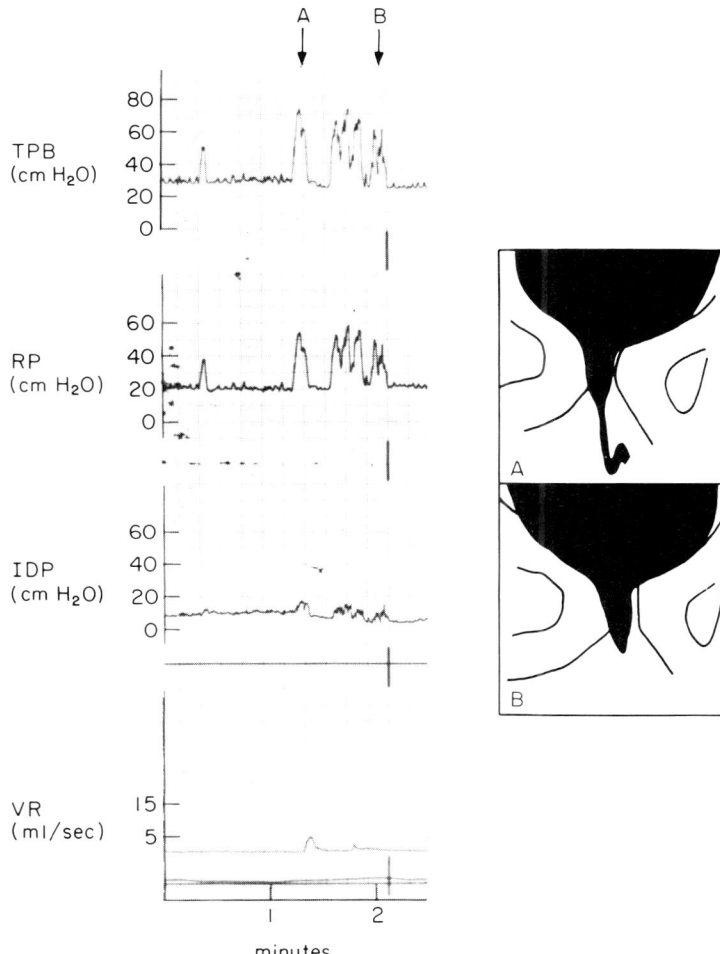

Fig. 3.9. Autonomous bladder. Voiding is by abdominal straining (A). There is a narrowing at the level of the external sphincter and obstruction ultimately becomes complete at this level despite continued straining (B) (isolated distal sphincter obstruction). (TBP = total bladder pressure, RP = rectal pressure, IDP = intrinsic detrusor pressure, VR = void rate.) Reproduced with permission from Rickwood (1984).

results from overactivity of alpha-adrenergically innervated smooth muscle in the proximal urethra but this view is open to question (Nordling 1983).

The capacity of these bladders is limited by SWI or by reduced detrusor compliance (or both) and their ability to empty by the presence of isolated distal sphincter obstruction.

Intermediate bladders (Fig. 3.10)

These can exhibit any combination of the properties found in hyper-reflexic and autonomous

Table 3.4. Congenital neuropathic bladder.

Factors limiting functional bladder capacity

Over-active detrusor reflex activity
Reduced detrusor compliance
Sphincter weakness incontinence

Factors limiting bladder emptying

Nonsustained detrusor contractions
Detrusor–sphincter dyssynergia
Isolated distal sphincter obstruction

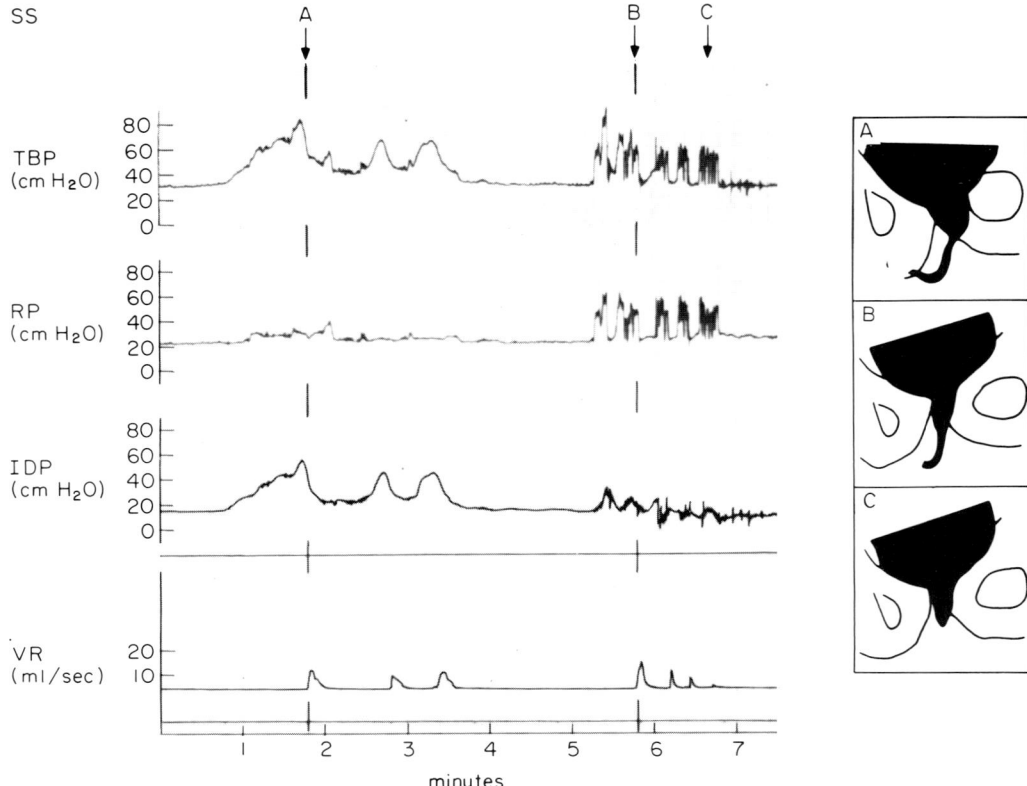

Fig. 3.10. Intermediate bladder. Voiding occurs both by reflex detrusor contractions (A) and by abdominal straining (B). There is isolated distal sphincter obstruction (C). (TBP = total bladder pressure, RP = rectal pressure, IDP = intrinsic detrusor pressure, VR = void rate.) Reproduced with permission from Rickwood (1984).

bladders. They are the commonest type associated with congenital lesions of the cord and also the least 'well behaved'; reduced detrusor compliance is common as are gross SWI and outlet obstruction.

The factors which may limit the ability of congenital neuropathic bladders to store and void urine are summarized in Table 3.4. It is important to realise that in any one patient several factors may be operative.

Peripheral neurology and bladder dysfunction

There is little correlation between the type of bladder dysfunction and the extent or site of congenital cord lesions but there is a good correlation with sacral neurological signs:

1 *Anocutaneous reflex:* this is positive in patients with hyper-reflexic bladders. In its absence there may be some reflex activity in the detrusor but this is likely to be weak.
2 *Pelvic floor tone:* gross SWI is unusual if there is good tone in the pelvic floor but common if the perineum is quite flaccid.
3 *Sacral sensory sparing:* sensory sparing to pain and temperature is usually associated with good bladder and urethral sensation.
4 *Sacral motor sparing:* here there is usually the ability to voluntarily contract the external urethral sphincter and sometimes the detrusor also.

All patients with normal bladder control have sacral motor and sensory sparing.

Bladder dysfunction and the upper renal tracts

Secondary upper renal tract complications are far more common in patients with congenital rather than acquired lesions of the cord and the factors responsible are:

1   *Bladder outlet obstruction:* this is the most important factor and it is rare to find upper renal tract complications in its absence.
2   *Vesicoureteric reflux:* this is very common and is found in 20% of myelomeningocele patients at birth.
3   *Reduced detrusor compliance.*
4   *Urinary tract infection:* the importance of this as a cause of renal damage in spina bifida patients has probably been exaggerated in the past although infections in the presence of vesicoureteric reflux should certainly be treated.

Management

General

The objectives are, in order of priority:

1   *maintenance of renal function:* the bladder outlet obstruction must be treated and it is now customary to deal with this prophylactically rather than to await complications;
2   *dryness:* this is ideally achieved without use of urinary appliances (penile urinals or indwelling urethral catheters).

If these objectives are to be fully realized it is necessary that:

1   the bladder should have adequate functional capacity for the needs of the individual patient (and requires to be greater in those confined to a wheelchair than for those who walk well);
2   the bladder should empty;
3   voiding should be voluntary.

The first and third requirements relate purely

Table 3.5.   Congenital neuropathic bladder: treatment.

Failure to fill	Failure to empty
Overactive detrusor reflex Medication (anticholinergic) 　Propantheline 　Oxybutynin 　Imipramine Surgery 　Sacral rhizotomy	Medication (alpha-adrenolytic) (Autonomous and intermediate bladders only) 　Phenoxybenzamine 　Indoramin Surgery 　Endoscopic sphincterotomy (males) 　Internal urethrotomy (females) Other 　Indwelling urethral catheter 　Intermittent catheterization
Reduced detrusor compliance Medication (smooth muscle inhibitors) 　Imipramine 　Oxybutynin Surgery 　Bladder augmentation (caecum, sigmoid colon)	
Sphincter weakness incontinence Medication (alpha-adrenergic) 　Ephedrine 　Phenylpropanolamine 　Imipramine Surgery 　Bladder neck suspension 　Bladder neck tightening 　Prosthetic sphincter	**Voiding at will** *Abdominal compression/straining* (Autonomous and intermediate bladders only) *Intermittent catheterization*

to the ideal of appliance-free dryness. The second, although mainly concerned with maintaining renal function, also bears on continence in that residual urine reduces the *effective* capacity of the bladder (for example, if functional capacity is 300 ml and residual urine is 250 ml, then effective capacity is only 50 ml). Sensation of fullness of the bladder is useful but is by no means essential to become dry; well motivated patients compensate for lack of it by voiding 'by the clock'.

Treatment must be *realistically* related to the patient's overall physical and intellectual status. Factors such as poor mobility, spinal deformity, intellectual impairment, etc. may affect management at least as much as the nature of the bladder dysfunction itself.

Management in relation to bladder dysfunction

The desirable features of bladder performance may be summarized as Fill, Empty and Void at Will and the various individual forms of treatment are listed under these headings in Table 3.5.

Surgical treatment for overactive detrusor reflex is reserved for cases not responding adequately to medication. The use of alpha-adrenergic stimulants to treat SWI is only effective where this is relatively mild. Gross SWI may require surgical treatment, but this should be limited to carefully selected (usually ambulant) cases. The prosthetic urinary sphincter (Fig. 3.11) is probably the best treatment for gross SWI but this device is expensive.

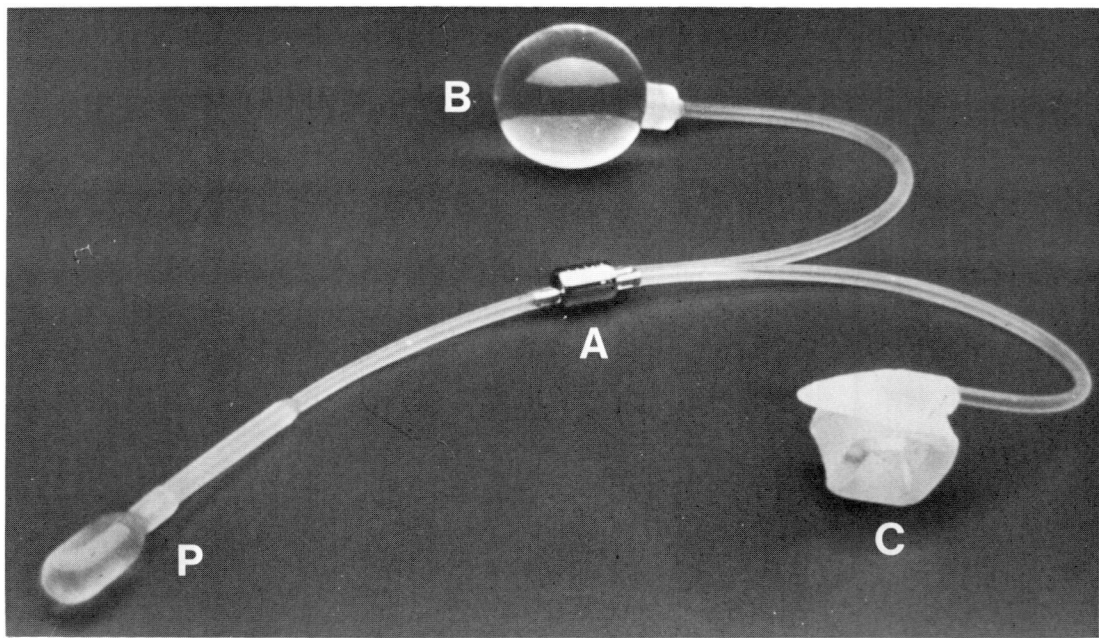

Fig. 3.11. The American Medical Systems Inc. prosthetic urinary sphincter. The cuff (C) fits around the bladder neck (or bulbar urethra as an alternative in males) and is normally inflated to compress the urethra and prevent urine leakage. The pressure in the cuff is regulated by the balloon reservoir (B). The cuff is deflated by compressing the pumping chamber (P), which lies in the scrotum or labia. This removes the fluid in the cuff to the balloon reservoir. The patient then voids by abdominal straining. The cuff then refills automatically, movement of fluid in the system being regulated by the control assembly (A).

Use of alpha-blocking agents such as phenoxy-benzamine to treat Isolated Distal Sphincter Obstruction has been largely supplanted by Intermittent Self-Catheterization. Endoscopic sphincterotomy in males is effective in relieving both detrusor–sphincter dyssynergia and isolated distal sphincter obstruction. Vigorous internal urethrotomy is similarly effective in girls.

Patients with autonomous and intermediate bladders who void by a deliberate act to raise intra-abdominal pressure may do this by straining (Valsalva manoeuvre) if the motor level lies at or below D12, or by direct compression over the bladder (Credé manoeuvre) when the level is above D12. Clean Intermittent Self-Catheterization (CISC) is the only way in which patients with hyper-reflexic bladders can void at will and may be the preferred method in those with autonomous or intermediate bladders when straining or compression leaves an appreciable residual urine. CISC has been a most useful advance since it combines emptying the bladder with voiding at will. To keep a patient dry also requires adequate functional bladder capacity and some 50% of those on CISC require adjuvant medication to achieve this. The technique of CISC is clean, not sterile. There is a risk of introducing infection but bacteruria in the absence of symptoms or vesicoureteric reflux can usually be ignored. Older patients can practise CISC independently, but many of the more severely physically or intellectually disabled find this impossible. CISC is not realistic for such cases, nor indeed is the general goal of appliance-free continence.

Because bladder dysfunction is often complex and because treatment to improve capacity may be at the expense of emptying (and vice versa) it is frequently necessary to use methods of treatment in combination. Schemes of management using abdominal compression/straining or CISC as the means of voiding at will are illustrated in Figs. 3.12 and 3.13.

These schemes have been effective in maintaining renal function or reversing established

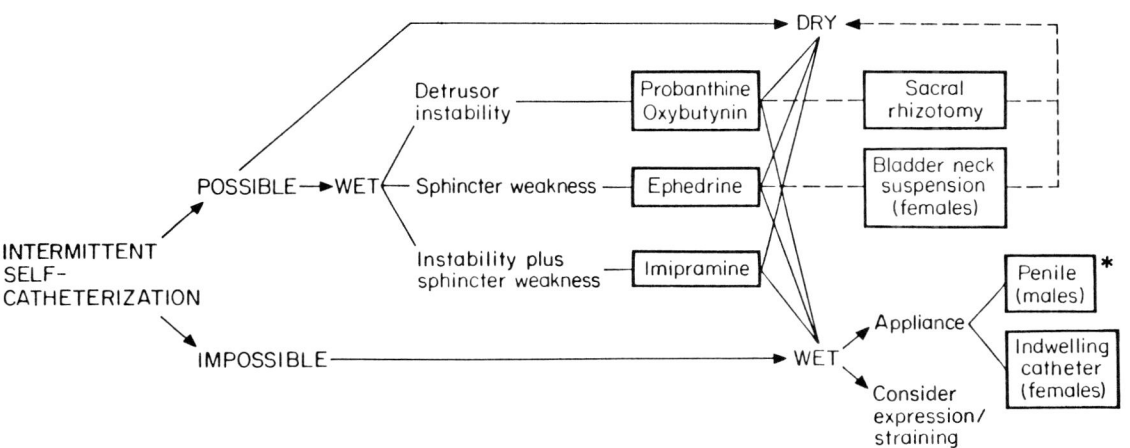

* plus spincterotomy if there is any bladder outlet obstruction

Fig. 3.12. Management using intermittent self-catheterization as the means of voiding at will. Surgical treatment of detrusor instability (reflex contractions) or sphincter weakness is limited to selected patients who do not respond adequately to appropriate medication. Self-catheterization may be impossible by virtue of low intelligence, severe spinal deformity in females or good urethral sensation in males with incomplete cord lesions. (Reproduced with permission from Rickwood 1984.)

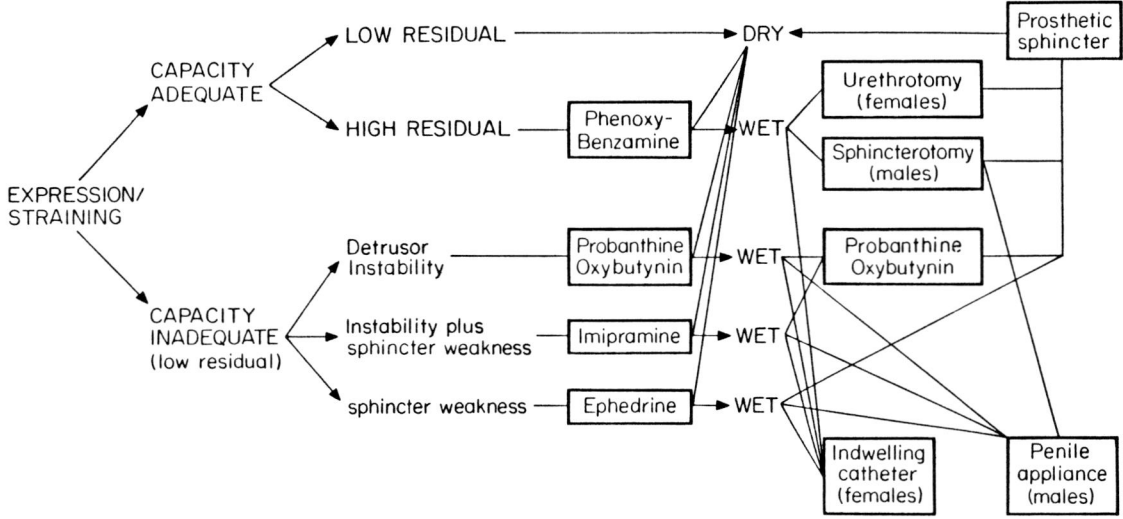

Fig. 3.13. Management using abdominal compression or straining as the means of voiding at will (autonomous and intermediate bladders only). The prosthetic urinary sphincter is reserved for selected cases; any bladder outlet obstruction or detrusor instability (reflex contractions) must be dealt with before insertion of this device. Reproduced with permission from Rickwood (1984).

complications (Fig. 3.14), but only some 50% of patients achieve appliance-free continence with CISC or medication employed singly or in combination. In ambulant patients this proportion can be considerably increased by judicious use of surgery to treat SWI.

For the more severely disabled, urinary appliances are the only realistic solution to incontinence. Most males over 7 years can be fitted with some form of penile urinal of which the condom sheath (Fig. 3.15) is usually the most reliable. Long-term indwelling urethral catheterization for females enjoys an undeservedly poor reputation. This method is most effective in maintaining renal function (and reversing established complications) and of treating urinary incontinence. It causes a number of practical problems, but most of these are readily solvable by appropriate measures (Rickwood *et al.* 1983).

Bowels

Nearly all patients with a neuropathic bladder also have a neuropathic bowel (or, to be more precise, a neuropathic rectum and anal canal). Fortunately this condition is not life threatening nor need its investigation require anything more elaborate than a pin. Management is straightforward and effective although experience suggests that many patients are never properly advised.

The objective is to secure evacuation of the bowel when, and only when, the patient wishes. The key to this is the anocutaneous reflex.

A positive reflex indicates that the anal sphincter is competent and that the rectum retains reflex activity. Bowel evacuation is obtained by stimulating a reflex rectal contraction and this is most conveniently effected by a bisacodyl (Dulcolax) suppository, usually given on alternate days. This should act within 30 minutes. If there is delay beyond this, bisacodyl rectal solution is a more rapidly acting alternative. Because bisacodyl is more effective when the motions are somewhat soft, and because the anal sphincter is competent, a high residue diet is beneficial.

When the anocutaneous reflex is absent there is no rectal reflex activity and the anal sphincter is incompetent. If the motor level is above D12

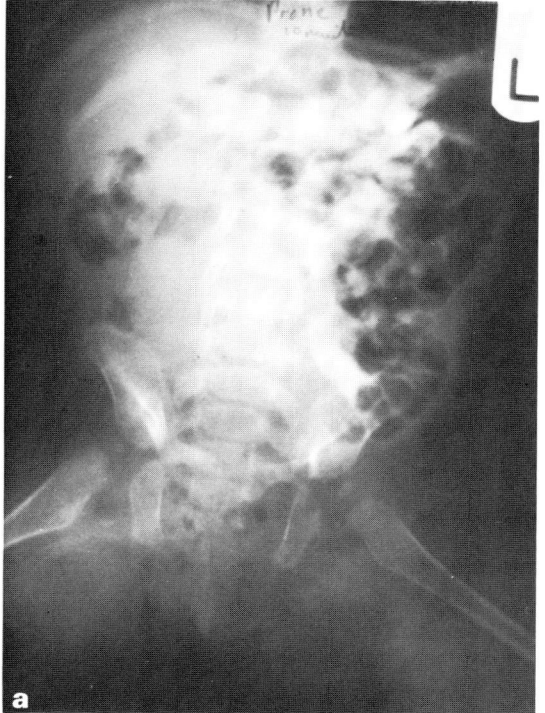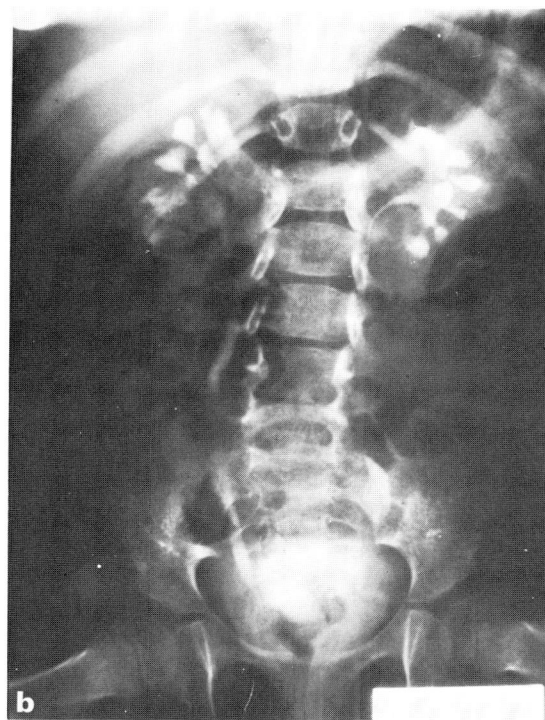

Fig. 3.14 (a) Female neonate with thoracolumbar myelomeningocele. The IVP shows gross bilateral hydronephrosis (associated with bilateral vesicoureteric reflux).
(b) IVP 3 years after internal urethrotomy showing resolution of the hydronephrosis; the reflux also ceased.

the bowels should be managed by daily digital evacuation of faeces. Those patients with a motor level at or below D12 can evacuate the bowels by abdominal straining although it is often necessary to complete this process by digital evacuation of the rectum. Because the anal sphincter is incompetent, the motions should be firm and high residue diets are not advisable.

These regimens are best commenced in infancy and it should be rare for faecal soiling to be a problem by school age. Naturally many of the more severely intellectually and physically disabled will never be able to cope with their bowels independently but this is no reason for altering the basic plan of management.

Sexual function in males

Nearly all males with a positive anocutaneous reflex achieve satisfactory reflex erections by handling the penis. Although ejaculation is usually possible, the quantity and quality of the ejaculate is generally poor.

Approximately half those patients with an absent anocutaneous reflex, but a neurological level below the sympathetic outflow, obtain erections which result from psychogenic rather than from tactile stimuli. These tend to be inadequate and poorly sustained and if ejaculation occurs at all it is liable to be retrograde into the bladder.

If there is no anocutaneous reflex and the neurological level lies above the lumbar sympathetic outflow, penile erections scarcely ever occur.

There is a risk that endoscopic urethral sphincterotomy will adversely affect erections and this applies especially to those patients with no anocutaneous reflex (Philp *et al.* 1983).

It is unlikely that many male patients with congenital lesions of the spinal cord will become fathers.

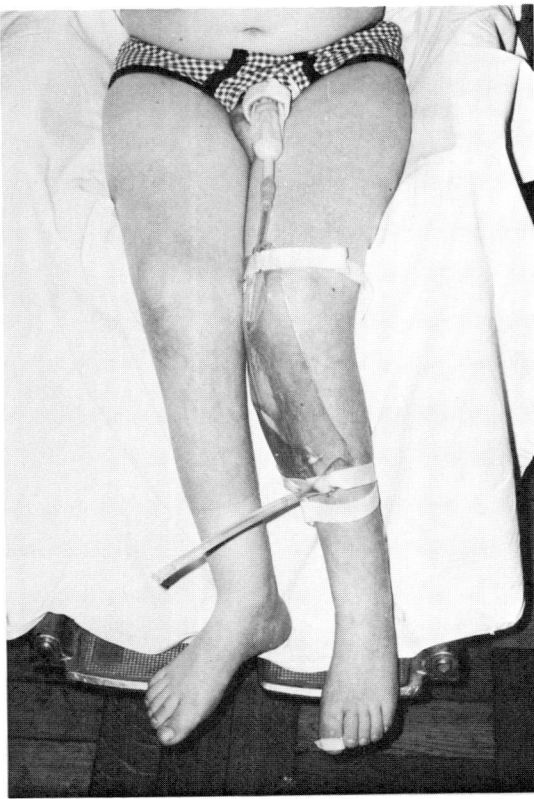

Fig. 3.15. Condom penile urinal.

Pressure sores

General

Pressure sores are uncommon in spina bifida patients during childhood but become a significant problem in adolescence and adult life. They may be considered in 3 main categories:

1 *Superficial sores on the legs in nonambulant patients* These result from combinations of deformity, ill-fitting footwear and poor circulation. Common sites are around the malleoli and over the dorsum of the feet and toes. They cause no general ill health and little functional disturbance.

2 *Sores on the weight-bearing areas of the feet in ambulant patients* These derive from a combination of deformity and analgesia. The usual sites are the heel and beneath the heads of the 1st or 5th metatarsals. The underlying bone is almost always involved and these sores cause major functional disability.

3 *Pelvic pressure sores* (sacral, ischial, trochanteric and post-trochanteric) mainly occurring in patients confined to a wheelchair and more especially in those with a major spinal deformity. The underlying bone is involved more often than not and septic arthritis of the hip may complicate trochanteric, post-trochanteric and sometimes ischial sores. They cause both functional disability and chronic ill-health and may be life threatening, immediately from overwhelming sepsis or more remotely from the development of secondary amyloid disease.

Management

Principles

In theory pressure sores are entirely avoidable by attention to skin care and by provision of special beds, wheelchair cushions etc. Important as these measures are, it is improbable that they will ever eliminate sores. Spina bifida patients are especially at risk by virtue of their deformities plus the effects of hydrocephalus on their intellectual function.

The basic principles of management are:

1 *Removal of pressure* If there is only one sore this poses no particular problems, but when there are multiple pelvic pressure sores it is necessary to employ one of the special beds marketed for this purpose. Net and low-loss air beds are comparatively cheap and as effective as various more expensive alternatives.

2 *Excision of necrotic tissue* Topical desloughing agents are of no value nor are antibiotics. Necrotic tissue must be excised surgically, a tedious process sometimes requiring

several sessions. The procedure includes removal of infected, necrotic bone; sacral sores often do not begin to heal until the coccyx has been excised.

3 *Avoidance of packing* Packing is a form of pressure in itself and serves to perpetuate sores or even to enlarge them.

Almost all sores will heal on a conservative regimen based upon these principles. Unfortunately this may take many months while the skin which ultimately forms over the defect is of poor quality and is liable to further breakdown. For these reasons surgical repair is often indicated.

Surgery of pressure sores

Surgical repair is only practicable in the case of pelvic pressure sores. Successful results are obtained by adhering to certain details:

1 *Timing* Repair should not be undertaken in the acute stage of a sore but should be delayed until the lesion is clean and beginning to heal with active granulation tissue.

2 *Preoperative treatment* Because repairs are liable to be contaminated with faeces, a low-residue diet is given for a week before and a week after operation. It is customary to prescribe a prophylactic wide-spectrum antibiotic immediately before and for some 10 days after the repair.

3 *Excision of the sore* Sores in the healing stage usually have a well defined pseudocapsule making it possible to ensure complete excision. All abnormal skin around the sore should be excised and also any underlying infected or prominent bone.

4 *Repair of the defect* Even where it is possible to close the defect by direct suture this is inadvisable since it leaves a suture line over the site of the sore. The skin around suture lines is unstable and liable to break down under pressure. Skin flap repairs are preferable because the suture line can be placed away from the immediate area of the sore. The recent trend has been away from random flaps, incorporating skin and

subcutaneous tissue only, towards myocutaneous flaps. These allow safe mobilization of large areas of skin and have the further advantage of incorporating underlying muscle to bolster the repair. The myocutaneous flap based on tensor fascia lata is particularly useful for the repair of trochanteric, post-trochanteric and sometimes ischial sores. Transposition flaps may leave a secondary defect; this is of no consequence provided that it is not over a pressure area. Skin grafting of a secondary defect is best left for 3 weeks after the repair. All repairs should be drained.

5 *Postoperative care* It is unwise to have the patient sit too early. It has been the author's practice to keep the patient in bed for 6 weeks after the repair and then only to return to sitting for long periods by stages over the following 2 weeks.

Septic arthritis of the hip should be treated by resection of the head and neck of the femur. It is not usually necessary to perform subsequent repair of the skin defect.

Pressure sores on the weightbearing areas of the foot are not amenable to repair. Correction of foot deformities is an important prophylactic measure. Although these sores usually heal on a conservative regimen, the recurrence rate is high and below-knee amputation may be advisable in this circumstance.

Spina bifida in adult life

Despite every effort, only some 50% of myelomeningocele patients treated actively from birth have survived to full maturity. Most deaths have occurred within the first five years of life and the commonest causes have been infection of the central nervous system in infancy and shunt malfunction later. Renal failure has been comparatively rare. Mortality has been related to the extent of the neural plaque, rising from 29% in those with sacral lesions to 58% in those with thoracolumbar lesions. These figures mainly relate to the situation some years ago and the present prognosis for babies with myelomeningocele undergoing active treatment is much improved.

The abundant literature on spina bifida relates principally to children. Less is known of the status of these patients in adolescence and almost nothing of the problems they encounter in adult life. The material which follows derives from the author's experience of 204 spina bifida patients followed from the age of 16 years for periods of up to 8 years (with a mean of 4 years).

were obese, a problem not related to neurological level and almost entirely confined to females.

Forty per cent of patients had compromised upper renal tracts in the form of hydronephrosis, renal parenchymal damage, stones or combinations of these. This was related to neurological level, with the incidence rising from 26% in the L5–S4 group to 53% in the above D12 group, and to whether urinary diversion had been performed or not. The upper renal tracts were

Table 3.6. Spina bifida patients: status age 16 years.

	Motor neurological level				Asymmetrical lesions (n = 5)	Closed lesions (n = 16)
	Above D12 (n = 55)	D12 – L2 (n = 29)	L3 – L4 (n = 68)	L5 – S4 (n = 31)		
Major spinal deformity	91%	80%	30%	23%	100%	6%
Mobility — wheelchair only	98%	76%	16%	—	20%	—
Shunted hydrocephalus	85%	62%	51%	26%	60%	6%
Mean I.Q.	78	84	88	94	86	102
Full physical independence	24%	52%	81%	87%	60%	94%

Status in midadolescence

In Table 3.6 certain general features of these patients are set out in relation to motor neurological level. It will be observed that physical and intellectual disabilities were almost linearly related to the extent of the neurological deficit, with the line separating severe from moderate handicap running fairly clearly between L2 and L3, indicating whether quadriceps function was present or not. Nearly all nonambulant patients with a level at or below L3 had quadriceps power 3 or less. Patients with a grossly asymmetrical neurological deficit (all examples of hemimyelomeningocele) fared rather worse than might have been anticipated while patients with 'closed' lesions fared comparatively well in all respects.

Deformities of the feet were present in nearly all cases while many of those with a level above L3 also had deformity or limited range of movement of the hips and knees. A quarter of patients

normal in 85% of those without a diversion, but in only 26% of those with a diversion. Although this is partly a reflection of the fact that in many cases diversion had originally been performed for renal tract complications, there is no doubt that diversion is itself an adverse factor in that complications were present in 19 out of 34 patients who had undergone the procedure purely to treat incontinence. The incidence of renal damage in patients with 'closed' lesions was surprisingly high (62%).

While only 5% of patients had normal bladder and bowel control, the problems of urinary and faecal incontinence were adequately managed in all but a small minority of the remainder.

Progress in adult life

Some idea of the problems encountered may be gained from hospital admissions, bed occupancy and operative procedures (Table 3.7).

Table 3.7. Spina bifida patients aged 16 years and over: hospital admissions, bed occupancy, operative procedures.

	Admissions (No.)	Bed occupancy (days)	Operative procedures (No.)
Genitourinary	102	1172	45
Pressure sores	35	2464	18
Shunt complications	32	308	16
Orthopaedic	9	205	7

Death

The mortality rate approximated to 1% annually, one third due to shunt complications, one third to renal failure (so far only in patients with urinary diversion) and one third to causes unrelated to spina bifida.

Deformity and orthopaedic surgery

One girl developed scoliosis at the age of 17 years. In the remaining 203 cases existing deformities have remained static and no new deformities have occurred. Four ambulant patients required a below-knee amputation for pressure sores, 5 nonambulant patients had deformed and useless digits removed and one correction of claw toes. This was the entire extent of orthopaedic surgery.

Shunt complications

Complications occurred in only 8 out of the 112 patients with shunts, including 3 who died as a result. It is probable that many of these patients were no longer shunt-dependent, although it would be unwise to assume this purely on the grounds that no revisionary surgery was required for many years.

Genitourinary complications

Fresh or further deterioration of the renal tracts occurred in 46 patients, including 3 who died of renal failure. Twenty-two of these did not have a urinary diversion, 19 being males with previously normal upper renal tracts. The majority of surgical procedures were for upper renal tract complications. Endoscopic sphincterotomy in male patients had completely resolved hydronephrosis in all but one case.

Pressure sores

Thirty patients had developed pressure sores, mainly in the pelvic region. By their very nature pressure sores took up a disproportionate share of bed-occupancy and mainly involved the more severely disabled patients.

Conclusion

If the present trend continues most of these patients will reach middle age or even beyond. The major factor limiting life-expectancy is the state of the upper renal tracts and this applies to many whose handicaps are otherwise quite slight. Those with a urinary diversion look likely to fare much worse than those who have escaped this procedure. Because the majority of complications are symptomless until irreversible renal damage has developed, close and continued urological supervision is vital.

Next in order of priority comes the problem of pressure sores. Experience indicates that these are often handled indifferently by community nurses, by general practitioners and even by hospitals not used to the problem. Adequate facilities and expertise for treating pressure sores must be available in any unit caring for older spina bifida patients.

In childhood shunt complications loom large but present evidence suggests that this is not so in adults. Although continued supervision is advisable it seems unlikely that these patients will prove to be a major burden to adult neurosurgical units.

The requirement for orthopaedic surgery in adult patients is minimal. This sharply contrasts with the situation in childhood although it may be observed that many procedures have been performed in children with limited ambulation and who go on to use a wheelchair exclusively in adult life. It is possible to identify such patients with some precision from their motor neurological level and here orthpaedic endeavours might best be limited to retaining an adequate range of movement of the hips and knees and straightening feet sufficiently for shoes to be worn (*see* Chapter 4).

References

ALTWEIN J.E., JONAS U. & HOHENFELLNER R. (1977) Long-term follow-up of children with colon conduit urinary diversion and ureterosigmoidostomy. *Journal of Urology*, **118**, 832–6.

BARSON A.J. (1970) The vertebral level of the termination of the spinal cord during normal and abnormal development. *Journal of Anatomy*, **106**, 489–95.

LONTON A.P. (1977) Location of the myelomeningocele and its relationship to subsequent physical and intellectual abilities in children with myelomeningocele associated with hydrocephalus. *Zeitschrift für Kinderchirurgie*, **22**, 510–9.

LORBER J. (1972) Spina bifida cystica: results of treatment of 270 consecutive cases with criteria for selection for the future. *Archives of Disease in Childhood*, **47**, 854–73.

LORBER J. & SALFIELD S.A.W. (1981) Results of selective treatment of spina bifida cystica. *Archives of Disease in Childhood*, **56**, 822–30.

MIDDLETON A.W. & HENDREN W.H. (1976) Ileal conduits in children at the Massachusetts General Hospital from 1955 to 1970. *Journal of Urology*, **115**, 591–5.

NORDLING J. (1983) Influence of the sympathetic nervous system on the lower urinary tract in man. *Neurourology and Urodynamics*, **2**, 3–26.

PHILP N.H., THOMAS D.G. & RICKWOOD A.M.K. (1983) The effect of anteromedian sphincterotomy on penile erections in patients with neurogenic bladder. *Paraplegia*, **21**, 301–4.

RICKWOOD A.M.K. (1984) The neuropathic bladder in children. In Mundy A.R., Stephenson T.P. & Wein A.J. (Eds.) *Urodynamics, Principles, Practice and Application*. Churchill Livingstone, Edinburgh and London.

RICKWOOD A.M.K., PHILP N.H. & THOMAS D.G. (1983) Longterm indwelling urethral catheterisation for congenital neuropathic bladder. *Archives of Disease in Childhood*, **58**, 310–4.

SHARRARD W.J.W. (1976) General orthopaedic management and operative treatment of spina bifida. In Brocklehurst G. (Ed.) *Spina Bifida for the Clinician*, Chapter 9. Heinemann (William) Medical Books Ltd, London.

SMITHELLS R.W., SHEPPARD S., SCHORAH C.J., SELLER M.J., NEVIN N.C., HARRIS R., READ A.P. & FIELDING D.W. (1981) Apparent prevention of neural tube defects by periconceptional vitamin supplementation. *Archives of Disease in Childhood*, **56**, 911–8.

Chapter 4
The Orthopaedic Management of Spina Bifida —
General Considerations

W. J. W. SHARRARD

The pathology of the spinal lesion

The spinal lesion in spina bifida presents in one of several forms: meningocele, open myelomeningocele or closed myelomeningocele (Sharrard 1966, Chapter 3).

Meningocele

This occurs in only 8% of lesions. It can be diagnosed with confidence only after surgical treatment when no neural tissues are found in the herniated meningeal sac. Orthopaedically, the lower limbs are undeformed and show normal movement at birth. If the lesion is operated upon sufficiently soon after birth, later paralysis or deformity does not develop.

Open myelomeningocele

This is the commonest variety of lesion and occurs in 87% of lesions. The lower part of the spinal cord and the cauda equina are exposed as a neural plaque. If left untreated, healing, usually accompanied by infection, takes place slowly but usually with additional damage to the neural structures. If treated by early surgical closure, further neural damage may be prevented (Sharrard *et al.* 1963). The extent of the lesion, topographically and neurologically, varies greatly. Lesions extending from the lower thoracic spine to the sacrum are likely to be associated with severe paraplegia. Sacral lesions are usually accompanied by paralysis affecting only the lower sacral neurological segments and lumbosacral lesions show intermediate levels of paralysis. Paralysis of some degree is almost invariably present at birth and may be associated with various deformities of the lower limbs.

The precise anatomy of the neural lesion and its relationship to the clinical manifestations defies analysis by dissection. Stark & Baker (1967) described four types of lesion. In *type I* the neural defect involved the terminal part of the spinal cord so that neurological function was intact down to a certain level below which there was impairment or loss of motor, sensory and reflex activity. In *type II* the spinal cord was normal down to a certain level; there was then a gap with total paralysis in one or more neural segments and, beyond this, an isolated functioning portion of cord showing spontaneous abnormal motor function. In *type III* a portion of the cord or its roots was absent but some descending tracts passed by the defective region; this type is present in some closed lesions. In *type IV* the distal spinal cord was not abnormal but neurological changes arose from abnormalities at a higher level.

Closed myelomeningocele

This is less often diagnosed at birth and is sometimes designated as spinal dysraphism (James & Lassman 1962). A number of subdivisions of pathological lesion may be represented such as lipoma of the cauda equina, diastematomyelia, filum terminale syndrome, dermal sinus or abnormal root or cord formation (Chapter 3). There may or may not be paralysis or deformity at birth, but there is a tendency for paralysis to develop or to increase with time and growth, and surgical treatment to correct any possible elements causing pressure or traction on neural tissues may be needed. Sometimes, bladder paresis, a partially paralysed foot or a foot deformity such as talipes equinovarus may be the presenting feature.

The nature of the paralysis

The nature of the paralysis in spina bifida in its various manifestations differs in several important ways from other childhood paralyses such as in poliomyelitis, cerebral palsy, muscular dystrophy or hereditary neuropathies.

Motor paralysis

Classical descriptions of motor paralysis divide the manifestations of motor defect into upper or lower motor neuron lesions. Upper motor neuron lesions are characterized by exaggerated flexes and spasticity in some muscles and muscle groups and weakness in others, usually accompanied by abnormalities of motor control. They are usually due to cerebral lesions. Peripherally, the muscles and their nerves are macroscopically normal. Except for patients with a very severe quadriplegic lesion, movements can be produced by volition in the limbs, with varied facility. Lower motor neuron lesions are characterized by specific muscle weakness with partial or total loss of action related to the extent of the nerve fibres that supply the muscle but with good control and no spasticity in such muscle fibres as are preserved.

The paralysis in spina bifida is mainly due to a lesion of the spinal cord and its nerve roots. The aspects of the paralysis that are due to nerve root or anterior horn cell lesions are typical of lower motor neuron paralysis in that the affected muscle fibres are totally inactive. The paralysis due to lesions of the spinal cord presents features that are neither those of a typical lower motor

lesion nor of an upper motor neuron lesion. The tendon reflexes are not increased but are normal or absent. The affected muscles are not voluntarily active but have tone and show spontaneous movements, either intermittent flickers of activity or mass movements in response to sensory stimuli. This motor activity arises in spinal cord segments that are intact but divorced from connection with pyramidal tracts or upper centres. Electromyography shows repeated bursts of spontaneous activity in alpha motor neuron.

Superimposed upon the spinal cord lesion there may be abnormal upper motor neuron activity in those who have hydrocephalus, so that a mixed neurological picture of lower, upper and intermediate motor neuron paralysis may be present.

The neurological deficit in spina bifida is present before birth and there will have been correspondingly diminished motor activity in the lower limbs *in utero*. This, in turn, affects limb posture and muscle growth in the developing limbs and is primarily responsible for the deformities that are present at birth. A correlation has been established in many infants between the type of deformity and the distribution of the paralysis at birth (Sharrard 1962, 1964a).

Sensory deficit

With the exception of peripheral nerve injuries, which are uncommon in the lower limb in childhood, no other type of paralysis in childhood shows such an extensive sensory loss as occurs in spina bifida. The pattern of sensory loss commonly, but not invariably, corresponds to the distribution of the motor deficit and is usually complete for all modalities of sensation. Its presence is of major importance in the management of the lower limbs in spina bifida, particularly in relation to deformities of the feet and the prevention and treatment of neurological ulceration in the foot and in the gluteal region.

Bladder and bowel paralysis (Chapter 3)

Bladder paralysis has important consequences in orthopaedic management. Secondary effects on the renal tract by infection or hydronephrosis, if not well managed, may affect the general health of the child and limit the feasibility of orthopaedic procedures, especially major ones such as anterior spinal fusion. A check on renal function and on the presence of urinary infection must precede any orthopaedic operation.

Hydrocephalus (Chapter 3)

The presence of hydrocephalus causing cerebral damage affects the neurological state in the lower limbs, as mentioned above, and may result in difficulties in balance and delay in walking additional to the effects of the peripheral paralysis. If sufficiently prolonged or severe, and especially if there has been meningitis as well, mental deficit and its associated problems may render any attempts at rehabilitation in walking futile. At any time, acute hydrocephalus, either spontaneous or secondary to shunt blockage or cerebral infection may threaten life and its treatment takes precedence over any orthopaedic procedure.

The progress and prognosis of the paralysis

The paralytic state that is present before and immediately after birth varies between the extremes of total paraplegia and paralysis confined to some of the intrinsic muscles of the feet. Its further progress depends on subsequent events.

If immediate and successful closure of the spinal lesion has been made without further damage to neural elements or the development of infection, about half of all open myelomeningoceles will maintain the same neurological level of lesion for at least the first 5–10 years of life. Some may lose one or two root levels, or even become severely paralysed after showing evidence of adequate muscle action immediately after birth. This may be either because of operative trauma, or because of infection or vascular changes in the affected neural tissues.

Even after satisfactory early operative closure of the lesion, an infant who, immediately after birth, showed what appeared to be good or even vigorous activity in most or all of its lower limb muscles may develop a gradual loss of spontaneous activity and, after a year, muscle activity may only be found in response to sensory stimuli and often in the form of a mass movement. When the child is old enough to respond to commands to move the limbs, it is apparent that there is no voluntary control of some or even almost all of the lower limb muscles.

This apparent loss of neurological function is not necessarily due to additional damage to neurological tissues. Activity in the limbs in a normal new-born baby is probably not under higher cerebral or 'voluntary' control but is mediated at spinal cord level. It is not until the pyramidal tracts have become myelinated that true voluntary activity occurs. The movements in the lower limbs in a myelomeningocele child in whom the lumbosacral segments are generally intact but divorced from connection with proximal tracts may seem to be normal at birth but the defect in their innervation manifests during the first year of life.

In children with a minor degree of paralysis, for instance in association with a small sacral myelomeningocele, a spina bifida occulta or a lipoma of the cauda equina, a slow true increase in the root level of paralysis may develop during the first few years of life because of tethering of the neural tissues and the effects of growth. Such patients need to be seen regularly to discover any neurological change for which further surgery on the spinal lesion may be needed.

In most children, the pattern and level of paralysis that is present at the end of the first 18 months of life does not alter during childhood. As puberty approaches, the upper limbs and

trunk increase in size and bulk disproportion-
ately to the size and strength of the lower limbs
and, thus, the effective paralysis increases.

In general, the prognosis for independent
walking bears a strong relationship to the root
level of voluntary activity in the lower limb
muscles. If there is innervation down to the
fourth lumbar root level or below it, useful
walking ability is likely to be present and this can
usually be assessed at or after the second year of
life. If the quadriceps in both lower limbs can be
shown to have strength greater than MRC grade
3 (antigravity) there is a strong chance that
walking ability will be adequate and measures to
correct deformity and to sustain the best possible
action in the lower limb musculature during
childhood will be worth-while.

Deformity

The main mechanism of lower limb deformity is
the same as in other forms of paralysis in
childhood (Sharrard 1967). Paralysis of one
muscle group in the presence of activity in its
opposing muscles leads to deformity directed
towards the active muscle. The stronger muscle
and tendon shows diminished growth and the
deformity becomes fixed (Chapter 6). Bony
deformity may follow after soft tissue deformity
has become established (Chapter 6).

Birth deformity

Congenital absence of innervation of muscles *in
.utero* may lead to deformities at birth
corresponding with the paralytic picture
(Sharrard 1964a) though lack of normal fetal
limb movements may also allow deformity to
develop from uterine pressure (Stark &
Drummond 1971). A number of specific
patterns of birth deformity and paralysis can be
recognized (Sharrard 1979). For example, in
babies showing good innervation of muscles
supplied by the first four lumbar neural segments
with paralysis below that level, the hips are

flexed, adducted, externally rotated and
dislocated, the knees show recurvatum
deformity and there is calcaneovarus deformity
of the feet (Fig. 4.1). Sometimes muscles that
have been active *in utero* and have produced
birth deformities become secondarily paralysed
after birth. There may then be deformity but
total paralysis or muscle activity not clearly
related to the deformity that is present.

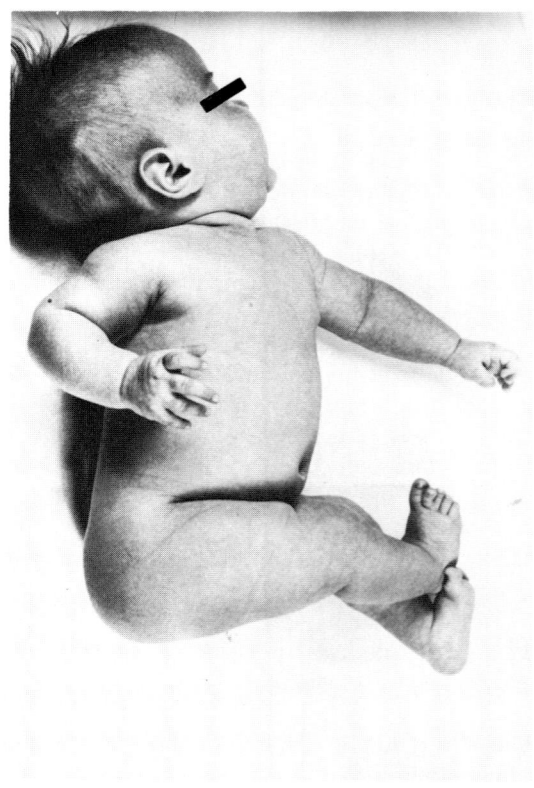

Fig. 4.1. Birth deformity in a child with innervation from the
first four lumbar neural segments.

Deformity during childhood

Progressive deformity may develop at any time
during childhood. For example, a baby in whom
there was no deformity at birth and a pattern of
muscle activity that seemed to be normal may
develop deformity as the result of alteration in

the distribution of the paralysis. In closed myelomeningocele lesions this is particularly likely to occur (Fig. 4.2). In general, once a paralytic deformity starts to develop, it shows a slow but steady increase in spite of splintage or physiotherapy if there is significantly unbalanced muscle activity.

The rate of increase of deformity depends partly on the degree of muscle imbalance and partly on the rate of growth of the child. Younger children usually show more rapid increase in deformity. As puberty approaches, deformity, except in the spine, progresses less rapidly and becomes static when growth ceases.

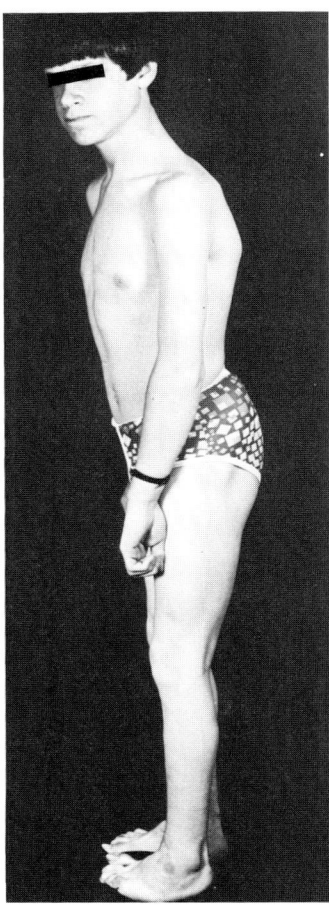

Fig. 4.2. Deformities of the feet developing in childhood in spina bifida occulta.

Spinal deformity (Chapter 7)

Deformity of the spine in spina bifida may arise from two potential causes: abnormality of vertebral form or development and the effects of trunk paralysis. In contrast with the situation in the lower limbs, vertebral abnormality is probably the more important cause.

In many patients, the main and only abnormality is absence of the posterior elements in the region of the bifid spine. In such patients, no significant deformity appears during the first 8–10 years of life. After this age, more rapid growth of the spine, particularly of the vertebral bodies, causes an increasing lordosis. If the lesion is extensive and the paralysis marked, severe lordoscoliosis develops and may seriously impair sitting posture in a patient already confined to a wheelchair.

In some patients, there may be other bony spinal abnormalities such as hemivertebrae, wedged vertebrae or fused vertebrae which, in themselves, may give rise to spine deformity in the form of scoliosis, lordoscoliosis or kyphosis. A variety of myelomeningocele lesion, not commonly seen, is hemimyelocele (Duckworth *et al.* 1968, Chapter 3) in which there is little or no deformity or paralysis in one lower limb but typical paralysis in the other limb. There is always a diastematomyelia and one or more hemivertebrae at or near the site of the spinal lesion. Scoliosis is likely to become severe. Such deformity may be present or show increase in younger children, but it increases markedly with the advent of puberty and causes increased disability in a child who is already handicapped by lower limb paresis or paralysis. Moreover, management by bracing, jackets or supports is made much more difficult in many patients because of sensory loss.

A deformity almost unique to patients with spina bifida is severe congenital kyphosis. It is usually associated with a wide and severe open myelomeningocele in which the erector spinae lies far laterally and becomes a perverted flexor of the spine. Such kyphoses can be corrected partially at birth by vertebral resection at the time of spine closure (Sharrard 1968) but the procedure is not now recommended because of the very poor general prognosis in such children. A few less severely affected children may survive and develop increasing kyphosis during childhood for which kyphus resection (Sharrard & Drennan 1972) may be indicated.

Assessment in the newborn

The examination of a child born with a myelomeningocele lesion involves paediatric, neurological and orthopaedic assessment. Paediatric assessment should determine the general health of the infant, the presence of any other congenital abnormalities and the fitness of the child for surgical treatment. Because of bladder paralysis before birth, attention will need to be paid to the adequacy of renal function, since some babies already show hydronephrosis at birth. The general neurological assessment should determine the state of neurological maturity of the infant, the presence of hydrocephalus and the size, nature and state of the spinal lesion with reference to the

feasibility of surgical closure of the defect. Orthopaedic examination needs to determine the general level of innervation of the lower limbs and the presence of deformity. Sometimes the orthopaedic surgeon may be able to make this assessment at the initial admission but, if not, it can be made after closure of the spinal lesion. Some general idea of sensory response can be obtained by pin-prick examination starting in sacrally-innervated segments and passing to lumbar-innervated regions until a response occurs. Limb movement does not necessarily indicate that the sensation is being appreciated, since it may be eliciting only reflex muscle activity. If the baby cries, it is possible that the pin is being felt but sensory testing is not entirely reliable at birth, or in infancy.

Precise assessment of muscle activity is difficult but, if the child is awake and moving its upper limbs, any spontaneous movements in the lower limbs may indicate the overall motor innervation. It is usually possible to determine and record the presence or absence of activity in most muscle groups or individual muscles in the lower limbs and to determine a root level of innervation by appreciation of the root supply of

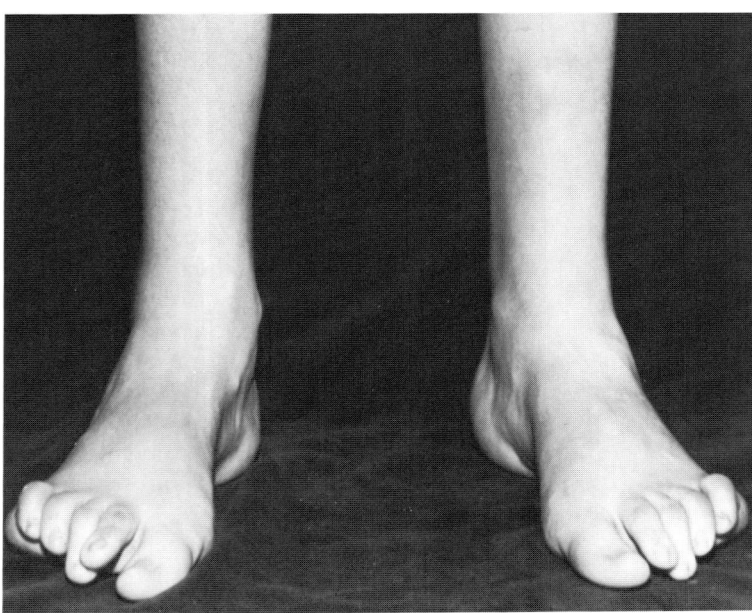

Fig. 4.3. Pes cavus and claw toes in a child with sacral myelomeningocele.

the lower limb muscles (Sharrard 1964a). Additional information may be obtained by percutaneous faradic stimulation of muscles or nerves which will define whether a muscle is innervated or not, irrespective of the presence of spontaneous activity in it. A description of the type and extent of deformity of the hips, knees and feet, supplemented if possible by a clinical photograph, should be made. There is often a correlation between the type of deformity and the pattern of neurological involvement. Radiographs should be taken of the lumbar spine, pelvis and lower limbs.

From this assessment, a general prognosis can be obtained. Brocklehurst (1976) described six groups of lesion.

Group A. A robust infant with no hydrocephalus and a sacral myelomeningocele or a superficial lesion in the cervical or thoracic region with no detectable neurological deficit in the lower limbs or sphincters. Urgent surgical treatment of the spinal lesion is indicated to prevent meningitis and loss of neurological function. The child will require regular orthopaedic review of the feet for future intrinsic foot muscle weakness and claw toe deformity (Fig. 4.3) that may need correction by simple tendon transfers.

Group B. A robust infant with an open lumbar or sacral lesion, no hydrocephalus and at least evidence of hip flexion, knee extension and perhaps ankle dorsiflexion indicative of lumbar innervation down to the third, fourth or fifth root level. There may be hip deformities including dislocation and calcaneovarus foot deformities (Fig. 4.1). Successful treatment by appropriate orthopaedic procedures and management of the renal tract should result in a patient able to walk to a limited or greater extent and with means to maintain social continence (Fig. 4.4). Urgent treatment of the spinal lesion is indicated.

Group C. A robust infant with evidence of prenatal hydrocephalus, an open thoracolumbar myelomeningocele with little or no spontaneous movement in the lower limbs and/or reflex muscle activity. The prognosis is poor whatever is done for the spinal lesion at birth and treatment can be surgical or medical for the lesion itself. If the child survives, a wheelchair existence is inevitable in adolescence (Fig. 4.5) even if very limited walking with extensive calipers may be possible during childhood.

Group D. A robust infant with an unusual variety of lesion such as hemimyelocele, lipoma of the cauda equina, or spinal dysraphism. All

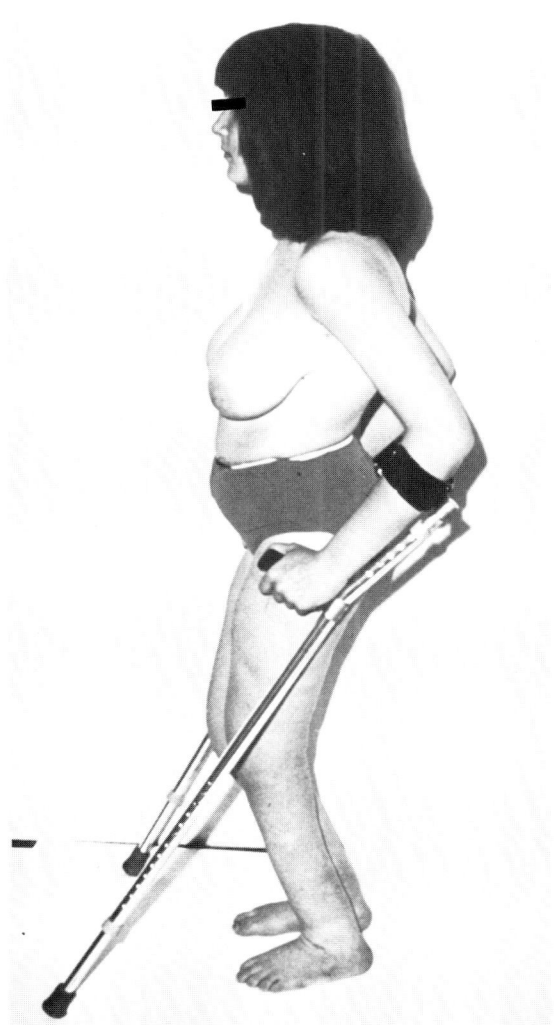

Fig. 4.4. Complete paraplegia in a child with thoracolumbar myelomeningocele.

necessary treatment as required for the neurological and orthopaedic lesions should be given.

Group E. A puny infant with a myelomeningocele and other congenital abnormalities of a moderate or severe nature. The prognosis is very poor and surgical treatment of the spine is not indicated.

Group F. A puny infant with a myelomeningocele and central nervous deficit possibly aggravated by hypoxia at birth. Only conservative management is appropriate and an early death is likely.

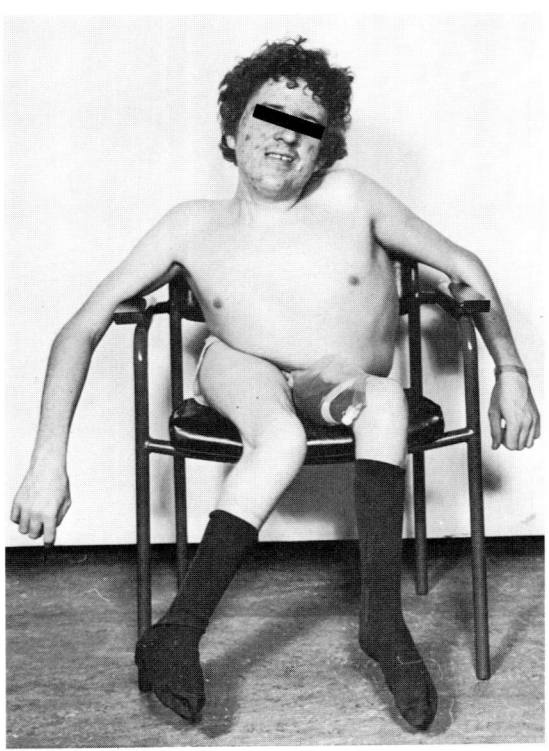

Fig. 4.5. End result in a patient born with partial paralysis and birth deformities similar to those in Fig. 4.1.

Assessment during childhood

Muscle activity and deformity can be assessed more accurately in an older child when the action of muscles can be recorded as being under voluntary control, reflex or a mixture of both. Faradic stimulation often gives additional information about muscle activity that is present but not under voluntary control. Electromyography can be used but, in general, does not provide as much useful information to guide orthopaedic management as does faradic stimulation. The assessment of lower limb deformity and paralysis needs to be made at least six-monthly throughout childhood up to the age of 10. After the first year, the neurological pattern of paralysis becomes more obvious and the presence of voluntary and reflex activity in individual muscles can be assessed with increasing accuracy and confidence as the child becomes older.

Orthopaedic management in the first year of life

Immediate orthopaedic treatment such as splintage that might be appropriate for congenital deformities in otherwise normal children cannot be applied in the newborn period because of the prior need for closure of the spinal lesion and nursing in an incubator. In some patients, hydrocephalus may require treatment by drugs or shunting. Only when the child has recovered well from the initial treatment of its more urgent neurosurgical and medical problems may attention be given to orthopaedic measures (American Academy of Orthopaedic Surgeons 1972, Menelaus 1980). Lesser and relatively mobile foot deformities can be managed conservatively by passive stretching or simple conservative means until an established pattern of paralysis can be defined. More severe and fixed foot deformities such as talipes varus may benefit from early surgical releases similar to those undertaken in normal children but tendons should be lengthened rather than divided in case they are needed for transfer at a later time.

Hip deformities, too, can be managed by passive movements and simple splints unless they are severe and fixed with dislocation of the hips. If so, a decision may need to be made as to whether to attempt reduction of the dislocations (Sharrard 1983). If there is evidence of strong muscle action, especially in the hip flexors and adductors with considerable fixed flexion and adduction deformity, only surgical release of the adductors and flexors can achieve reduction and this is best done during the second six months of life. If the hips reduce fairly easily after adductor release, a tendon transfer to provide abductor and extensor power such as posterolateral iliopsoas or external oblique transfer (Chapter 8) will be needed if recurrent dislocation is to be avoided. If hip reduction proves to be difficult, or muscle activity is limited, it may be better to accept the dislocations if they are bilateral and to rely on muscle and tendon lengthenings alone to correct unacceptable hip deformity. Unilateral dislocation should be treated wherever possible, since unequal limb length and hip deformity will make future management difficult whatever the level of innervation.

Orthopaedic management in childhood

Milder deformity that was present at birth but has not increased or has only worsened slowly can be corrected by suitable musculotendinous releases and limited tendon transfers. Before the age of 5, it is better to release or lengthen short tendons and muscles than to embark on other than single tendon transfers.

More severe deformity that has not been corrected in the first year of life, or which has been incompletely corrected, needs radical surgery and such tendon transfers as are necessary to achieve balanced muscle action. Deformity that becomes apparent as growth and activity take place may need surgical measures depending on the pattern of paralysis. It is not advisable to rely on physiotherapy or splintage to correct progressively increasing deformity due to active muscles, whether under voluntary control or acting reflexly, until fixed deformity and muscle imbalance have been corrected surgically.

At the hip, the aim should be to achieve stable hips, preferably concentrically in joint, with no fixed adduction or abduction deformity and not more than 20 degrees of flexion deformity. At the knee, fixed recurvatum or fixed flexion of more than 20 degrees should be corrected. At the ankle, correction must be made of equinus deformity of more than 10 degrees and of any fixed calcaneus deformity. At the foot, any fixed varus, valgus or plantaris deformity must be corrected and toe flexion deformities liable to sustain pressure from footwear should be treated. A plantigrade foot in which weight is borne on at least half of the area of the heel and sole is the primary aim in a foot that has complete or partial loss of sensibility. It is better to achieve a well-corrected foot during the first 5 or 6 years than it is in adolescence, when there may be established bony deformity.

Calipers and surgical footwear can be prescribed once deformity has been corrected and when the child is making attempts to stand. In some children, this may be during the second year of life; in others, it may not be until the age of 3 or 4 years. The extent of support that is needed will depend on the extent of the paralysis. If there is sufficient hip abductor and extensor activity, hip calipers will not be necessary and if there is good quadriceps activity bilaterally, calipers to support the knee should not be needed. However, it is often useful to give more extensive support than may seem to be necessary in a younger child who is trying to establish walking balance and to diminish the extent of caliperage later. A weak or flail ankle or foot will need irons and boots with heel sockets and appropriate T-straps and drop-foot or calcaneus stops. Although moulded plastic or cosmetic supports can be used, they are difficult to mould to a smaller foot and may cause pressure on an anaesthetic foot. While the foot is still growing fairly rapidly, they may need frequent replacement. For the more severely paraplegic child, hip–knee–ankle orthoses or one of the variety of swivel walkers will allow limited upright walking which is valuable for the maintenance of bone development and strength and to avoid spontaneous fractures.

When a fracture occurs in the paralysed and insensitive limb of a spina bifida child, it often does so without obvious trauma. The affected part of the limb becomes swollen and red, there may be a moderate pyrexia and there is an elevated white cell count. Initially, there may be minimal radiographic changes, especially if there has been only a slight slipping of an epiphysis. Osteomyelitis is often mistakenly diagnosed; antibiotics may be given and surgical incision of the swelling may even be made before further radiographs after a week show the characteristic extensive callus formation. Plaster cast treatment is unnecessary and may lead to pressure sores. A crepe and wool bandage with Cramer wire or other stiffening is sufficient. Healing is rapid and weight-bearing in calipers can be resumed after 3–4 weeks at the most.

Spinal deformity is rarely a problem in the absence of congenital bony deformity during this period of life. Milwaukee or other types of trunk bracing are poorly tolerated and usually ineffective in spina bifida with congenital scoliosis or kyphosis. If severe vertebral kyphosis, hemivertebrae or vertebral wedging is present in early childhood, it is best treated by early local spine fusion.

Orthopaedic management in adolescence

After a spina bifida child passes the age of 10, some important changes occur in his development and progress. As puberty is reached, the adolescent growth spurt results in a disproportionate increase in bulk and size of the trunk relative to the lower limbs, which show only a relatively small increase in length and size. Of even greater importance is the finding that the strength of the lower limb muscles does not increase in proportion to the total increase in weight. In consequence, the child with innervation to, for example, the third lumbar root level who has been able to walk independently to a limited extent with the aid of fairly extensive hip–knee–ankle orthoses finds it increasingly difficult to do so and takes to a wheelchair existence for most or all of his or her daily activities.

Nevertheless, the aim should be to make the child as independent as possible. If, as is usual, the strength of the upper limbs is adequate, he or she should be able to transfer from wheelchair to bed or chair or to a vehicle. If he or she cannot do so, a course of instruction at a paraplegia centre may be needed. It is children with this level or innervation, and who may have a fairly extensive bony spinal defect, who are very likely to develop a progressive and severe lordoscoliosis with the onset of puberty (Fig. 4.6). Pelvic obliquity, which usually accompanies the scoliosis, results in a sitting posture in which excessive pressure is applied to a limited area of the buttock with the development of ulceration over one ischial tuberosity or greater trochanter.

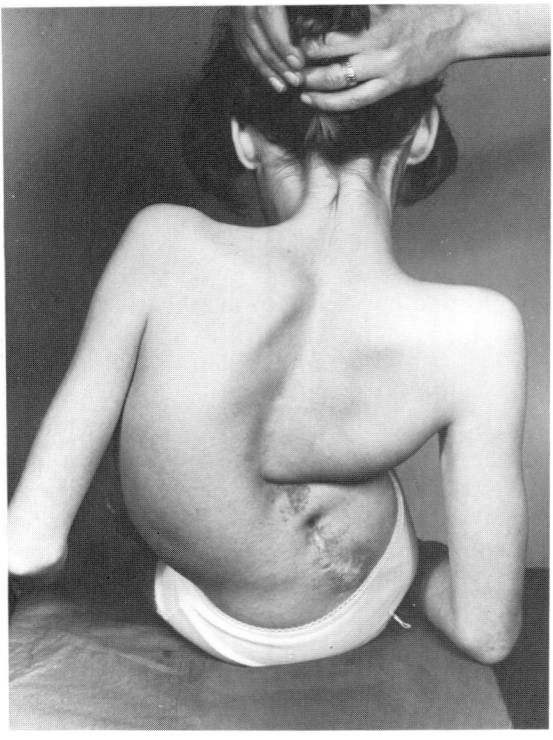

Fig. 4.6. Adolescent patient with myelomeningocele. Severe lordoscoliosis with abnormal sitting posture.

Sitting balance may become disturbed so that the child, unless supported by the arms of a chair or wheelchair, falls sideways, and has to support himself with one hand, leaving only one upper limb free for manipulative actions. The scoliosis may lead to pain from pressure of ribs on the pelvic brim or to diminished respiratory capacity. For any or all of these reasons, corrective spine fusion, often by combined anterior and posterior approaches, frequently is indicated. The child with innervation to the fourth or fifth lumbar level who is able to walk with ankle orthoses or supportive footwear but who has weakness in the gluteus maximus and calf muscles cannot sustain a good upright gait and tends to walk with flexed hips and knees. Attempts to improve the walking posture by reverting to full knee–ankle orthoses makes the appearance better but seldom increases walking speed or effectiveness, and may even diminish overall function.

The child with innervation down to the upper sacral segments is usually able to continue to walk with minimal aids but the increase in weight which is being borne on an area of the foot which does not increase correspondingly results in a greatly increased pressure per unit area. If there is any abnormal distribution of pressure on the sole of the foot because of residual deformity, particularly calcaneus deformity, a serious neural pressure ulcer may develop (Fig. 4.7). Fortunately, provided that bone infection is avoided or treated early, most ulcers, even if large, can be healed by the application of a skin-tight plaster cast with no weightbearing (Lang-Stevenson *et al.* 1985). Once the ulcer has healed, the deformity that gave rise to the ulcer must be treated by a suitable surgical procedure to restore a better distribution of weight on the sole of the foot. Amputation is not often needed except where there is deep bony sepsis or severe circulatory deficiency.

Up to the age of adolescence, most spina bifida children will have been supplied with supportive or corrective footwear which often takes the form of a surgical boot, and orthoses that may

not necessarily be of the cosmetic type. Because of growth and the need for adjustment in length, the classic type of orthosis with boot or shoe sockets may have been more suitable. At adolescence, there is naturally a desire by the child to be given a cosmetic type of orthosis and to have a shoe rather than a boot. It may be possible to dispense with orthoses altogether, especially if a certain amount of rigidity and stability has developed in the ankle and foot joints. Alternatively, one of the variety of triple arthrodesis, especially of the Lambrinudi or Elmslie type, may be performed.

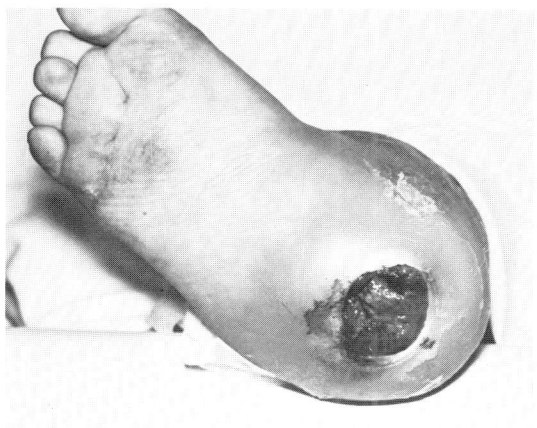

Fig. 4.7. Neuropathic ulcer in an adolescent foot with calcaneus deformity.

Obesity is an especial problem at this time. Dietary measures to combat this tendency are important in those who are still able to walk independently, but those who are confined to a wheelchair should perhaps not become too thin, since they may then be more liable to develop buttock ulceration.

Preparation for adult life needs to take account of future employment relative to the degree of motor impairment and the educational level of the child. When growth ceases, progressive deformity is rarely seen and the general level of locomotor function becomes static. Orthopaedic supervision can be confined to the continuing provision of orthoses and footwear and the management of ulcers should they develop. Renal and urinary function need continued intermittent review for any deterioration.

The techniques of the surgical management of deformities of the spine, hip, knee and foot are detailed in Chapters 7, 8, 9 and 10 respectively. Further details regarding the overall management of these patients can be obtained from American Academy of Orthopedic Surgeons (1972) and Menelaus (1980).

References

American Academy of Orthopedic Surgeons (1972) Symposium on myelomeningocele. C.V. Mosby Co., St. Louis.

BROCKLEHURST G. (1976) Spina Bifida for the Clinician. *Clinics in Developmental Medicine No. 57.* Heinemann (William) Medical Books Ltd, London.

DUCKWORTH T., SHARRARD W.J., LISTER J. & SEYMOUR N. (1968) Hemimyelocele. *Developmental Medicine and Child Neurology,* **Suppl. 16,** 69–75.

JAMES C.C.M. & LASSMAN L.P. (1962) Spinal Dysraphism. The diagnosis and treatment of progressive lesions in spina bifida occulta. *Journal of Bone and Joint Surgery,* **44B,** 828–40.

LANG-STEVENSON A.I., SHARRARD W.J.W., BETTS B.P. & DUCKWORTH T. (1985) Neuropathic ulcers of the foot. *Journal of Bone and Joint Surgery,* **67B,** 438–42.

MENELAUS M. (1980) *The Orthopaedic Management of Spina Bifida Cystica.* Second edition. Churchill Livingstone, Edinburgh.

SHARRARD W.J.W. (1962) The mechanism of paralytic deformity in spina bifida. *Developmental Medicine and Child Neurology,* **4,** 310–3.

SHARRARD W.J.W. (1964a) The segmental innervation of the lower limb muscles in man. *Annals of the Royal College of Surgeons of England,* **35,** 106–22.

SHARRARD W.J.W. (1964b) Posterior iliopsoas transplantation in the treatment of paralytic dislocation of the hip. *Journal of Bone and Joint Surgery,* **46B,** 426–44.

SHARRARD W.J.W. (1966) Mortality, Paralysis and Deformity in Spina Bifida Cystica. ChM Thesis, University of Sheffield.

SHARRARD W.J.W. (1967) Paralytic deformity in the lower limb. *Journal of Bone and Joint Surgery,* **49B,** 731–47.

SHARRARD W.J.W. (1968) Spinal osteotomy for congenital kyphosis in myelomeningocele. *Journal of Bone and Joint Surgery,* **50B,** 466–71.

SHARRARD W.J.W. (1979) *Paediatric Orthopaedics and Fractures.* Second edition. Blackwell Scientific Publications Ltd., Oxford.

SHARRARD W.J.W. (1983) Management of paralytic subluxation and dislocation of the hip in myelomeningocele. *Developmental Medicine and Child Neurology,* **25,** 374–6.

SHARRARD W.J.W. & DRENNAN J.C. (1972) Osteotomy-excision of the spine for lumbar kyphosis in older children with myelomeningocele. *Journal of Bone and Joint Surgery,* **54B,** 50–60.

SHARRARD W.J.W., ZACHARY R.B., LORBER J. & BRUCE A.M. (1963) A controlled trial of immediate and delayed closure of spina bifida cystica. *Archives of Diseases of Childhood,* **38,** 18–22.

STARK G.D. & BAKER G.C.W. (1967) The neurological involvement of the lower limbs in myelomeningocele. *Developmental Medicine and Child Neurology,* **9,** 732–44.

STARK G.D. & DRUMMOND M. (1971) The spinal cord lesion in myelomeningocele. *Developmental Medicine and Child Neurology,* **Suppl 25,** 1–14.

Chapter 5
Medical Aspects of the Dystrophies, Myopathies and Atrophies

J. Z. HECKMATT, V. DUBOWITZ

Introduction

This chapter is devoted to medical aspects of the neuromuscular disorders. These are of particular interest and importance to the orthopaedic surgeon, frequently presenting with a specific problem such as difficulty with gait or deformity: congenital dislocation of the hips, talipes or scoliosis. The diagnosis of an underlying neuromuscular disorder is important because management of any orthopaedic problem may differ radically from the usual management in an otherwise healthy child. In particular the child's overall potential, prognosis and speed of development has to be taken into account.

Aspects of diagnosis and investigation will be dealt with first, then specific disorders in more detail. Some disorders of little relevance to the orthopaedic surgeon, such as the metabolic myopathies, will not be discussed. More complete texts are available (Dubowitz 1978, Dubowitz 1980).

Diagnosis of neuromuscular disease

Clinical aspects

History

The history of the child's general level of activity and motor development should be taken. If there seems to be underlying weakness, determine whether it appears to be improving, static or worsening. Enquire into the developmental

history including fetal movements, presence of poly- or oligohydramnios, birth asphyxia, abnormalities of limb movement or tone during early infancy and any difficulties with sucking, swallowing or breathing.

In an older child establish the ages at which he could sit independently, pull to standing, stand and walk independently; whether walking was stable and if getting up from the floor was easy. Time of first smiling, reaching out for objects, speaking single words and sentences reflect intellectual development. Even if many details are forgotten, parents usually remember when their child first walked and spoke sentences.

In the family history, presence of an affected relative may reveal pattern of inheritance and under some circumstances indicate disease severity. In congenital myopathy there may be associated deformities. In congenital myotonic dystrophy the mother is affected and is likely to have mild symptoms and signs.

Examination

The young child should be encouraged to do as much as possible without attempting to undress or restrain him, observing the gait, ability to get down onto the floor and rise again. Getting him to build a tower of cubes shows manipulation and shoulder girdle power. He should be encouraged to try to jump, hop and climb steps, and if able to do so easily is unlikely to have significant lower limb weakness. At this stage he should be undressed for a more detailed examination. In children over 5 years a more detailed assessment of power of individual muscle groups is often possible.

When examining infants, establish the range of facial movements and visual alertness. Hypotonia is indicated by adoption of a frog posture and weakness by absence of antigravity power. Limb movements should be observed, if necessary provoked by stimulation. General tone and power is assessed by pulling on the hands showing head control and holding the infant in ventral suspension.

In older children assess facial weakness by noting the appearance at rest and the ability to screw up the eyelids and bury the eyelashes, to show the teeth, pout and whistle. The shoulder girdle should be examined for ability to abduct fully and any tendency of the scapula to rise upwards.

Tendon jerks may be reduced but are only consistently absent in severe spinal muscular atrophy (Werdnig–Hoffmann disease). Tongue fasciculation at rest is seen in severe and intermediate spinal muscular atrophy. Finger tremor is invariably present in the intermediate type but more variable in the mild type. Tremor may also be usefully picked up as a disturbance of the baseline on the ECG.

Toe walking usually with restriction of ankle dorsiflexion is seen early in Duchenne muscular dystrophy. In peripheral neuropathy there may be a drop foot gait. In children with the mild type of spinal muscular atrophy the feet tend to evert and be externally rotated (Moosa & Dubowitz 1973).

The range of joint movement should be measured, and any tightness of the iliotibial bands assessed. In dystrophic children there is a tendency for contractures. In some floppy infants and children excessive joint laxity may occur as an isolated phenomenon.

The spine should always be examined. Scoliosis is very common in those confined to a wheelchair (Chapter 6) but may also occur in children who are ambulant. Rigidity of the spine with limited flexion or a fixed lumbar lordosis may sometimes occur.

Investigations

The three most useful investigations are serum enzymes, electrodiagnostic studies and muscle biopsy. In general the first two are screening and the muscle biopsy more definitive investigations.

Serum enzymes

Various enzymes have been measured in the past, particularly the transaminases, but the most specific is the serum creatine (phospho)kinase (CPK or CK). It is present in heart and skeletal muscle and not present in other tissues except brain.

Serum CK activity is markedly elevated in the Duchenne, Becker and limb girdle dystrophies. This is especially so early on when clinical signs are absent or minimal. In the Duchenne type serum CK activity is at least ten times greater than the upper limit of the normal adult range (Fig. 5.1).

Serum CK activity is also elevated in about half the cases of congenital muscular dystrophy and acute polymyositis (Fig. 5.1). In most other disorders serum CK activity is normal or only minimally elevated. However, moderate elevation is sometimes seen in the mild type of spinal muscular atrophy. Serum CK activity is also elevated in female carriers of muscular dystrophy.

Electrophysiological investigations

Nerve conduction velocity This measurement is performed using surface electrodes. Velocity reflects size and degree of myelination of the largest nerve fibres. Myelination is incomplete in infancy and velocity is half that of the adult increasing to the adult level between 3 and 5 years.

Electromyography This is useful as a screening test and can also help to distinguish neuropathy from myopathy. A concentric needle electrode is

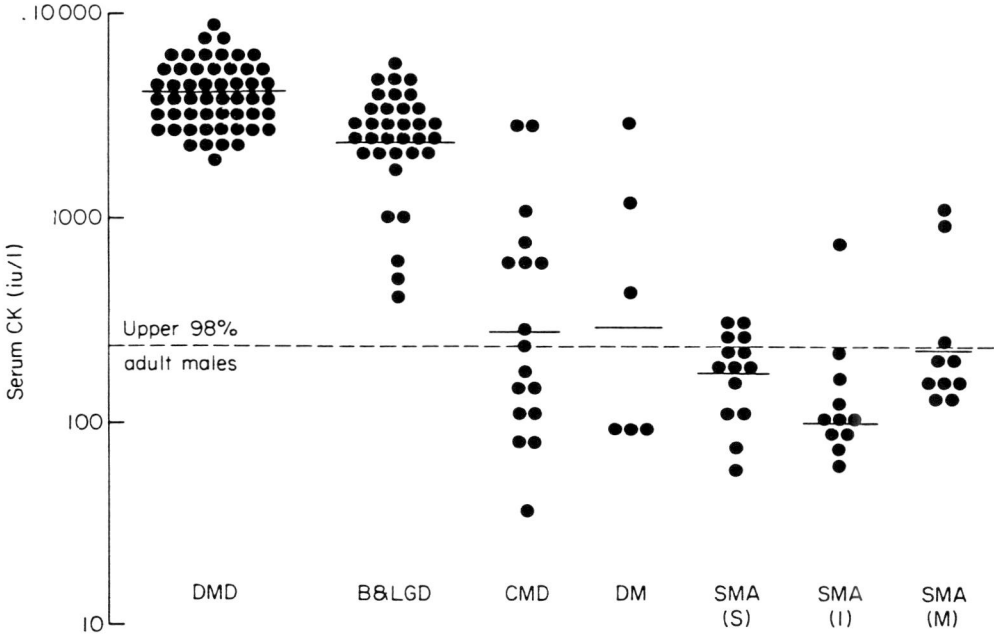

Fig. 5.1. Serum CK activity in 146 children, all referred as new cases to the authors' muscle clinic, values represented on a log scale. Upper limit of adult range for men 200 iu/l (dotted line), with grossly elevated levels in Duchenne muscular dystrophy (DMD), and most of those with limb girdle and Becker dystrophy (B & LGD). Activity in congenital muscular dystrophy (CMD) and new cases of dermatomyositis (DM) elevated in about half. Activity in severe and intermediate spinal muscular atrophy (SMA [S] and [I]) is normal or only minimally elevated while activity in the mild type (SMA [M]) is occasionally moderately elevated.

placed within the muscle and electrical activity produced by contraction is displayed on an oscilloscope and relayed through a loudspeaker.

In myopathy there is reduction in amplitude of the electrical activity and the individual motor units appear ragged or 'polyphasic' and sound crackly in the loudspeaker. In neuropathy the pattern is of isolated high amplitude individual units separated by a flat base line. There may also be fibrillation potentials at rest. The EMG of myotonia deserves special mention, in which there are spontaneous bursts of potentials firing rapidly and waxing and waning giving a characteristic 'dive-bomber' effect over the loudspeaker.

Ultrasound imaging

The application of ultrasound imaging to the

diagnosis of neuromuscular disease is a new concept (Heckmatt *et al.* 1982). The principle, as applied to muscle, is a comparison of echo intensity reflected from the surface of bone against that reflected from the overlying muscle substance. In normal children muscle appears relatively echo-free while bone stands out clearly as a strong echo. In children with diseased muscle increased echo is reflected from within the muscle substance while bone echo is reduced (Fig. 5.2).

Sensitivity of ultrasound to abnormality within muscle is broadly similar to the EMG and ultrasound is useful as a safe, noninvasive screening test. In congenital muscular dystrophy ultrasound is probably more sensitive than the EMG, showing marked increase in muscle echo even when the child's disability is relatively mild (Fig. 5.3).

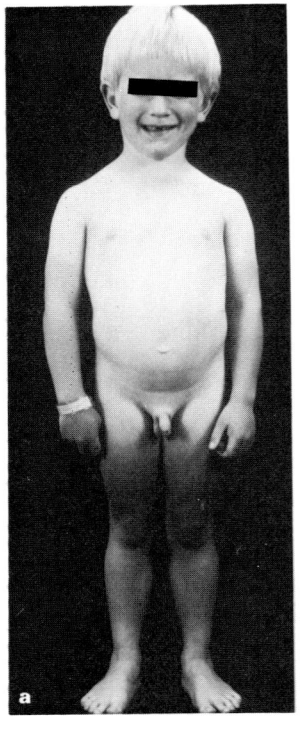

Muscle biopsy

Even if the clinical picture appears typical and abnormality is present on these preliminary investigations, it is important to perform a muscle biopsy to establish a definitive diagnosis. Techniques of fixing and processing muscle have undergone significant improvements in recent years (Dubowitz 1985). Techniques of taking muscle have also undergone considerable change and the biopsy can now be performed relatively atraumatically using the Bergström needle (Edwards *et al.* 1980), and the authors are so confident about the needle biopsy technique in patients of all ages, including neonates, that they virtually never carry out an open biopsy.

Needle biopsy has the advantage that the muscle can be taken through a small skin incision under local anaesthesia, requiring no sutures and leaving practically no scar. The technique is simple and quick and can be done as a side-room or outpatient procedure. So long as the site of biopsy is properly chosen there is no

Duchenne (4 years)

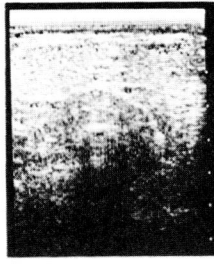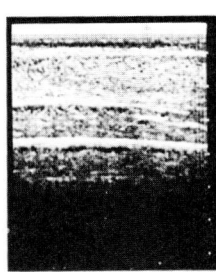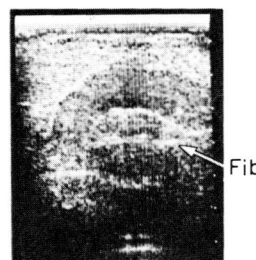

Normal

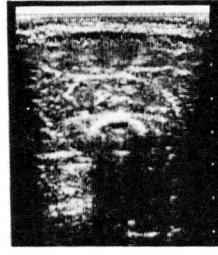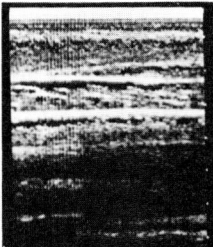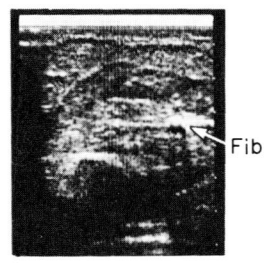

Thigh   Calf

b

Fig. 5.2. (a) Four-year-old boy with Duchenne muscular dystrophy.
(b) Realtime linear array ultrasound scans of the thigh and calf compared with a boy who presented with motor problems due to ligamentous laxity. In the boy with Duchenne dystrophy there is an increase in intensity of echo reflected from the muscle.

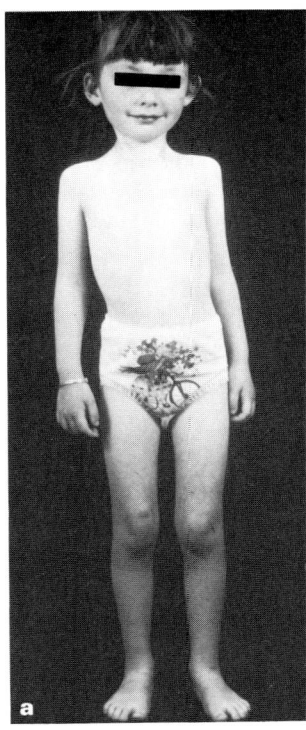

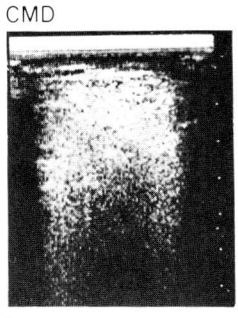
CMD

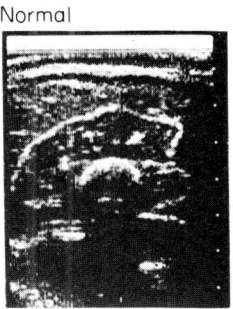
Normal

b

Fig. 5.3. (a) Four-year-old girl with congenital muscular dystrophy who initially presented with congenital dislocation of the hips. Difficulty with mobilization following splinting and reconstructive surgery to the hips led to further investigation. EMG performed at referring hospital was normal.
(b) Ultrasound scan of the muscle performed by ourselves was unequivocally abnormal, showing marked increase in echo reflected from the muscle and almost complete loss of bone echo.

risk of complications such as haematoma or damage to vital structures.

In children the authors routinely biopsy the anterior quadriceps in the midline at mid-thigh level. This area is free of major vessels and nerves. Occasionally we biopsy the deltoid muscle, but only in older children when the quadriceps is not likely to be involved or has been completely replaced by severe chronic disease. Edwards *et al.* (1980) reported successful biopsy of a number of different muscles in adult patients. The Bergström needle provides specimens of good size adequate for diagnosis and detailed quantitation. Smaller needles, such as the 'Tru-cut', have been tried, but they do not provide specimens of as good size. The technique is described in detail in the appendix to this chapter (p. 79).

Before introducing the needle biopsy technique in children in 1978 the authors conducted a feasibility study comparing needle and open biopsy in a series of 24 children, taking both through the same incision. The needle biopsies were later analysed 'blind'. The authors made an identical diagnostic interpretation from needle and open biopsies in 22 of the 24. In the remaining two the needle biopsies were too small for analysis.

In a review of 675 diagnostic needle biopsies done in children, between April 1978 and October 1982, 657 were successful (97.3%). Overall the needle biopsies were as good as open biopsies that had been performed in previous years, being well preserved, well orientated and of adequate size (Heckmatt *et al.* 1984).

Processing of biopsy samples is performed purely on frozen sections and several histological and histochemical stains are routinely done. Together, these stains provide a comprehensive picture of pathology within the muscle. The haematoxylin and eosin (H & E) stain shows the general histological pattern within the muscle.

The Verhoeff van Gieson (VVG) stain shows up connective tissue. The Gomori trichrome stain demonstrates abnormal structures such as 'nemaline rod bodies' and the 'ragged red' fibres of mitochondrial myopathy. The oxidative enzyme stain (NADH–TR) shows central and minicores; the ATPase stain demonstrates the two fibre types, fibre type grouping and myofibrillar loss. The periodic acid Schiff (PAS) stain shows glycogen and the oil-red-O stain lipid. The acid phosphatase stain demonstrates degenerating and regenerating fibres along with any active inflammatory cells. Two important cytoplasmic enzymes can be demonstrated histochemically, phosphorylase (deficient in McArdle's disease, glycogenosis type 5) and phosphofructokinase (deficient in glycogenosis type 7).

The muscular dystrophies

The muscular dystrophies are a group of genetically determined disorders characterized by progressive degeneration of skeletal muscle and without associated structural abnormality in the central nervous system. They are an important group both numerically and in terms of severity. The following disorders are included:

Duchenne muscular dystrophy;
limb girdle muscular dystrophy;
Becker muscular dystrophy;
facioscapulohumeral dystrophy;
myotonic dystrophy.

The first three are discussed as a group and the clinical features are summarized in Table 5.1.

Duchenne muscular dystrophy

Duchenne muscular dystrophy is the most rapidly progressive and the most common childhood neuromuscular disorder with about 2000 children affected in the UK (Gardner-Medwin 1980). It is X-linked recessive and affects only boys.

Parents are usually unaware of any problem in the first year of life. About 50% present in the second year with walking and speech delay. Alternatively presentation may be with abnormalities of gait such as toe walking, a tendency to fall often and unexpectedly with reluctance to walk and 'laziness'. The diagnosis is frequently missed at this stage, but can be easily confirmed by measurement of serum CK. In the majority of boys diagnosis is usually made between 3 and 6 years.

Early signs can be subtle, with no overt abnormality of gait, although there is usually difficulty rising from the floor with a Gowers' manoeuvre and inability to jump and run properly (Fig. 5.4).

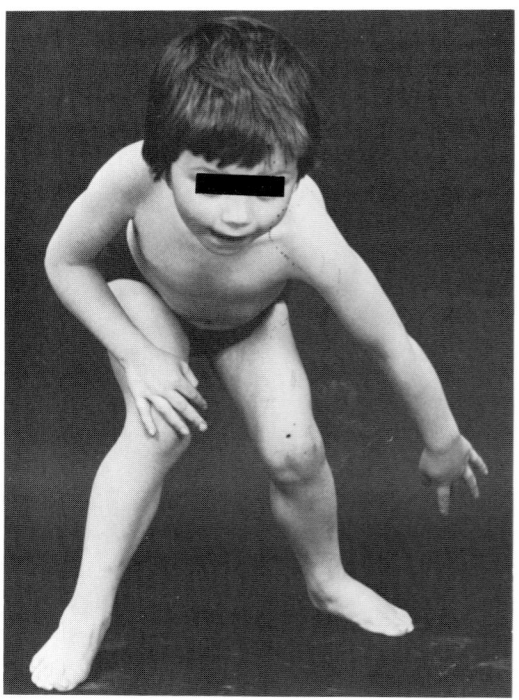

Fig. 5.4. Four-year-old boy with Duchenne muscular dystrophy. Note early Gowers' manoeuvre placing a hand on his knee as he rises from the floor.

The muscle weakness is relentlessly progressive although at first there is often a brief period of improvement. The ability to walk is lost on average at 9 years with a range from 6 to 12 years (Dubowitz 1978). Death is in the teens or early twenties (*see* below).

Table 5.1. Differential features in the various dystrophies.

	Duchenne	Becker	Limb-girdle	Facioscapulo-humeral	Congenital dystrophy	Myotonic Congenital onset	Myotonic Adult onset	Spinal muscular atrophy (mild)
Presentation	Early child-hood	Mid/late childhood	Variable ≡ Duchenne or Becker	Adolescence/adult life — occ. childhood	Birth or infancy	Birth	Childhood/adolescence/adult life	Early childhood
Progression	Loss of mobility by walking 6-12 yrs	Still walking adolescence ± adult life	Variable. Usually milder than Duchenne.	Slow, occasionally rapid.	None	None	Slow	None
Clinical features	Prox. weakness, toe walking, equinus, unable to run or jump well. Big calves common. 50% very big calves. walk late.	Mainly pelvic girdle weakness (mild at first). Often very big calves.	Variable severity. Calf hypertrophy less common.	Shoulder & facial weakness ± pelvic weakness later	Floppy infant + contractures ± facial weakness	Poly-hydramnios, birth asphyxia, talipes, facial diplegia, floppy. Myotonia absent at first.	Progressive facial involvement & myotonia. Some prox. weakness	Proximal weakness. External rotation & eversion of feet. Calf hypertrophy less common.
Non-muscle complications	± Mental handicap	—	—	—	Occ. mental handicap	Usually mental handicap	Many (text)	No mental handicap, often bright
SCK at presentation	Very high	Usually very high	Usually very high	Normal	50% high	Normal	Normal	Normal or mod. raised
Genetics	X-linked recessive	X-linked recessive	Autosomal recessive	Autosomal dominant	Autosomal recessive	Autosomal dominant (always mother)	Autosomal dominant	Autosomal recessive
Carrier detection	SCK	SCK	—	Clinical	—	Clinical (EMG)	Clinical (EMG)	—
Antenatal diagnosis	Abort all males	? needed	—	—	Poor fetal movements (late)	Poly-hydramnios (late)	—	—

There are a certain number of specific aspects worth considering in detail.

Abnormalities of posture and gait

Equinus deformity of the feet with Achilles tendon contracture is a common and early deformity. As weakness progresses there is a tendency for hip, knee and iliotibial band contractures to develop. With increasing weakness the boys stand with an exaggerated lumbar lordosis.

As the child begins to lose mobility there is commonly a tendency for asymmetry of stance. Early signs of asymmetry may develop when walking is still good, the weaker limb having slightly greater contractures.

Scoliosis is the most serious and rapidly progressive deformity once the child is in a wheelchair (Chapter 6). It may not be noticed at first and is frequently only obvious when the point of instability (about 30°) is reached or exceeded.

Management

There is no effective drug treatment for muscular dystrophy which prevents progression. A large number of drugs have been tried, particularly in Duchenne muscular dystrophy, with many claims that have proved false when a properly controlled trial has been carried out (Dubowitz & Heckmatt 1980).

Physical therapy is, on the other hand, very important. While the child is still ambulant, regular passive stretching of the ankles is required to prevent Achilles tendon tightness and wearing of night splints should be encouraged. Specific stretching of iliotibial bands should be practised from early on. It is important to prevent asymmetrical contractures.

Prolongation of the ability to walk Spencer and Vignos (1962) reported a series of 15 boys in whom they had performed Achilles tenotomy plus tensor fascia lata release followed by provison of knee–ankle–foot orthoses to prolong ambulation. Siegel *et al.* (1968) reported a similar series of 21 boys in whom, in addition to the other procedures, they sometimes released tight hip flexors. Hsu (1976) reported a similar rehabilitation programme but included tibialis posterior transfer. Since 1977 the authors have routinely rehabilitated boys with Duchenne muscular dystrophy using special lightweight knee–ankle–foot orthoses which allow mobility to be rapidly regained. Brief details of our techniques are given here, and further details can be obtained elsewhere (Hyde *et al.* 1982, Heckmatt *et al.* 1985).

Boys are rehabilitated at the point they have lost useful independent walking and are just about to go or have recently gone into a wheelchair (Fig. 5.5a). Following rehabilitation boys walk in the orthoses with stability and confidence, frequently less liable to fall than in the previous year. Prolongation of walking benefits the boys psychologically and also prevents the development of scoliosis (Chapter 6), contractures and deformities.

Almost all have equinus of the ankles, and to ensure proper support from the orthoses require Achilles tenotomy. The technique of Siegel *et al.* (1968) is used, which involves cutting the tendon through a small skin incision. No stitches are needed. However, the authors do not release iliotibial bands, nor do they perform any further procedures. From the first postoperative day the boy stands and walks in plaster casts. These maintain the ankles at right angles, the knees straight and extend proximally to give support under the ischia (Fig. 5.5b). The plasters are removed on the third postoperative day and the orthoses are cast. The plasters are re-applied and the boy walks in these for a further 7 days until the orthoses are ready. He spends a further week in hospital learning to walk in the orthoses (Fig. 5.5c).

The authors never intervene while the boy still has useful independent walking. However, it is important not to leave things too late. They are usually unable to rehabilitate those who have

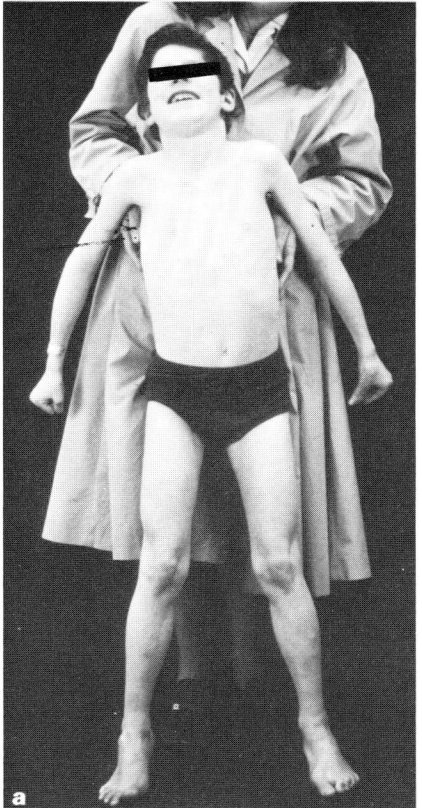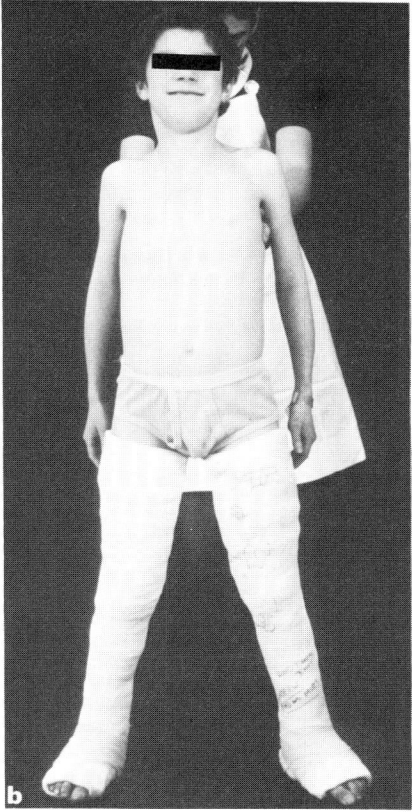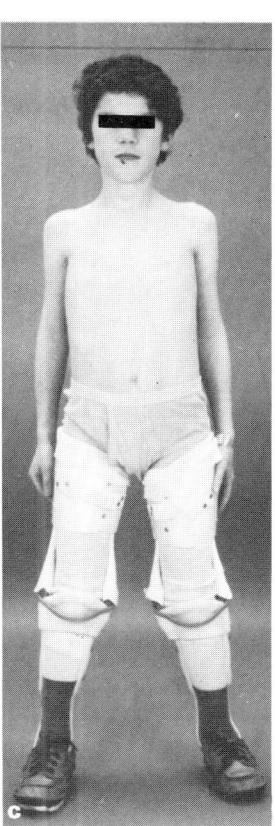

Fig. 5.5. Eleven-year-old boy with Duchenne muscular dystrophy.
(a) Unable to walk independently for the previous 7 weeks.
(b) Standing following bilateral transcutaneous Achilles tenotomy in full length ischial weightbearing plaster-of-Paris casts.
(c) Standing one week later in lightweight knee–ankle–foot orthoses.

been confined to a wheelchair for more than 3 months, because of weakness and contractures. Presence of asymmetrical contractures with an early fixed scoliosis also prevents rehabilitation.

Aspects of orthotic design are important. They are constructed of moulded polypropylene with aluminium alloy side members and are much lighter than the conventional steel and leather type. They have a rigid ankle support at 90°, the foot plate extending to the metatarsal heads but not beyond. They have a lip at the upper end to give good support under the ischial tuberosities. Boys remain dependent upon the orthoses providing support under the ischium and the length of the orthosis has to be adjusted regularly.

In a recent review of the authors' last 57 consecutive patients rehabilitated in lightweight orthoses, 47 achieved good independent walking in their orthoses. Of these 47, 27 have now stopped walking after periods ranging from 8 months to 48 months (mean 21 months) and 20 are still walking 9–29 months following rehabilitation. Ten never walked, but seven of them failed because of serious delay in the provision and bad design of the orthoses (Heckmatt *et al.* 1984).

Management of scoliosis While the child is still ambulant contractures, and in particular asymmetry of stance, should be avoided as much as possible with regular passive stretching.

Prolongation of walking with orthoses is a further important step in prevention, encouraging a symmetrical stance, ensuring mobility of the spine as the boy walks and a lordotic posture which helps stabilize the spine.

Maintenance of proper posture in the wheelchair is also important. The seat of the wheelchair should be firm, which encourages the boy to sit squarely, and the back should be of a sling design with a 15° recline which supports the spine. It is wise to check with regular X-rays at the slightest suspicion of scoliosis in all non-ambulant boys. A lightweight anterior-opening polypropylene brace should be fitted at the first sign. The development of obesity, common at this stage, can be a serious problem limiting the child's tolerance of a brace and should be prevented by prophylactic diet control.

With the introduction of new surgical techniques to control scoliosis, stabilization of a progressive curvature is feasible. The Luque technique offers advantages of virtually immediate postoperative mobilization and permanent freedom from a brace (Chapter 6).

Limb girdle muscular dystrophy

Limb girdle muscular dystrophy is an autosomal recessive disorder and affects both males and females. Clinical severity is very variable and it may be similar to Duchenne or the milder Becker dystrophy. In an isolated affected male it may be impossible to distinguish the milder type of limb girdle from Becker dystrophy.

Becker muscular dystrophy

This is a distinct form of muscular dystrophy very similar in clinical appearances and distribution of weakness to the Duchenne type but milder in severity. It is also X-linked recessive. Onset is generally later than Duchenne with normal early development but presentation in childhood, adolescence or adult life.

Presentation is with progressive muscle weakness, principally of the pelvic girdle. Generally the weakness is relatively mild with ability to jump and run only moderately impaired early on. Muscle cramps on exertion, sometimes associated with haemoglobinuria, is another common presentation. Calf hypertrophy may be present and can become quite marked in later years. Mobility is preserved until the teens or adult life.

We have had considerable success with prolongation of walking in a few teenagers who went off their feet. In one case this allowed the boy to remain at normal school, complete his studies, and gain entrance to university.

Differential diagnosis

Clinical severity and rate of disease progression are the most useful indications. When differentiating between the Duchenne and Becker dystrophies, severity in affected relatives is an important guide. Ability to walk beyond the age of 12 years or survival beyond the age of 30 years suggests a milder type of dystrophy than Duchenne.

Differentiation can also be made at presentation on the basis of severity. If the boy is able to jump easily or hop he is likely to have a milder disorder than Duchenne dystrophy. Objective quantitative assessment of muscle force and function is also useful (Scott *et al.* 1982).

Other aspects of muscular dystrophy

Intelligence

In Duchenne muscular dystrophy intelligence is impaired with a shift to the left of the normal distribution curve. The mean IQ is in the region of 85 as compared with the normal of 105 on the Wechsler scale. The intellectual handicap affects verbal more than performance IQ (Leibowitz & Dubowitz 1981). Intelligence is sometimes impaired in the other dystrophies.

Genetic counselling

Duchenne muscular dystrophy is an X-linked recessive disorder. It is thought, on the basis of the Haldane hypothesis, that one third of cases arise as spontaneous mutations. Thus the mother of an isolated case has a 2/3 risk of being a carrier and any of her sisters and daughters a 1/3 risk. However, the mother is an obligate carrier if she has an affected brother, nephew or uncle (through a direct female line). She is also very likely to be a carrier if she has two affected sons.

Measurement of serum CK activity helps to further define the risk of carrier status with about 2/3 of obligate carriers having a serum CK activity elevated above the normal range. For further refinement the actual level of CK activity can be used to calculate risk and this can be combined with genetic information to provide a final more accurate estimate of the risk (Emery 1976).

There is no means currently available of accurately telling if a male fetus is affected. The only option is to abort all male fetuses. Hopefully developments in the near future will allow a DNA probe to be developed which will accurately define carrier status and whether a male fetus is affected (Lancet 1983).

The situation is similar with Becker dystrophy. One important difference is that affected males may have children. A man with Becker dystrophy will not have an affected son but all his daughters will inherit his single abnormal X chromosome and therefore be obligate carriers. In limb girdle dystrophy the risk for brothers and sisters being affected is 25%. The disease is unlikely to be passed on to the next generation unless the affected person or carrier marries a carrier of the gene, which is more likely in consanguinous marriages.

Most females with muscular dystrophy have the autosomal recessive type but to date at least seven with a muscular dystrophy similar to Duchenne/Becker types have been found to have a balanced translocation of the X chromosome involving a break at the Xp21 site. On this basis the locus for the Duchenne gene has been established and recent work with DNA probes close to this locus have established that the Becker gene is located in the same region as well (*see* review by Roses *et al.* 1983).

Respiratory involvement

There is always some respiratory muscle weakness in Duchenne muscular dystrophy and this increases when the boy becomes wheelchair bound. It is usually a respiratory infection which directly causes death, after the boy has been in a wheelchair for some years. Progression of scoliosis aggravates respiratory impairment. Diaphragmatic function is relatively preserved until late. Respiratory involvement of itself rarely gives rise to any symptoms.

In Becker and limb girdle dystrophy respiratory involvement generally parallels overall severity of the disease. Occasionally in limb girdle dystrophy diaphragmatic involvement may be more severe (Newsom-Davis 1980).

Cardiac involvement

There is progressive involvement of cardiac muscle in Duchenne muscular dystrophy with replacement by connective tissue. This proceeds apace with decline in overall function and is rarely symptomatic (Hunter 1980). However, children in the advanced stages of the disease may die suddenly and unexpectedly during what appears to be a mild intercurrent infection. This is presumably a result of arrhythmia or other form of cardiac dysfunction.

Investigations

In Duchenne muscular dystrophy serum CK activity is very high in the early stages, at least 10 and up to 50 times the upper limit of the adult range. A normal or only moderately elevated activity should thus exclude the diagnosis (Fig. 5.1). CK activity is already high in infancy and even at birth so that screening is quite feasible from a drop of blood taken with the Guthrie, though screening is not yet widely practised (Zellweger & Antonik 1975). This is because of the lack, as yet, of any therapeutic agent to arrest the disease.

The EMG shows characteristic myopathic changes though it may be normal in early cases. Muscle biopsy shows unequivocal abnormalities, even in infancy, with variability in fibre size, internal nuclei, degenerating and regenerating fibres, cellular infiltrates, and proliferation of connective tissue and later also adipose tissue.

The findings in the limb girdle and Becker dystrophies are very similar and differentiation cannot be made on the basis of any of these investigations.

Facioscapulohumeral dystrophy

The muscle weakness is principally in the shoulder girdle and facial muscles. The patient usually complains of difficulty carrying objects and accomplishing tasks which require elevation of the arms above shoulder height.

The inheritance is autosomal dominant and the severity is very variable even amongst affected members in a single family. In mild cases there is minimal facial weakness with inability to bury the eyelashes and to show fully the teeth. On abduction of the arms the scapulae rotate upwards, giving the shoulders a characteristic terraced appearance when viewed from the front. In severe cases there is overt facial weakness with marked proximal weakness of shoulder and pelvic girdles, and early loss of ambulation.

Fixation of the scapulae by surgery allows better shoulder abduction (Chapter 6).

Investigations

The serum CK activity is frequently normal, the EMG may show myopathic changes, and mus-

cle biopsy may show various types of change including overt dystrophic change. However, the most common abnormality is the presence of small isolated angular fibres amongst relatively normal-looking muscle. The degree of pathological changes may be mild compared with overall disability.

Myotonic dystrophy

This is an important and probably one of the commonest neuromuscular disorders, with approximately 3000 affected individuals in the United Kingdom. There are two distinct types, a commoner adolescent or adult-onset type and a congenital type, and the inheritance is autosomal dominant. Harper (1979) gives a full account of this complex disorder.

Adult type

The diagnosis is frequently missed because patients deny symptoms and rarely present with myotonia. Myotonic dystrophy is a multisystem disorder and frequently presents with a complication such as presenile cataracts, malabsorption or constipation, breathing or swallowing difficulties, dementia, infertility or cardiac arrhythmia.

The term 'myotonia' refers to a state of delayed relaxation or sustained contraction of muscle. This is best elicited by asking the patient to make a fist and then open the hand as rapidly as possible, observing the characteristic delay in straightening the fingers. This stiffness can be relieved to a certain extent by repeatedly opening and closing the hand. Sustained contracture can be demonstrated by percussing the muscle directly, which produces a characteristic dimpling. On direct questioning patients may complain of difficulty releasing objects and there is often some associated clumsiness.

Even in early cases there is some facial weakness with inability to close the eyes fully, bury the eyelashes, and show the teeth (Fig. 5.6). In estab-

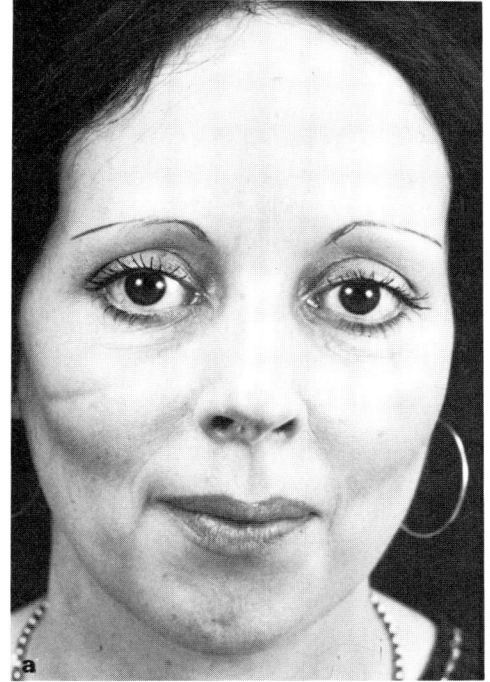
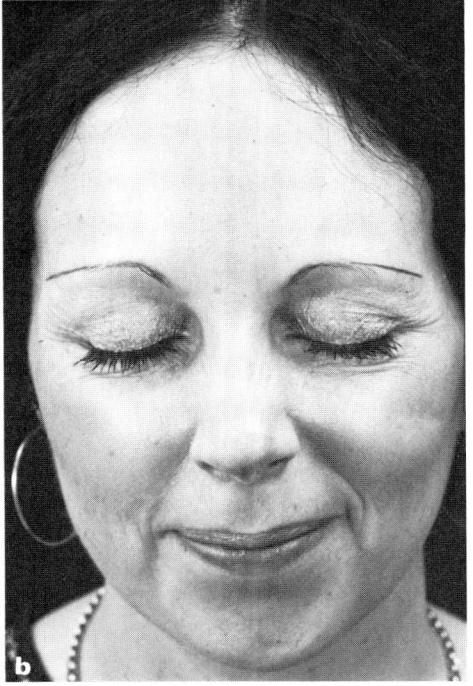
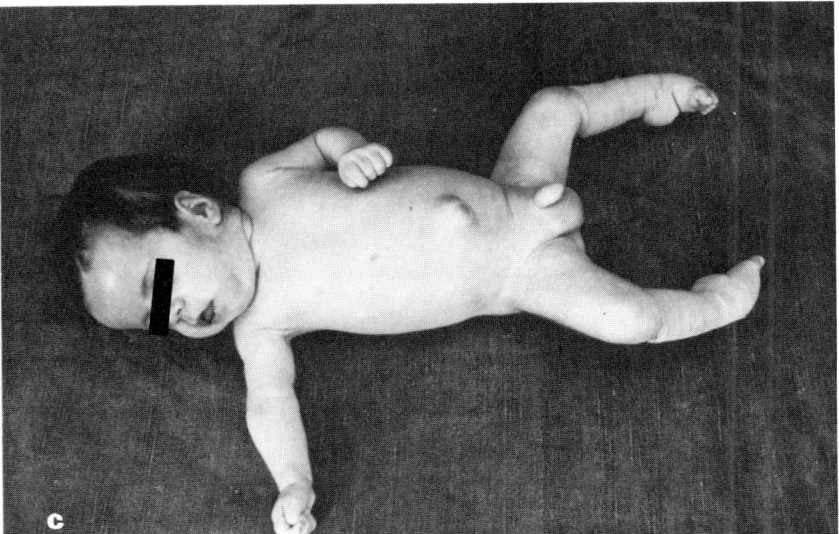

Fig. 5.6 (a) Twenty-nine year-old woman with myotonic dystrophy showing mild facial weakness and (b) difficulty burying eyelashes.
(c) Her son who was asphyxiated at birth but successfully resuscitated; note characteristic talipes equinovarus.

lished cases the facies have a characteristic appearance with facial weakness, wasting and ptosis.

One particularly hazardous complication of this disorder is an adverse reaction to general anaesthetic. This type of reaction usually occurs in early, mild and previously undiagnosed cases (and an unsuspecting anaesthetist).

Congenital type

In the congenital type the mother, not the father, carries the gene. In general she may be unaware of any problem in herself, although there will usually be subtle early signs and the EMG may reveal characteristic myotonic discharges. In the infant there is no evidence of myotonia clinically or on electrophysiological testing until later childhood. To clarify the diagnosis it is frequently helpful to enquire about a family history of muscular stiffness and presenile cataract; and to examine other relatives who may show signs of the disease.

During pregnancy there is polyhydramnios and a history of poor fetal movements. Birth asphyxia is common and there may be persistent ventilatory failure. Fixed talipes equinovarus is present commonly at birth (Fig. 5.6). The infant is hypotonic but antigravity power is sometimes preserved; there is severe facial weakness and ptosis.

A number of these infants do not survive the neonatal period because of the severe respiratory problems. Indeed, it is with the advent of better resuscitation and more widespread intensive care facilities that more of these infants are being diagnosed. In those that survive, intellectual and motor milestones are delayed, though most eventually gain the ability to walk.

The talipes should be managed initially by regular daily passive stretching. Once the child is able to take weight on the legs any residual deformity may be corrected surgically. Early surgery before the child is ready to stand is likely to result in recurrence of the deformity.

Disorders of the lower motor neuron

The spinal muscular atrophies

The spinal muscular atrophies are a group of hereditary proximal and symmetrical muscular atrophies associated with degeneration of anterior-horn cells of the spinal cord and in severe cases of the bulbar motor neurons. Inheritance is autosomal recessive.

The classification of these disorders is most practically divided into three subtypes (Dubowitz 1978):

severe: unable to sit unsupported;
intermediate: able to sit, unable to stand;
mild: able to stand unaided.

The clinical spectrum is a continuum and a few patients fall between these categories. Nevertheless it is useful to try and draw a distinction between the subtypes because of important differences in prognosis and incidence of complications.

The early clinical history of these disorders is similar in all three subtypes, with a period of apparently normal development followed by an insidious, or occasionally relatively acute, onset of weakness and then a plateau during which the weakness remains relatively static. Age of onset is variable and its exact timing may be difficult. Timing of onset is not an absolute guide to classification. However, onset *in utero* usually indicates the severe type.

Severe (Werdnig–Hoffmann disease)

Onset is in fetal life or infancy with paralysis of the legs and severe weakness of the arms. Respiratory muscles are involved with marked intercostal weakness but better preservation of diaphragm function so that the chest wall moves paradoxically with respiration. The legs are held in a frog posture and antigravity power is lost. The arms are typically held internally rotated at the shoulders in a 'jug handle' position; there is usually some antigravity power at the elbows but none at the shoulders. Tongue fibrillation is frequently present. Tendon jerks are always completely absent. The facies are normal and there is no intellectual involvement; the infant is bright and alert.

The degree of skeletal muscle weakness tends to remain static and prognosis is dependent upon degree of respiratory involvement. In general, death occurs from intercurrent infection before the age of 3 years, though many of the more severe ones die within the first year and an occasional child may survive beyond 3 years.

Intermediate severity

The onset is generally after the first 6 months of life. Usually the child learns to sit but never acquires the ability to walk.

Weakness is most severe in the lower limbs and trunk with power in the upper limbs better preserved and antigravity. The pattern of respiratory involvement is similar to the severe type but milder in degree.

There is a fine tremor of the fingers which is often quite striking and sometimes associated with a worse tremor of the hands. There may be tongue fasciculation. The tendon jerks are lost, and the facies is normal. There is often hypermobility of the hands and feet but the large joints tend to develop contractures. There is no intellectual impairment, and frequently these children are very intelligent.

Mild severity (Kugelberg-Welander disease)

The onset is usually in the second year of life with achievement of the ability to stand and usually walk but not to run. Those who have an earlier onset walk late. The degree of disability is variable; some may have only minimal difficulties. On examination there is proximal muscle weakness. The stance may be abnormal with external rotation and eversion of the feet (Moosa & Dubowitz 1973). A finger tremor may be detectable, and the tendon jerks are very variable. Some patients may be very difficult to differentiate from those with muscular dystrophy.

Investigations

The serum creatine kinase activity is normal or only minimally elevated except in the mild type where elevation may be up to five times the upper limit of the adult range (Fig. 5.1). Nerve conduction studies are valuable in the severe type, showing a reduced amplitude response in the muscle because of the extensive denervation. Nerve conduction velocity in the intermediate and mild types is normal. The EMG in most cases shows typical neurogenic changes. Muscle biopsy shows extensive denervation with large groups of atrophic fibres and signs of reinnervation with groups of normal sized or large fibres (Dubowitz 1985). Muscle biopsy may look normal in infants who have the severe type of spinal muscular atrophy with a recent onset ('pre-pathological' change, Dubowitz 1978). It is not possible to gauge severity or prognosis from appearance on the muscle biopsy.

Management and prognosis

There is still confusion about prognosis in spinal muscular atrophy. Some authors have reported a better outlook in the intermediate and mild types with survival and minimal progression (Dubowitz 1964, Munsat et al. 1969, Schwentker & Gibson 1976), but Russman et al. (1983) in a review of 57 patients disagreed, reporting serious progression of the disease in their patients, although only patients with the severe type actually died. To resolve these apparent differences it is important to distinguish between progression of the disease itself and progression of the complications. In general, the degree of weakness tends to remain static, while the complications, particularly contractures and scoliosis, are progressive. An active physical programme which allows the child to achieve his full potential helps prevent complications. Russman and coauthors gave no details of any rehabilitative management of their patients.

Attainment of mobility   In the second year of

life those who can sit but are unable to stand should be encouraged to use a standing frame. Some, by standing in this way, will gain sufficient power to walk independently or with lightweight orthoses, generally of the knee–ankle–foot type. Others who are weaker can achieve useful mobility in a swivel walker. As in Duchenne muscular dystrophy standing helps prevent contractures and scoliosis.

Children with the intermediate type have stronger upper than lower limbs and it is tempting to try to achieve mobility with elbow crutches and braces. Great attention must be paid to overall posture as use of elbow crutches encourages flexion, which allows hip contractures and an unstable kyphosis. If the child has sufficient trunk and pelvic girdle power, better posture and mobility is achieved in lightweight knee–ankle–foot orthoses. Children with the mild type and with limited walking ability may also benefit considerably from this type of orthosis.

Dislocation of the hips is common in the intermediate type. It may be better to concentrate initially on getting the child standing, rather than attempting to reduce the hips with splinting or surgery which may lead to increasing weakness and contracture.

Scoliosis is the most serious deformity occurring in all those with the intermediate type because of the constant sitting posture and spinal muscular weakness. A lightweight close-fitting anterior-opening polypropylene brace should be applied to support the spine as soon as the child is sitting, even if no scoliosis is detectable. In those under one year who are very weak, a more flexible plasterzote jacket with some neck support may be more acceptable. The provision of the brace must be seen as prophylactic. Once the scoliosis is established ($>30°$) it is impossible to prevent progression. Unless some mobility with walking or frequent and prolonged standing is achieved the scoliosis is usually progressive and a spinal fusion around the time of puberty virtually inevitable (Schwentker & Gibson 1976, Hensinger & MacEwen 1976, Evans *et al.* 1981,

Shapiro & Bresnan 1982a). The new Luque technique should be of particular value (Luque 1982).

The hereditary peripheral neuropathies

Hereditary motor and sensory neuropathies

These are divided into at least five subgroups (Dyck 1975):

1   hypertrophic neuropathy (peroneal muscular atrophy);
2   neuronal type of peroneal muscular atrophy;
3   hypertrophic neuropathy of infancy;
4   hypertrophic neuropathy with excess phytanic acid (Refsum's disease);
5   peripheral neuropathy with spastic paraplegia.

Hypertrophic neuropathy: type 1 (peroneal muscular atrophy)

Presentation is with foot deformity and an abnormal gait. The child is frequently reported to be awkward and clumsy. Physical signs vary in severity but there is pes cavus, or less commonly pes planus, a bilateral drop foot gait and distal muscle wasting. The peripheral nerves may be palpably enlarged or firm. There may be tremor of the hands. In childhood there are rarely any detectable sensory changes but in adults there may be distal loss of vibration sense and light touch.

Electrophysiological studies show marked slowing of nerve conduction velocity, in all peripheral nerves, to the region of usually <20 metres/second. Inheritance is autosomal dominant. It is frequently possible to pick up unequivocal slowing of nerve conduction in one of the parents, even in the absence of any symptoms or clinical signs (Vanasse & Dubowitz 1981).

Neuronal type of peroneal muscular atrophy: type II

The clinical features are very similar though there is more wasting of the leg muscles, severe weakness of ankle plantar flexion and a greater tendency to pes planus. A sensory deficit is more commonly found. The hands may be severely involved with clawing of the fingers.

Electrophysiological studies show normal or only minimally slow nerve conduction velocity but frequently a striking reduction in the amplitude of the motor action potential in the legs.

Though autosomal dominant, it is usually not possible to identify a symptom-free parent by electrophysiological testing.

Dejerine-Sottas (hypertrophic neuropathy of infancy)

This disorder presents in infancy with delayed motor development. There is loss of tendon jerks and it is often possible to find some distal sensory loss when the patient is older. Ataxia, shortness of stature and scoliosis may be found. There is an initial improvement but sometimes later deterioration. The peripheral nerves are frequently enlarged and palpable. Electrophysiological studies show slowing of nerve conduction.

Hypertrophic neuropathy with excess phytanic acid (Refsum's disease)

This is a very rare disorder in the United Kingdom. There is a severe motor and sensory neuropathy in association with retinitis pigmentosa, ataxia, hearing loss, cardiomyopathy, pupillary abnormalities, lens opacity and ichthyosis of the skin. Serum phytanic acid levels are elevated.

Peripheral neuropathy with spastic paraplegia

The spastic paraplegia dominates the clinical picture, distal limb weakness develops later and nerve conduction velocity may be slightly slowed.

Friedreich's ataxia (spinocerebellar degeneration)

This is an autosomal recessive progressive disorder with an onset in childhood or adolescence. There is pes cavus, distal wasting and awkwardness of gait. Typically, tendon jerks are lost and plantar responses extensor. Scoliosis, cardiomyopathy and cerebellar ataxia occur.

Deformities in the peripheral neuropathies

Scoliosis occurs more frequently in Friedreich's ataxia and in the other severe neuropathies with limited mobility and ataxia.

Foot deformity is common in all and may be severe. Early pes cavus should be treated with regular passive stretching and wearing of night splints. A drop foot gait can be managed by provision of lightweight polypropylene ankle–foot orthoses. When foot deformity is severe, hampers mobility and power is generally good, corrective surgery should be considered.

Hereditary sensory neuropathy

This term encompasses a group of disorders. An autosomal dominant type (HSN type 1), an autosomal recessive type (HSN type 2), dysautonomia (HSN type 3, Riley Day syndrome), and HSN type 4. A full account is available (Dyck & Ohta 1975).

All have certain features in common to a variable degree. An apparent indifference to pain, chronic foot ulceration, osteolysis with phalangeal resorption, recurrent stress fractures, episodes of cellulitis, lymphangitis, osteomyelitis and paronychia. Charcot joints may occur. Autonomic symptoms accompany the last two types with excessive sweating in type 3 and inability to sweat in type 4. On examination there is distal sensory loss of some or all modalities, particularly light touch and pain. Sensory nerve conduction is impaired.

The inflammatory disorders

Dermatomyositis/polymyositis

Dermatomyositis is an inflammatory disorder of muscle which presents with the combination of skin lesions and general symptoms. The diagnosis is difficult to sustain without the presence of muscle weakness. General symptoms are important and common and the authors' rule is: muscle weakness + misery = dermatomyositis, until proven otherwise.

Clinical features

The onset may be acute but is usually more insidious, coming on over a period of a few months. There is weakness and frequently other symptoms such as pain, tenderness and aching of the muscles. Parents may notice a general stiffening of gait and there is a tendency for joint contracture. Sometimes the first abnormality noticed is a change in personality with a general reluctance to take part in activity. The muscle weakness is usually generalized but may more specifically involve the palate, pharynx, larynx and the muscles of respiration with hoarseness, nasal speech, difficulty in swallowing and, in severe cases, risk of ventilatory failure.

Subcutaneous and intramuscular calcification are peculiar to dermatomyositis, usually a late manifestation but very occasionally a presenting feature. The calcification may occur as small discrete subcutaneous lumps, substantial plaques or large lumps which tend to liquify and ulcerate. Calcification in soft tissues around joints tends to lead to contracture.

The rash occurs on the face, particularly around the eyelids, over the dorsum of the fingers, hands, forearms and occasionally the trunk. Generally the violet coloured activity of the rash is tremendously variable and does not always follow activity in the muscle. Ulceration of the skin, particularly in the region of the axillae, is common, presumably a result of vasculitis.

Investigations

Serum CK activity is elevated in approximately half the patients. The EMG is almost always abnormal with reduced amplitude and increase in the number of polyphasic potentials. Fibrillation potentials may be present at rest. Muscle biopsy may show cell necrosis, chronic inflammatory infiltration and perifascicular atrophy. A comparatively normal biopsy, however, does not exclude the diagnosis.

Management

Drug therapy Childhood dermatomyositis is very steroid sensitive and remission should be induced with prednisolone in a dose of 1 mg/kg/day. As soon as improvement occurs, without waiting for full remission, usually within 1–3 weeks, the daily dose can be gradually reduced in 2.5 or 5 mg steps on a weekly or two-weekly basis, tailoring the rate of reduction against the child's clinical progress. Use of doses in excess of 1 mg/kg/day to induce remission is unnecessary and likely to lead to steroid toxicity. The authors' treatment regimens are set out in detail elsewhere (Dubowitz 1976, Miller *et al.* 1983).

Physical therapy Physical therapy is as important as drug therapy. Mobility should be actively promoted and contractures treated and prevented. Contractures that have occurred at the time of presentation usually resolve as the disease comes under control. More serious is the development of contractures secondary to immobility. Once established, these are usually impossible to resolve. Prevention with regular passive stretching is vitally important.

The congenital myopathies

These are a group of disorders characterized by structural abnormalities of the muscle fibres and were unknown as distinct entities until the introduction of modern histochemical techniques. They generally present as the floppy infant syndrome or later with skeletal muscle weakness. It can be difficult to distinguish them from each other on clinical grounds alone, although with experience certain patterns are emerging. Congenital myopathies discussed here are:

central core disease;
minicore disease;
nemaline myopathy;
myotubular myopathy;
congenital fibre type disproportion;
'minimal change' myopathy.

Central core disease

This is generally a mild myopathy. There is proximal muscle weakness and mild facial weakness with difficulty burying eyelashes completely and showing the teeth fully. Inheritance is autosomal dominant and families have been reported with associated deformities such as dislocation of the hip (Ramsey & Hensinger 1975), kyphoscoliosis and pes cavus (Isaacs et al. 1975).

Muscle biopsy usually appears virtually normal on routine histological stains (H & E, VVG, Trichrome) but the oxidative enzyme stain shows striking 'core'-like areas. There is frequently type 1 fibre predominance (Dubowitz 1985).

Nemaline myopathy

Nemaline myopathy is a very variable disorder which may present as a floppy infant with quite severe weakness and respiratory involvement or later in childhood or adolescence. Sometimes disability is only minimal. Though skeletal muscle weakness may be mild, respiratory involvement is quite common and there is also a risk of progressive scoliosis which aggravates the respiratory difficulty.

The genetic pattern seems to be variable; some cases are clearly dominant and others seem autosomal recessive with affected siblings and healthy parents. The majority of cases appear isolated. Kondo and Yuasa (1981) reviewed the whole question of genetics and favoured autosomal dominant inheritance as a general rule but our own experience does not support this (Heckmatt & Dubowitz 1983).

Muscle biopsy shows variability in fibre size and isolated small fibres. On the trichrome stain there are small red rod-shaped bodies, frequently concentrated in the smaller fibres.

Myotubular myopathy

In myotubular myopathy the abnormal muscle fibres superficially resemble fetal myotubes. The clinical severity and inheritance patterns of this myopathy are variable and we can recognize three subtypes:

1 a severe X-linked recessive type presenting with birth asphyxia and persistent ventilatory failure from birth;
2 an infantile or juvenile type, presenting with skeletal muscle weakness, frequently with a negative family history;
3 an adult type, generally milder in severity, about 50% of cases being autosomal dominant.

Myotubular myopathy may be distinguished clinically on the basis of severe facial weakness, ptosis and external ophthalmoplegia. Swallowing and respiratory difficulties may be encountered, particularly in the severe X-linked and juvenile types. On muscle biopsy the abnormal fibres have a prominent central nucleus surrounded by an area devoid of myofibrils showing up as 'holes' on the ATPase stain and central aggregation of stain on the oxidative enzyme and glycogen reactions. A similar clinical and pathological state has been described where the abnormal fibres are virtually all type 1 and reduced in size. Some regard this as a separate entity ('type 1 hypotrophy with central nuclei'), although it is probably the same disorder.

Minicore disease

This is a separate disorder from central core disease and the oxidative enzyme stain shows multiple small 'holes' or core-like areas within the muscle fibres. Severity of weakness is usually greater than central core disease with the patient presenting as a floppy infant. There may be mild ptosis and facial weakness. The condition is probably autosomal recessive.

Congenital fibre type disproportion

This disorder is particularly associated with skeletal deformities such as congenital dislocation of the hips, scoliosis and club foot (Brooke 1973). The diagnosis has to be confirmed pathologically and biopsy shows hypertrophied type 2 fibres and small type 1 fibres with no other abnormality. Though considered as a congenital myopathy, there is no structural abnormality within the muscle fibres.

Minimal change myopathy

Quite frequently, in children who appear to have a congenital myopathy, biopsy fails to show a definitive abnormality within the muscle fibres although the appearance of the muscle is abnormal with variability in fibre size and internal nuclei (Dubowitz 1978). Clinical problems may be relatively severe despite mild change on the biopsy.

Respiratory muscle involvement and scoliosis in congenital myopathy

Both may be severe and disproportionate to the degree of skeletal muscle weakness. This is in contrast to muscular dystrophy where scoliosis only becomes a problem when the child is in a wheelchair. Significant respiratory involvement is a late event.

Management

Scoliosis may be difficult to manage because application of a brace may seriously reduce mobility. Fortunately, some of these children have sufficient pelvic girdle power to remain ambulant while wearing a brace. The primary curve frequently affects the thoracic spine, and it should be possible to fit a satisfactory brace so long as the apex of the curve is at the level of T6 or below. If the scoliosis is severe, unstable or a brace cannot be tolerated, spinal fusion may be the best option.

Respiratory involvement There may be an almost selective diaphragmatic involvement in these patients. This may be complicated by sleep apnoea, because the diaphragm is the main driving force to respiration during ('REM') sleep. In a young child sleep apnoea may be a very difficult problem to manage without a tracheostomy and night ventilation with a suitable positive pressure ventilator. In late adolescence or adult life the patient may accept sleep in a cuirass negative pressure ventilator and tracheostomy can be avoided.

Miscellaneous disorders

Congenital muscular dystrophy

Though similar to other dystrophies in appearance of the muscle, congenital muscular dystrophy clinically resembles the congenital myopathies. Presentation is usually at birth with weakness and hypotonia. Some with milder disease present in childhood with delay in motor milestones but eventually become ambulant and cope reasonably well. There is a striking association with contractures and deformities. Contractures may be severe and multiple, presenting at birth with arthrogryposis, or occur later as a result of immobility (Banker *et al.* 1957, Pearson & Fowler 1963, Donner *et al.* 1975, Jones *et al.* 1979). Intelligence is usually normal but an association with mental retardation has been reported from Japan (Fukuyama *et al.* 1960, Kamoshita *et al.* 1976) and Finland (Santavuori *et al.* 1977).

There may be respiratory involvement but without the paradoxical chest wall movement seen in the severe type of spinal muscular atrophy. Facial weakness and difficulties with swallowing or chewing can occur.

Serum CK is elevated in about 50% of patients (Fig. 5.1). The EMG is usually myopathic but can be surprisingly normal. Muscle biopsy shows dystrophic change with replacement of muscle by fat and connective tissue. The degree of change may be marked but bears no relationship to prognosis or clinical severity.

In our experience the muscle weakness is nonprogressive and there is improvement with time. McMenamin *et al.* (1982) in a review of 24 patients reported disease progression in virtually all. However, no mention was made of any attempts at rehabilitation. Undoubtedly, without rehabilitation, contractures and deformities worsen and the disease appears 'progressive' (Jones *et al.* 1979).

Every effort should be made to try and get the child mobile, correcting and preventing contractures with regular passive stretching and using, if necessary, lightweight orthoses to promote walking. Dislocation of the hips is quite common. Great caution should be taken with attempting to realign the hips. Prolonged immobilization and reconstructive surgery is likely to lead to increased weakness and contracture (Jones *et al.* 1979). It is better to concentrate on promoting ambulation.

Arthrogryposis

The term arthrogryposis refers to the presence at birth of multiple joint contractures and deformities. It is not one single disorder but a symptom complex with an identical clinical picture produced by a number of different pathological processes. Joints are contracted and have limited mobility with hips, knees, shoulders and elbows all being affected to varying degrees. There is frequently severe equinus of the feet and fixed flexion deformities of the wrists and fingers.

The direct cause of arthrogryposis is immobility *in utero,* due either to adverse factors in the intrauterine environment or intrinsic abnormality affecting the fetus. For example, oligohydramnios may severely restrict the fetus. In the authors' experience it has been possible to implicate amniocentesis in some of these cases. Restriction may also be caused by a uterine abnormality such as a bicornuate uterus or large fibroid. Neuromuscular disease affecting the fetus can also lead to arthrogryposis with congenital muscular dystrophy probably the single most important causal entity. Evidence for denervation may be found although spinal muscular atrophy is a very rare cause. Central nervous system disorders of intrauterine onset with abnormalities of muscle tone and movement can be associated with arthrogryposis.

It is frequently impossible on clinical grounds to distinguish the various possible causal aetiologies and full investigation with electrophysiological studies and needle muscle biopsy with histochemistry is essential.

Management can be a difficult problem. The orthopaedic literature usually advises early surgery to correct deformity (Friedlander *et al.* 1968, Shapiro & Bresnan 1982b). In a major review Williams (1978) advocated:

1   early surgical release (in the case of the feet immediately after birth), followed by
2   prolonged plaster fixation and, later, other procedures such as tendon transfer.

All authors acknowledge the tendency for contractures to recur after surgery.

The authors advocate a different approach. Initially contractures should be passively stretched. This needs to be several times a day by the parents with regular back-up by the physiotherapist. Serial splinting should be avoided in general as this leads to a joint which is in a better position but still fixed. No surgery is performed until the child is ready, from the point of view of general development, to take advantage of the operation. In this way corrected joint position will be maintained by posture and multiple repeat operations avoided.

Ligamentous laxity

This is an important and common but rather ill-defined group of disorders. Severity is very variable, ranging from slight to extreme joint hypermobility. In severe cases there is progressive scoliosis and a tendency to subluxation of large joints. There is presumably a relationship with the rare Ehlers–Danlos syndrome but without the skin manifestations.

Presentation is often as a floppy infant but, in contrast with neuromuscular disease, full antigravity power is retained in the limbs. Milder cases may present with delay in motor milestones and lack of confidence with walking. Inheritance may be autosomal dominant with one of the parents being 'double-jointed' as a child.

The general trend is for improvement and it is important to try to get the child mobile, stabilizing the joints with lightweight orthoses, and protecting the back if necessary with a brace.

Rigid spine syndrome

Originally described by Dubowitz (1973), the predominant feature of this condition is marked limitation of flexion of the whole dorsolumbar and cervical spine due to shortening of the spinal extensor muscles or associated ligaments. There may be scoliosis which tends to be rather fixed. Other joints may be limited in particular elbows and occasionally ankles. The condition tends to be non- or slowly progressive and severe weakness does not occur. Biopsy of limb muscle shows myopathic change which is usually mild but biopsy of sacrospinalis may show striking fibrosis (Dubowitz 1978). This disorder is related to the X-linked recessive type of muscular dystrophy associated with cardiac involvement described by Emery & Dreifuss (1963). Surgical release of contractures may be necessary.

Malignant hyperthermia

Malignant hyperthermia occurs as an uncommon, catastrophic and often fatal complication of general anaesthesia. Suxamethonium and the potent inhaled anaesthetic agents have been implicated most consistently. The first indication of development of the condition may be the onset of jaw rigidity following administration of suxamethonium. The patient's temperature rises, sometimes with alarming rapidity, reaching 44°C or even higher. Generalized muscle rigidity occurs in about 80% of instances.

There is a generalized metabolic upset with tachycardia, tachypnoea, metabolic and respiratory acidosis. There may be muscle necrosis and this leads to hyperkalaemia, myoglobinaemia and the possibility of renal failure. Serum CK activity usually becomes grossly elevated.

The reaction is rare in adults over 50 years and uncommon in infants under 2 years. It frequently occurs in apparently healthy young individuals undergoing a relatively minor operative procedure. However, there is an association with musculoskeletal abnormality, in particular ptosis, strabismus, various hernias, kyphoscoliosis, a tendency to joint dislocation and foot deformity. Britt and Kalow (1970) reported 89 patients of whom 32 had musculoskeletal or congenital muscle abnormality and 22 (23%) had undergone an orthopaedic procedure. Inheritance is generally autosomal dominant and some extensive pedigrees have been reported, although isolated cases also occur.

Generalized muscle hypertrophy and focal muscle wasting may be found but only a minority of patients have overt myopathy (Isaacs & Barlow 1974). Family studies are important once a susceptible individual is identified. Definitive investigation involves demonstration of *in vitro* sensitivity of the patients muscle to halothane and if necessary other anaesthetic agents.

King and Denborough (1973) reported 4 unrelated boys who all had an unusual syndrome of short stature, undescended testes, thoracic kyphoscoliosis and pectus cavinatum. They also had an abnormal facial appearance with a small chin, low-set ears and an anti-mongoloid slant to the eyes. Parents were healthy though not studied in full. Inheritance may have been autosomal recessive.

Despite the presence of associated clinical features it is obviously difficult to anticipate and prevent the condition in routine clinical practice. It is important to enquire about possible hyperthermic episodes and unexplained deaths during anaesthesia in relatives. Serum CK is chronically elevated in some susceptible patients but this is not sufficiently consistent or definitive for effective pre-operative screening.

A detailed review of this disorder is available (Britt 1979).

Hysterical (nonorganic) disorders of movement

Clinicians are frequently afraid of diagnosing hysterical disorders. It is easy to be discouraged by reports of patients, originally thought to have a hysterical disorder, who turn out to have serious organic disease (Slater 1965, Rivinus et al. 1975). It might be argued that hysteria should only be diagnosed after thorough investigation and exclusion of all other possibilities.

Hysteria is not a diagnosis of exclusion, however, but should be made positively on clinical grounds, frequently because of bizarre and dramatic symptoms and signs inexplicable on an anatomical or physiological basis. Some diagnostic confusion may arise because hysteria can be associated with organic disease. Creak (1938) classified hysteria into three groups:

1 true conversion hysteria where anxiety is manifest as somatic symptoms;
2 hysteria prolongation of symptoms originally part of organic disease;
3 hysteria accompanying undoubted organic disease.

The bizarre and incomprehensible nature of the symptoms can produce considerable anxiety in the clinician. Gold (1965) emphasised how, if the clinician communicated this anxiety to the child, the abnormal mode of behaviour was reinforced and the pattern set for a prolonged and intractable illness. Dubowitz & Hersov (1976) described five patients where hysteria symptoms appeared to follow a relatively trivial organic illness. In each case the original symptoms were exacerbated by the doctor undertaking a protracted series of (often painful) investigations and, in some cases, prescribing prolonged period of immobilization or traction.

It is important therefore to recognize hysteria clinically and to initiate an appropriate course of management without recourse to extensive investigation. The majority of children usually have no predisposing psychological abnormality and can be returned to full health.

Dubowitz & Hersov (1976) recommend three essentials of management:

1 stopping any further investigations beyond the minimum necessary;
2 institution without delay of a well-planned programme of physical rehabilitation;
3 involvement of the psychiatric team to assess and deal quickly with any psychological stresses at school or home, to help the child give up his 'sick role' and to alter the parents' perception of their child as a chronic invalid to one of potential health.

Appendix

Technique of needle muscle biopsy

The Bergström needle consists of two concentric hollow cylinders. The outer cylinder has a pointed end and a side window and the inner has an open end with a cutting edge (Fig. 5.7). The procedure of quadriceps muscle biopsy is as follows: Children between 1 and 10 years are premedicated with chloral for sedation. The site of biopsy is routinely the quadriceps femoris in the midline at mid-thigh level. The biopsy is performed with the child supine, the examiner standing on the opposite side from the patient to the limb being biopsied and holding the needle in the opposite hand (i.e. right for left leg, left for right leg), the other hand being used to steady the muscle. Skin and subcutaneous tissue but not muscle is infiltrated with local anaesthetic and a small 5 mm incision is made in the skin with a number 11 scalpel blade.

the cutting edge, from the main muscle, is important otherwise the patient will experience an uncomfortable tearing sensation as the needle is withdrawn. The authors sharpen the cutting edges of their needles at least once every ten biopsies.

At completion of the procedure external pressure is applied on the thigh for 5 minutes to prevent any bleeding within the muscle. The wound is closed with a butterfly dressing and no sutures are used.

The biopsy samples are removed from the needle and orientated together on a cork disc under a dissecting microscope so all the fibres run perpendicular to the plane of view. They are then surrounded by a viscous medium such as

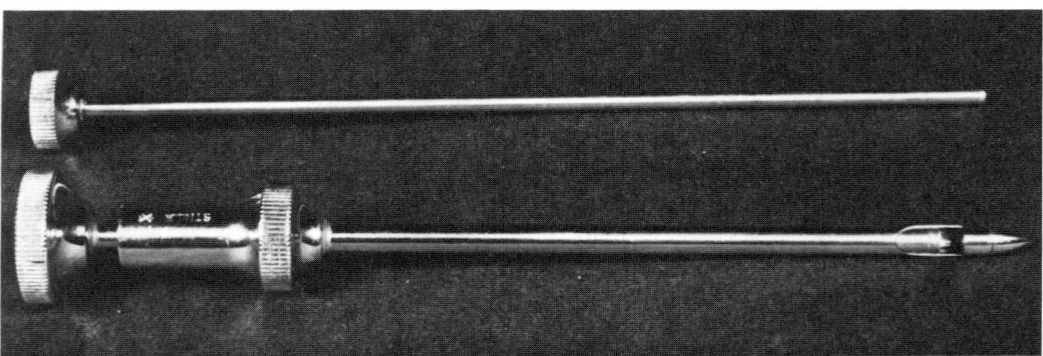

Fig. 5.7. Bergström muscle biopsy needle showing inner cylinder partially withdrawn and side window half open. Central plunger completely removed.

The needle is inserted into the muscle through the incision with the side window closed and facing laterally. Once in the muscle the central cylinder is withdrawn slightly, opening the window. With the free hand pressure is applied on the outside of the thigh, causing the muscle to bulge into the needle opening. The central cylinder is then pushed home and a small sample of muscle is taken with the guillotining action of the cutting edge. Without moving the needle within the muscle this action can be quickly repeated, allowing 2 or 3 separate samples to be taken. If necessary, further muscle can be taken by reinsertion of the needle through the same incision.

Complete separation of the muscle samples by

'Tissue Tek' and frozen by immersion in isopentane or 'Artane' which has been precooled in liquid nitrogen. The samples are then ready for cutting in transverse section on a cryostat. Full details of this aspect of the procedure are given by Dubowitz (1985).

References

BANKER B.Q., VICTOR M. & ADAMS R. (1957) Arthrogryposis multiplex due to congenital muscular dystrophy. *Brain*, **80**, 319–34.

BRITT B.A. (1979) Malignant hyperthermia. *International Anaesthesiology Clinics*, **17**, 63–96.

BRITT B.A. & KALOW W. (1970) Malignant hyperthermia: a statistical review. *Canadian Anaesthetists' Society Journal*, **17**, 293–315.

BROOKE M.H. (1973) A neuromuscular disease characterized by fiber type disproportion. In Kakulas B.A. (ed) *Clinical Studies in Myology*. Proceedings of the Second International Congress on Muscle Diseases, Perth, Australia, 1971, part 2. p.147–59 Excerpta Medica, Amsterdam.

CREAK M. (1938) Hysteria in childhood. *British Journal of Children's Disorders*, 35, 85.

DONNER M., RAPOLA J. & SOMER H. (1975) Congenital muscular dystrophy: a clinicopathological and follow-up study of 15 patients. *Neuropädiatrie*, 6, 239–58.

DUBOWITZ V. (1964) Infantile muscular atrophy: a prospective study with particular reference to a slowly progressive variety. *Brain*, 87, 707–18.

DUBOWITZ V. (1973) Rigid spine syndrome: a muscle syndrome in search of a name. *Proceedings of the Royal Society of Medicine*, 66, 219.

DUBOWITZ V. (1976) Treatment of dermatomyositis in childhood. *Archives of Disease in Childhood*, 51, 494–500.

DUBOWITZ V. (1978) *Muscle Disorders in Childhood*. W.B. Saunders Co., London and Philadelphia.

DUBOWITZ V. (1980) *The Floppy Infant*, 2nd ed. Clinics in Developmental Medicine No. 76. Spastics International Medical Publications/Heinemann, London.

DUBOWITZ V. (1985) *Muscle Biopsy: A Practical Approach*. Ballière Tindall, London and Philadelphia.

DUBOWITZ V. & HECKMATT J.Z. (1980) Management of muscular dystrophy. Pharmacological and physical aspects. *British Medical Bulletin*, 36, 139–44.

DUBOWITZ V. & HERSOV L. (1976) Management of children with non-organic (hysterical) disorders of motor function. *Developmental Medicine and Child Neurology*, 18, 358–68.

DYCK P.J. (1975) Inherited neuronal degeneration and atrophy affecting peripheral motor, sensory, and autonomic neurones. In Dyck P.J., Thomas P.K. & Lambert E.H. (eds) *Peripheral Neuropathy*, Vol. 2, p.825–67. W.B. Saunders Co., Philadelphia.

DYCK P.J. & OHTA M. (1975) Neuronal atrophy and degeneration predominantly affecting peripheral sensory neurones. In Dyck P.J., Thomas P.K. & Lambert E.H. (eds) *Peripheral Neuropathy*, Vol. 2, p.791–824. W.B. Saunders Co., Philadelphia.

EDWARDS R., YOUNG A. & WILES M. (1980) Needle biopsy of skeletal muscle in the diagnosis of myopathy and the clinical study of muscle function and repair. *New England Journal of Medicine*, 302, 261–71.

EMERY A.E.H. (1976) *Methodology in Medical Genetics – An Introduction to Statistical Methods*, p.92–5. Churchill Livingstone, Edinburgh.

EMERY A.E.H. & DREIFUSS F.E. (1966) Unusual type of benign X-linked muscular dystrophy. *Journal of Neurology, Neurosurgery and Psychiatry*, 29, 338–42.

EVANS G.A., DRENNAN J.C. & RUSSMAN B.S. (1981) Functional classification and orthopaedic management of spinal muscular atrophy. *Journal of Bone and Joint Surgery*, 63B, 516–22.

FRIEDLANDER H.L., WESTIN G.W. & WOOD W.L. (1968) Arthrogryposis multiplex congenita. A review of 45 cases. *Journal of Bone and Joint Surgery*, 50A, 89–112.

FUKUYAMA Y., KAWAZURA M. & HARUNA H. (1960) A peculiar form of congenital progressive muscular dystrophy: report of 15 cases. *Pediatria Universitatis Tokyo*, 4, 5–8.

GARDNER-MEDWIN D. (1980) Clinical features and classification of muscular dystrophies. *British Medical Bulletin*, 36, 109–15.

GOLD S. (1965) Diagnosis and management of hysterical contracture in children. *British Medical Journal*, 1, 21–3.

HARPER P.S. (1979) *Myotonic Dystrophy*. W.B. Saunders Co., London, Philadelphia & Toronto.

HECKMATT J.Z. & DUBOWITZ V. (1983) Congenital myopathies (including glycogenoses), in Emery A.E.H. & Rimoin D.L. (eds) *Principles and Practice of Medical Genetics*, Vol.1, p.367–91. Churchill Livingstone, Edinburgh.

HECKMATT J.Z., LEEMAN S. & DUBOWITZ V. (1982) Ultrasound imaging in the diagnosis of muscle disease. *The Journal of Pediatrics*, 101, 656–60.

HECKMATT J.Z., MOOSA A., HUTSON C., MAUNDER-SEWRY C.A. & DUBOWITZ V. (1984) Diagnostic needle muscle biopsy: A practical and reliable alternative to open biopsy. *Archives of Disease in Childhood*, 59, 528–32.

HECKMATT J.Z., DUBOWITZ V., HYDE S.A., GABAIN A.C., THOMPSON N. & FLORENCE J. (1985) Prolongation of walking in Duchenne Muscular Dystrophy with lightweight orthoses: A review of 57 cases. *Developmental Medicine and Child Neurology*, 27, 149-54.

HENSINGER R.N. & MACEWEN G.D. (1976) Spinal deformity associated with heritable neurological conditions: spinal muscular atrophy, Friedreich's ataxia, familial dysautonomia, and Charcot–Marie–Tooth disease. *Journal of Bone and Joint Surgery*, 58A, 13–24.

HSU J.D. (1976) Management of foot deformity in Duchenne's pseudohypertrophic muscular dystrophy *Orthopedic Clinics of North America*, 7, 979–84.

HUNTER S. (1980) The heart in muscular dystrophy. *British Medical Bulletin*, 36, 133–4.

HYDE S.A., SCOTT O.M., GODDARD C.M. & DUBOWITZ V. (1982) Prolongation of ambulation in Duchenne muscular dystrophy by appropriate orthoses. *Physiotherapy*, 68, 105–8.

ISSACS H. & BARLOW M.B. (1974) Central core disease associated with elevated creatinine phosphokinase levels. Two members of a family known to be susceptible to malignant hyperpyrexia. *South African Medical Journal*, 48, 640–2.

ISSACS H., HEFFRON J.J.A. & BADENHORST M. (1975) Central core disease: a correlated genetic, histochemical, ultramicroscopic, and biochemical study. *Journal of Neurology, Neurosurgery and Psychiatry*, 38, 1171–86.

JONES R., KHAN R., HUGHES S. & DUBOWITZ V. (1979) Congenital muscular dystrophy: the importance of early diagnosis and orthopaedic management in the long-term prognosis. *Journal of Bone and Joint Surgery*, 61B, 13–7.

KAMOSHITA S., KONISHI Y., SEGAWA M. & FUKUYAMA Y. (1976) Congenital muscular dystrophy as a disease of the central nervous system. *Archives of Neurology*, 33, 513–6.

KING J.O. & DENBOROUGH M.A. (1973) Anaesthetic-induced malignant hyperpyrexia in children. *Journal of Pediatrics*, 83, 37–40.

KONDO K. & YUASA T. (1980) Genetics of congenital nemaline myopathy. *Muscle and Nerve*, 3, 308–15.

LANCET (1983) Editorial: DNA probes for the Duchenne carrier. 2, 497.

LEIBOWITZ D. & DUBOWITZ V. (1981) Intellect and behaviour in Duchenne muscular dystrophy. *Developmental Medicine and Child Neurology*, 23, 577–90.

LUQUE E.R. (1982) Segmental spinal instrumentation for correction of scoliosis. *Clinical Orthopaedics and Related Research*, 163, 192–8.

MCMENAMIN J.B., BECKER L.E. & MURPHY E.G. (1982) Congenital muscular dystrophy: a clinicopathologic report of 24 cases. *Journal of Pediatrics*, 100, 692–7.

MILLER G., HECKMATT J.Z. & DUBOWITZ V. (1983) Drug treatment of juvenile dermatomyositis. *Archives of Disease in Childhood*, 58, 445–50.

MOOSA A. & DUBOWITZ V. (1973) Spinal muscular atrophy in childhood: two clues to clinical diagnosis. *Archives of Diseases in Childhood*, 48, 386–8.

MUNSAT T.L., WOODS R., FOWLER W. & PEARSON C.M. (1969) Neurogenic muscular atrophy of infancy with prolonged survival. The variable course of Werdnig–Hoffman disease. *Brain*, 92, 9–24.

NEWSOM-DAVIS J. (1980) Respiratory system in muscular dystrophy. *British Medical Bulletin*, 36, 135–8.

PEARSON C.M. & FOWLER W.G. (1963) Hereditary non-progressive muscular dystrophy inducing arthrogryposis syndrome. *Brain*, 86, 75–88.

RAMSEY P.L. & HENSINGER R.N. (1975) Congenital dislocation of the hip associated with central core disease. *Journal of Bone and Joint Surgery*, 57A, 648–51.

RIVINUS T.M., JAMISON D.L. & GRAHAM P.J. (1975) Childhood organic neurological disease presenting as psychiatric disorder. *Archives of Disease in Childhood*, 50, 115–9.

ROSES A.D., PERICAK-VANCE M.A., YAMAOKA L.H., STUBBLEFIELD E., STAJICH J., VANCE J.M., ROSES M.J. & CARTER D.B. (1983) Recombinant DNA strategies in genetic neurological diseases. *Muscle and Nerve* 6, 339–55.

RUSSMAN B.S., MELCHREIT R. & DRENNAN J.C. (1983) Spinal muscular atrophy — the natural course of disease. *Muscle and Nerve*, 6, 179–81.

SANTAVUORI P., LEISTI J. & KRUUS S. (1977) Muscle, eye and brain disease: a new syndrome. *Neuropädiatrie*, 8, (suppl), 553.

SCHWENTKER E.P. & GIBSON D.A. (1976) The orthopaedic aspects of spinal muscular atrophy. *Journal of Bone and Joint Surgery*, 58A, 32–8.

SCOTT O.M., HYDE S.A., GODDARD C. & DUBOWITZ V. (1982) Quantitation of muscle function in children: a prospective study in Duchenne muscular dystrophy. *Muscle and Nerve*, 5, 291–301.

SHAPIRO F. & BRESNAN M.J. (1982a) Current Concepts Review: Orthopaedic management of childhood neuromuscular disease. Part I: Spinal muscular atrophy. *Journal of Bone and Joint Surgery*, 64A, 785–9.

SHAPIRO F. & BRESNAN M.J. (1982b) Current concepts review: Orthopaedic management of childhood neuromuscular disease. Part II: Peripheral neuropathies, Friedreich's ataxia and arthrogryposis multiplex congenita. *Journal of Bone and Joint Surgery*, 64A, 949–53.

SIEGEL I.M., MILLER J.E. & RAY R.D. (1968) Subcutaneous lower limb tenotomy in the treatment of pseudohypertrophic muscular dystrophy. *Journal of Bone and Joint Surgery*, 50A, 1437–43.

SLATER E. (1965) Diagnosis of 'hysteria' *British Medical Journal*, 1, 1395–9.

SPENCER G.E. & VIGNOS P.J. (1962) Bracing for ambulation in childhood progressive muscular dystrophy. *Journal of Bone and Joint Surgery*, 44A, 234–42.

VANASSE M. & DUBOWITZ V. (1981) Dominantly inherited peroneal muscular atrophy (hereditary motor and sensory neuropathy type I) in infancy and childhood. *Muscle and Nerve*, 4, 26–30.

WILLIAMS P. (1978) The management of arthrogryposis. *Orthopedic Clinics of North America*, 9, 67–88.

ZELLWEGER H. & ANTONIK A. (1975) Newborn screening for Duchenne muscular dystrophy. *Pediatrics*, 55, 30–4.

Chapter 6
The Orthopaedic Management of the Dystrophies, Myopathies, Atrophies, Neuropathies and Ataxias

C. S. B. GALASKO

The orthopaedic management of patients with neuromuscular disorders is aimed at obtaining the optimum quality of life, within their disability, by preventing deformity or treating it when it has occurred. Deformities occur commonly in these conditions (Galasko 1977). The prevention and treatment of scoliosis may be associated with an increased life expectancy, but orthopaedic treatment will not affect the underlying neuromuscular disorder.

Development of deformity

The causes of deformity are shown in Table 6.1. The prime cause is muscle imbalance. The power of the muscle is relatively unimportant; it is the imbalance in power between the agonist and antagonist that produces the deformity. Imbalance may occur in overactive muscles (for example, cerebral palsy) as well as in weak muscles (for example, Duchenne dystrophy). If the muscles are fully balanced deformity is less likely to occur.

Table 6.1. Causes of deformity in neuromuscular disease.

Muscle imbalance

Gravity + weak musculature

Pressure (e.g. bed clothes) across a joint with weak musculature

Unequal growth of bone and fibrotic muscle

Initially the deformity is due to the muscle imbalance, and correction of the imbalance will correct the deformity. However, if the deformity has been present for some time secondary

changes develop. These are due to fibrosis and shortening of the joint capsule and ligaments on the contracted side of the joint. At this stage muscle balancing procedures alone will not correct the deformity; a soft tissue release of the contracted tissues is also required.

These mechanisms occur in the adult as well as the child, but the third stage of deformity occurs only in the growing child. If the muscle insertion is distal to a growth plate the bone will be 'bent' in the direction of the more powerful muscle.

Other mechanisms that may play a role in the development of deformity in neuromuscular disorders include:

1 the effect of gravity on weak musculature. This probably plays an important role in the development of spinal deformity;
2 extrinsic pressure, for example, tight bedclothes on a paralysed foot;
3 fibrotic muscle does not grow normally, and probably grows more slowly than the adjacent bone producing contractures.

It is not surprising, therefore, that deformities occur commonly in patients with neuromuscular disorders.

Prevention and treatment

Ideally, patients with these disorders should be treated with a multidisciplinary approach, the members of the team depending on the disease. For example, in spina bifida, a team could consist of a paediatric surgeon, neurosurgeon, urologist, orthopaedic surgeon, physiotherapist,

83

occupational therapist, orthotist and social worker; whereas in patients with dystrophies, myopathies and atrophies, the team requires a paediatric neurologist, clinical geneticist, orthopaedic surgeon, physiotherapist, occupational therapist, orthotist and social worker.

The value of the multidisciplinary approach is that it leads to an earlier and more precise diagnosis, a more accurate assessment of prognosis and the earlier recognition and treatment of deformities.

Assessment

Before embarking upon treatment these patients require a detailed assessment. This includes an assessment of the muscle power, the range of movement of each joint and measurement of any joint contractures. All deformities must be noted and the ability of the patient to cooperate determined. Most of the patients are children and their ability to cooperate depends on the intelligence of the child, his or her physical development, the psychological approach of the child and the family to treatment, and the age of the child. The assessment is usually carried out by the physiotherapist.

As part of the author's initial assessment he obtains an erect anteroposterior X-ray of the spine, an X-ray of the pelvis and lung function tests.

The deformities vary in the different disorders, possibly because different muscles are involved and they will be discussed separately.

Duchenne dystrophy

This is the commonest of the neuromuscular disorders considered in this chapter. The incidence at birth is 1 in 3000–3500 males and in the total population is approximately 3 per 100000. It is associated with progressive and rapid increase in weakness, the majority of boys losing their ability to walk independently between the age of eight and ten years (Chapter 5). Most die in their late teens from respiratory infection or cardiomyopathy. Discussion with the parents of boys attending the author's Muscle Clinic indicated that there are four main areas of concern where orthopaedic management may help: delay in diagnosis, loss of independent ambulation, scoliosis and foot deformity.

Early diagnosis

Many of the parents stated that the diagnosis was missed for months or years, even though the parents realized that their son's gait was abnormal, a waddling gait being characteristic. Difficulty with climbing stairs and running, and a tendency to fall often, at about the age of 3 or 4 years are other common complaints. The condition may cause lateness in onset of walking; about 50% of all affected boys do not walk until after 18 months of age (Walton 1983). In several instances the parents were initially reassured that their son would grow out of his stumbling gait and frequent falls. A diagnosis of flat feet or other benign condition was often initially made. Gardner-Medwin (1979) reported that in the United Kingdom the average age at diagnosis was 5.8 years, and in the United States the average time which elapsed between initial parental concern and ultimate diagnosis was 3.0 years (range 1.5–5.5 years) (Crisp et al. 1982). The average age of diagnosis of patients referred to our clinic (which is a tertiary referral clinic) is 5.2 years (range 1.5–9 years) with an average delay in diagnosis of 2.0 years (range 0–6 years). Moosa (1982) reported a family with six affected brothers aged from 15 months to 13 years. The diagnosis of Duchenne dystrophy was only made when the oldest boy was 13 years old even though his parents had first sought medical advice when he was five.

The diagnosis is unlikely to be missed if the possibility of muscle dystrophy is considered when a boy is late in walking (O'Brien et al. 1983), is clumsy or his walking deteriorates.

With a clumsy child – think dystrophy. A creatinine kinase estimation is a simple investigation.

Late diagnosis causes parental distress (Firth 1983), but more importantly may delay genetic counselling until the family have 2 or 3 affected sons.

Mobility

Many parents stated that the morale of their son deteriorated significantly when he lost the ability to walk independently. Provision of calipers can maintain weightbearing for several years (Fig. 6.1, Chapter 5, Spencer & Vignos 1962, Roy & Gibson 1970, Miller & Dunn 1982). However, the calipers must be fitted before the boy goes off his feet. It is not possible to mobilize a child with Duchenne dystrophy once he is chairbound. Calipers should be prescribed when the child is starting to have difficulty climbing stairs or getting out of a chair (Table 6.2). Once the calipers have been provided, the child uses them for 20–30 minutes each day, and as he starts to go off his feet he gradually becomes more dependent upon them.

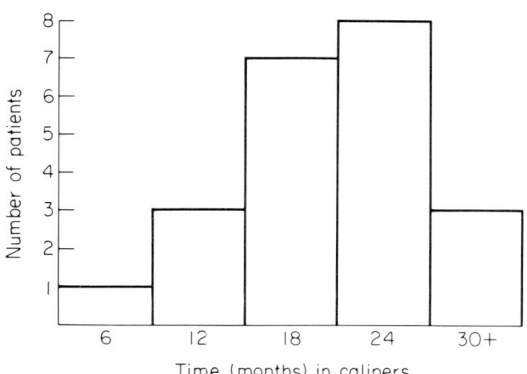

Fig. 6.1. The effect of calipers on prolonging ambulation in 22 patients with Duchenne muscular dystrophy. Eight patients were able to walk without any additional aid for a further two years and three patients for 30 months or longer.

Several types of calipers are available (Fig. 6.2), including cosmetic calipers where the moulded footpiece fits into the shoe, calipers with a patellar bearing lower leg piece and elasticated calipers. The former rely on a well moulded thigh piece, which is ischial bearing and

allows the patient to extend and stabilize his hips (Fig. 6.3), the dynamic caliper on an elastic strap which passes posterior to the hip joint producing a hip extension force (Nuzzo 1980).

Table 6.2. Functional assessment.

Grade	Functional ability
1	Walks; climbs stairs without assistance.
2	Walks; climbs stairs with aid of rail.
3	Walks; unable to climb stairs; able to get out of chair.
4	Walks unassisted; unable to get out of chair.
5	Walks with assistance or calipers.
6	Stands in calipers; unable to walk with assistance or calipers.
7	In wheelchair; can roll chair.
8	In wheelchair; able to perform bed and chair activities.
9	In wheelchair; sits erect with support. Minimal activities.
10	In bed; unable to perform activities of daily living.

Frequently, these patients lose the ability to walk independently after they have been confined to bed for an intercurrent illness, following an operation or as a result of injury. In general terms, these boys should never be confined to bed. Fractures should be treated by plaster of Paris or alternative lightweight casts and immediate mobilization (p. 95). If a child is operated on in the morning he should be stood with the help of the physiotherapist that afternoon. If surgery is carried out in the afternoon, he should be stood the following morning.

Not every child nor every family will accept calipers. They are cumbersome and slow down the patient and some centres prefer to prescribe a wheelchair to allow the boy to keep up with his peers. Learning to use calipers requires a lot of effort and unless the family cooperate the child will never succeed.

Scoliosis

This is the most important and most serious deformity that can occur in a child with

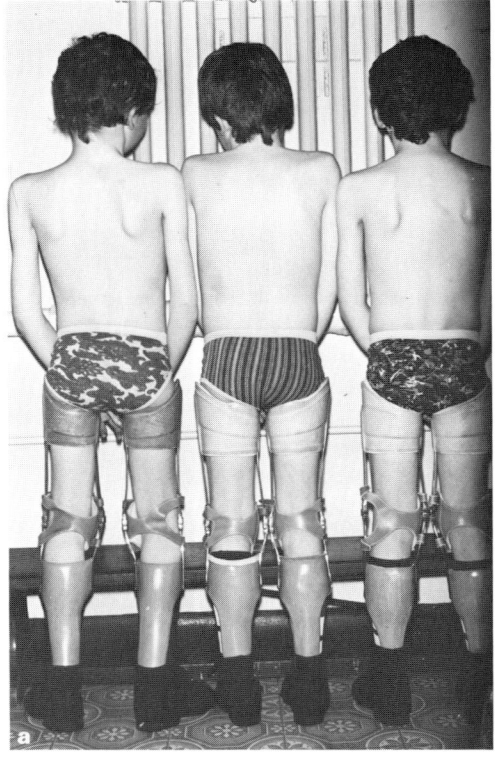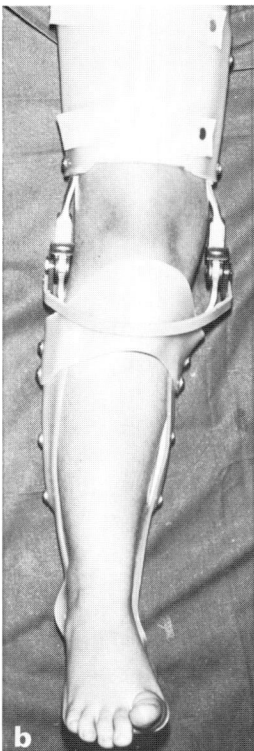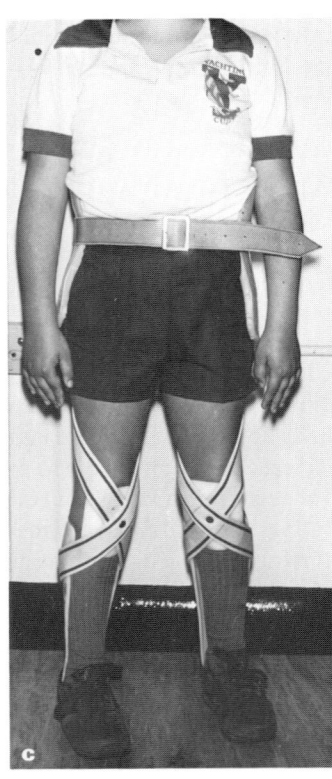

Fig. 6.2 Types of calipers.

(a) Cosmetic calipers. There is a moulded ischial bearing thigh portion, fitted to a moulded ankle–foot orthosis and connected via a knee hinge. This illustration shows three affected brothers. The diagnosis was made only after the third boy was born.

(b) Patellar bearing ankle–foot orthosis. The thigh piece is also ischial weight bearing. There is a modified knee hinge to allow easier release.

(c) Elasticated calipers, which also are patellar bearing.

neuromuscular disease. It is not just a cosmetic deformity, but is associated with significant disability. In Duchenne dystrophy, like many other neuromuscular disorders, the scoliosis eventually involves the pelvis and results in an increasing pelvic obliquity. The patient can no longer sit squarely and weight is increasingly taken on one buttock, and subsequently the lumbar spine (Fig. 6.4). Sitting becomes uncomfortable and the patient is confined to bed, not because of the underlying neuromuscular disease, but as a result of the progressive scoliosis. Hsu (1983) reported that progression of the curve beyond 40° was associated with diminished sitting tolerance and use of the arms and hands to prop the body up when seated.

The scoliosis tends to progress rapidly and continues to deteriorate after growth has ceased, perhaps due to the effect of gravity on the weakened trunk musculature.

Progressive scoliosis is associated with diminished lung function. As the curve deteriorates there is progressive pulmonary insufficiency. Treatment of the scoliosis does not improve the lung function but may prevent further deterioration due to the progressive deformity. Kurz *et al.* (1983) showed that pulmonary function (measured as forced vital capacity) correlated with the age of the patient and the degree of thoracic scoliosis. They found that the forced vital capacity (FVC) peaked at approximately the age when standing ceased and

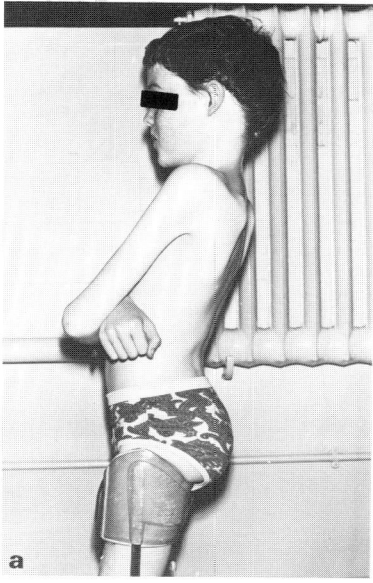 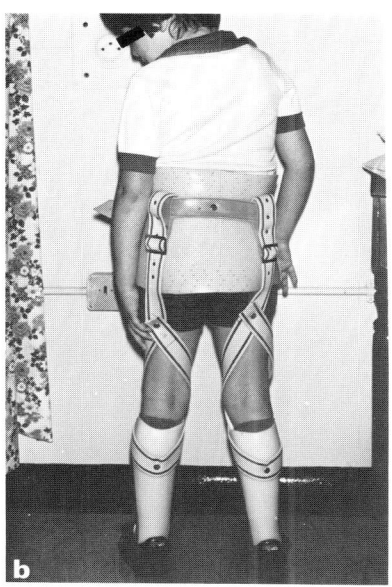

Fig. 6.3. (a) The ischial bearing moulded thigh piece allows the patient to extend and stabilize his hips.
(b) The elastic strap passes posterior to the hip joint producing a hip extension force.

then declined rapidly. Age and thoracic scoliosis together were better predictors of FVC than either one alone. Each one year of age had approximately the same negative influence on FVC that each 10° of thoracic scoliosis had; both decreased FVC by approximately 4%. As muscle strength decreased, and particularly as scoliosis developed, the respiratory reserve declined (Burke *et al.* 1971).

Obesity is another factor which may effect pulmonary function. It is important that the parents and the patient understand the complications of obesity. Furthermore, because of their loss of muscle bulk, their ideal weight is less than the normal for their height and age (Edwards *et al.* 1984).

Prevention

The scoliosis increases with increasing age (Fig. 6.5, Gibson & Wilkins 1975). There is a dispute whether hand dominance has any effect on the direction of the deformity, Johnson & Yarnell (1976) reporting a correlation, which Gibson & Wilkins (1975) did not find. Under the age of eight years scoliosis is uncommon. This is thought to be due to the lordotic posture adopted by patients who are still mobile (Fig. 6.6). Once the patient is confined to a wheelchair the curve deteriorates rapidly. Very rarely patients develop fibrotic extension contractures of the spine, with fixed lordosis and a mild scoliosis (Fig. 6.7, Gibson & Wilkins 1975). Provision of calipers not only maintains mobility but also seems to maintain the lordotic posture and slows the development of scoliosis (Fig. 6.8).

Standing for 2–3 hours per day in the calipers, swivel walker or standing frame (Fig. 6.9) even when the patient is no longer mobile, may protect the spine (Miller & Dunn 1982).

Many centres have tried to modify the wheelchair to maintain a lordotic posture. If the back of the chair is made to recline at about 20–25° and is made from soft material that surrounds the trunk when the child leans back it will support the spine and hold it straight (Chapter 5). Alternate designs include the use of a moulded

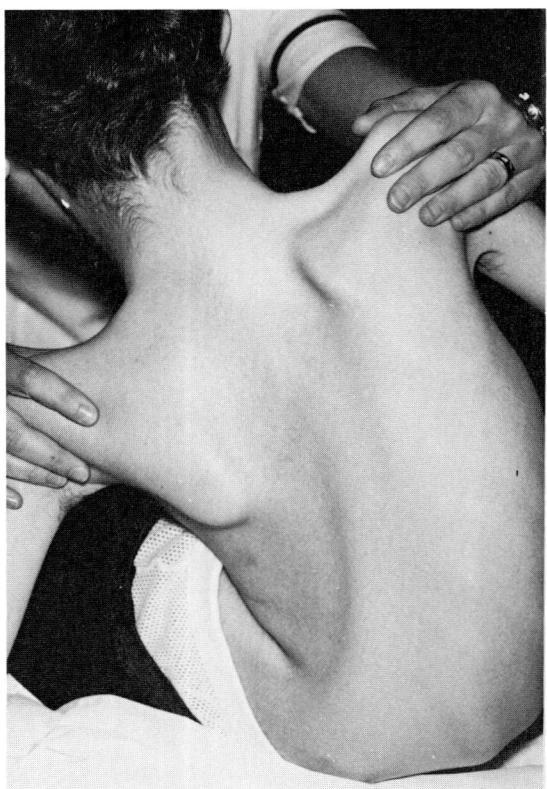

Fig. 6.4. A sixteen-year-old boy with Duchenne muscular dystrophy. He has progressive scoliosis. He is unable to sit unsupported, and when he sits his weight is taken on the lumbar spine. His pelvis is almost vertical.

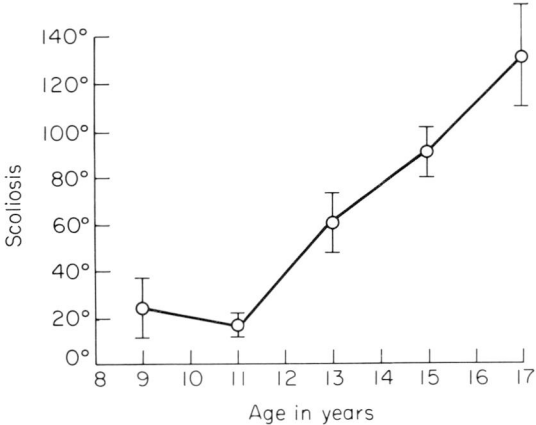

Fig. 6.5. The progression of scoliosis with increasing age in patients with Duchenne muscular dystrophy.

lumbar lordosis in the reclined back (Gibson *et al.* 1975). However, this design of chair has major disadvantages. Because the patient is reclining he is further away from his work surfaces both at school and at home. In practice, it has proved extremely difficult to raise the work surfaces to the patient's level, so that he has to lean forwards, adopting a kyphotic posture and putting his spine at risk. As a result, the use of these modified wheelchairs has been largely abandoned.

In some instances the arms of the wheelchair are removed to allow the child easier access to the wheels. This results in further lack of support to the trunk, the patient leaning to one or other side and this may start the scoliotic process (Fig. 6.10). It is essential that arm rests are fitted to the wheelchair to provide maximum support.

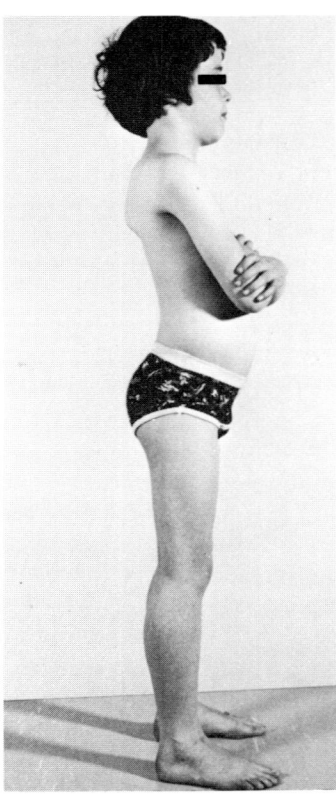

Fig. 6.6. Lordotic posture in an independently mobile boy with Duchenne muscular dystrophy.

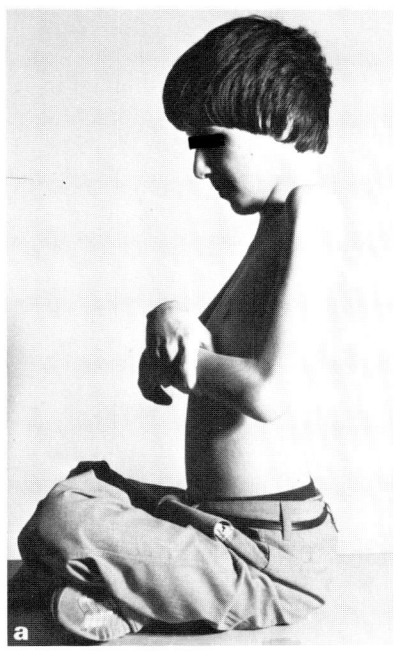
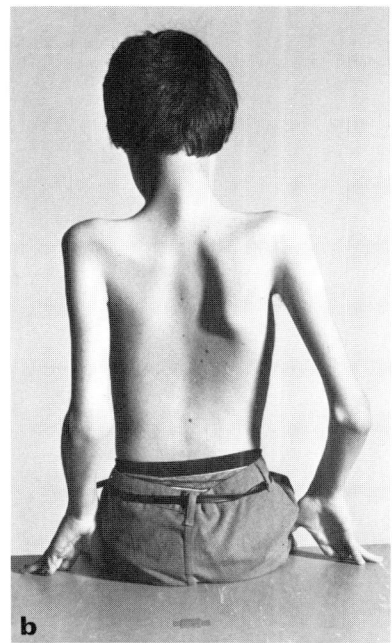

Fig. 6.7. Lordotic posture due to fibrotic extension contracture of the spine in a patient who is no longer ambulant.
(a) Lateral view.
(b) He has a mild scoliosis.

A variety of spinal orthoses have been tried. They may slow the scoliotic process, but there are inherent difficulties with these orthoses. Because the patients are sedentary they are more difficult to fit and tend to ride up, even if carefully moulded. They are often uncomfortable and if they are too well fitting may interfere with respiration. Many patients will not use them regularly. The author's results (Fig. 6.11) show that they slow the progression of the curve, but do not prevent it. This may be due to lack of patient cooperation.

Treatment

Once a scoliosis has developed, use of a modified chair or orthosis may slow the progression of the curve if it is less than 30°, but the curve tends to deteriorate rapidly once it is greater than 45—

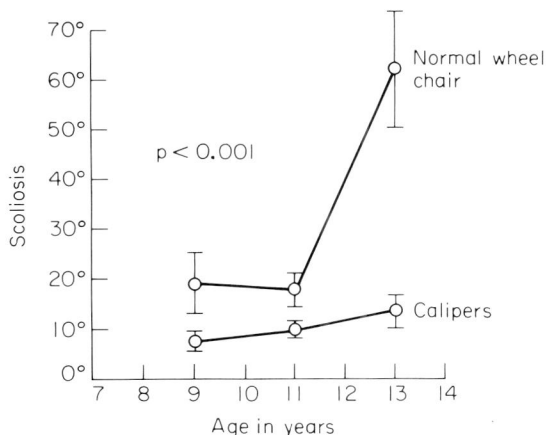

Fig. 6.8. The effect of calipers in preventing scoliosis in patients with Duchenne muscular dystrophy. Patients who wore calipers had a significantly smaller curve than patients confined to a wheelchair.

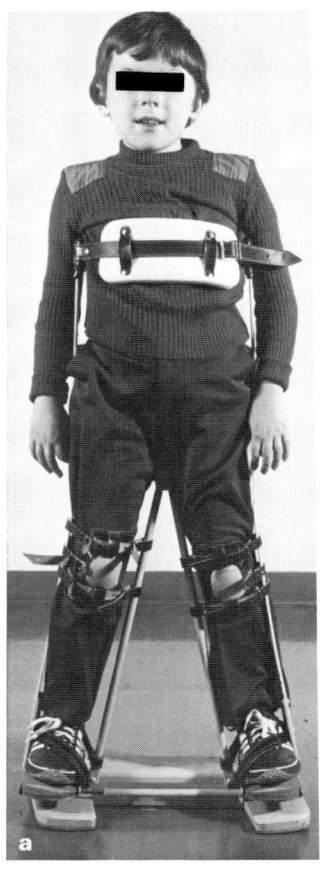 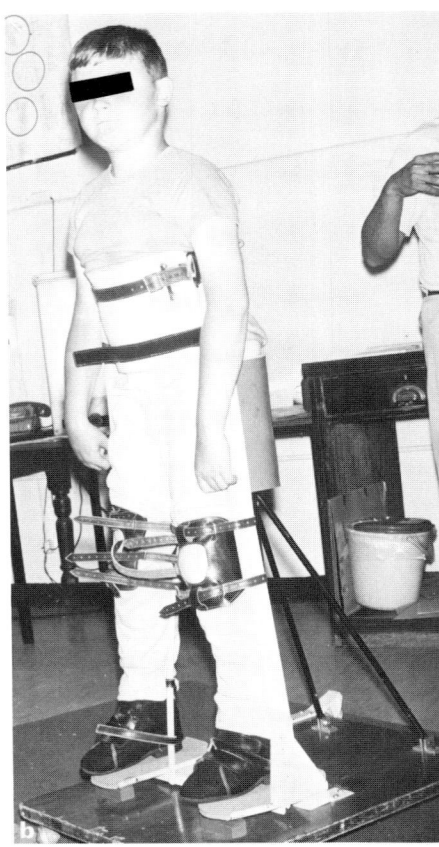

Fig. 6.9. (a) Use of a swivel walker as a standing frame in a patient with Duchenne muscular dystrophy, who is no longer able to stand with calipers.
(b) Modified swivel walker for use as a standing frame.

50°. Moulded chair inserts have been tried, but most patients with Duchenne dystrophy find them uncomfortable. Seeger *et al.* (1984) found that modular seats, spinal jackets and custom-moulded seats had no effect on rate of progression of the curve in patients of 14 years of age and older.

The optimum method of treatment for a progressive curve is surgical stabilization of the spine. However, in Duchenne dystrophy the patient may no longer be fit for surgery, because of progressive deterioration in lung function, by the time he has developed a major curve. Therefore, the concept of 'prophylactic' surgery has been developed, i.e. stabilization of the spine when the patient is still fit for major surgery even though the curve is relatively small. The optimum time

to stabilize the spine in a patient with Duchenne dystrophy is soon after he loses his ability to walk independently, when his lung function is adequate for major spinal surgery, before he has developed cor pulmonale or cardiomyopathy, and when his curve is still mobile and preferably less than 30–35°. Despite the risks of major spinal surgery in these children it is the author's opinion that such 'prophylactic' surgery is extremely worthwhile, in avoiding the problems associated with a late severe scoliosis.

The patients require a six monthly erect X-ray of their spine and six monthly lung function tests. Rapid deterioration in lung function suggests earlier stabilization of the spine. The author is concerned also about the cardiac status and ECGs and echocardiography are required prior to surgery. Providing their cardiac status is reasonable we have operated on patients whose forced vital capacity was down to 25% and even 23% of the expected normal for their age and armspan, although Swank *et al.* (1982), who reported 13 boys with Duchenne dystrophy who had undergone spinal fusion with Harrington instrumentation did not recommend surgery if the vital capacity was less than 40%, the patient had a nonfunctional cough, symptomatic cardiomyopathy or rapidly progressive deterioration in muscle strength.

The postoperative regimen is critical. They require nursing in an intensive care unit for at least 24 hours and the author prefers to intubate the patients for the first 12–24 hours and ventilate them for some hours. Analgesia is provided via an intravenous morphine drip, using a regimen of 0.1 mg/kg body weight in 40 ml normal saline given at 10 ml/hr. The drip rate is increased or decreased as required. For reasons as yet unexplained, they all develop a profound ileus and require nasogastric suction and intravenous feeding for three to four days.

Table 6.3 The effect of Luque segmental spinal stabilization in 11 patients with Duchenne muscular dystrophy.

	Range	Average
Age	11 yrs 8 mths – 15 yrs 8 mths	13 yrs 6 mths
Pre-op curve	10–82°	43°
Post-op curve	0–30°	17°
Correction	28.6–100%	49.3%

The author has stabilized the spine in 19 patients with Duchenne muscular dystrophy. The details of the first 11 are given in Table 6.3. The spine should be stabilized from D4 to the pelvis or sacrum and the operation is associated with profound blood loss (Chapter 7). The mean blood loss in 11 patients was 3397 ccs and Weimann *et al.* (1983) recorded a mean blood loss of 3067 ccs in 24 patients treated by posterior fusion from D4, 5, 6 or 7 to the sacrum with Harrington instrumentation. The author carries out a facet joint fusion, at the time of stabil-

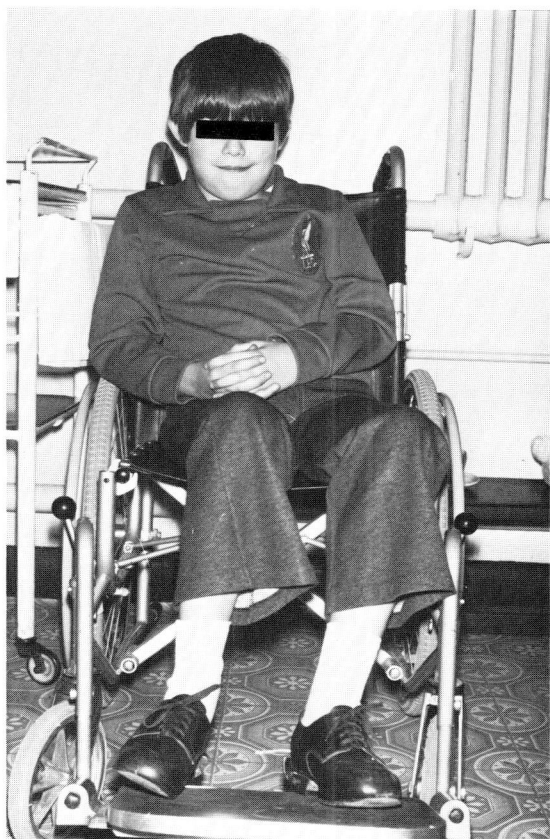

Fig. 6.10. Removal of armrests from a wheelchair. The patient is unable to maintain an erect posture and leans to one side, resting on the wheel.

ization. The effect of surgery on lung function is shown in Table 6.4. The X-rays of one patient are shown in Fig. 6.12. Even though the patients are confined to a wheelchair, surgical stabilization should be carried out with spinal cord monitoring. Despite their motor weakness, most

Table 6.4 The effect of D4-sacrum stabilization on pulmonary function in 11 patients with Duchenne muscular dystrophy. (Figures are mean and range.)

	Pre-op	Post-op (2 months)
% FEV1	39.6 (26–63)	42.0 (36–54.6)
% FVC	37.1 (23–57)	37.4 (31.2–52.2)
% PEFR	39.2 (27.5–51)	32.9 (28.2–36.3)

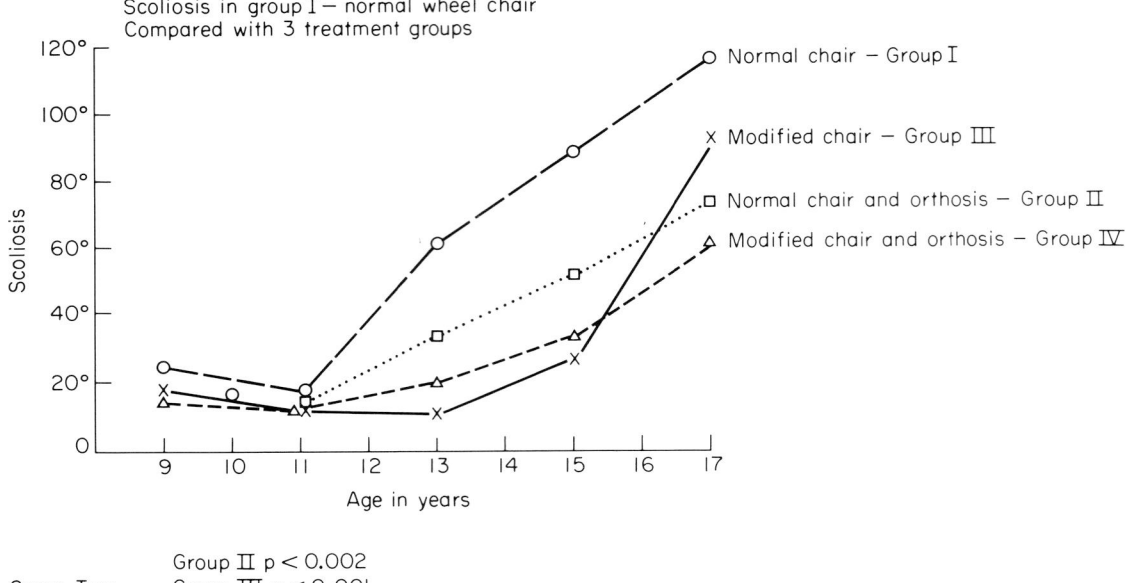

Fig. 6.11. The effect of spinal orthoses and a modified wheelchair on the progression of scoliosis in Duchenne muscular dystrophy. Although there is some slowing of the rate of progression of the scoliosis, these forms of treatment do not prevent the development of a severe deformity.

patients have normal sensation and normal bladder control.

The treatment of the gross curve (Fig. 6.4) is unsatisfactory. At this stage the patients are unfit for surgical correction. Attempts have been made to pad the chair or provide moulded inserts but these usually fail and often the patient cannot be sat without discomfort.

Foot deformity

Mobile patients

The development of an equinus deformity in a mobile patient makes walking even more difficult in a child with inherent muscle weakness (Fig. 6.13). Contractures should be avoided or minimized by physiotherapy in the form of gentle ankle stretching exercises and night splints. The stretching exercises must be carefully carried out to avoid a reflex contracture of the calf

muscles. The parents should be taught the exercises so that they can be carried out daily. If the Achilles tendon becomes tight, night splints should be provided.

Once an equinus or equinovarus deformity has occurred surgical correction should be considered (Williams *et al.* 1984). The deformity can usually be corrected by simple elongation of the Achilles tendon. However, it is essential not to overlengthen the tendon, as this may result in excessive dorsiflexion in the standing position with loss of balance. Some authors combine the elongation of the Achilles tendon with a 'prophylactic' transfer of the tendon of tibialis posterior to the dorsum of the foot (Shapiro & Bresnan 1982).

Postoperatively the limbs are immobilized in below knee plaster casts and the patients mobilized, with the aid of the physiotherapist, within 12–16 hours of surgery. The plaster of Paris casts are changed at 2–3 weeks, when the sutures are removed and casts are taken for night splints, which are used routinely after the plaster casts are finally removed at approximately six weeks.

Patients in calipers

Equinus or equinovarus deformities must be corrected before a patient is fitted with calipers. Following surgery the patient is mobilized with the plaster of Paris casts, within 12–16 hours. In this group of patients long leg plasters are usually required, and the patients are mobilized in their plasters until the calipers are ready. The casts for the manufacture of the calipers are made when the plaster casts are changed for removal of sutures.

Chairbound patients

Most of the equinus and equinovarus deformities develop after the patients have gone off their feet. (Williams *et al.* 1984, Fig. 6.14). Prog-

ressive equinovarus is often associated with pain which may be due to a stress fracture of an osteoporotic bone, pressure sores over bony prominences and inability to fit footwear. Attempts have been made to prevent the development of these deformities by providing adequate foot support by the wheelchair footplates, modifying the foot plate, the use of night splints and the provision of lightweight, moulded day foot–ankle orthoses which fit into the shoes and hold the feet in a neutral or slightly dorsiflexed position.

Modification of the footplates may make the chair slightly more inconvenient to use and some families do not like them. If this is the case day and night splints should be used. Removal of the footplates to allow the patients to use their feet to propel the chair leads to rapid progression of the deformity and should be avoided by providing powered chairs.

If the deformity is symptomatic surgical cor-

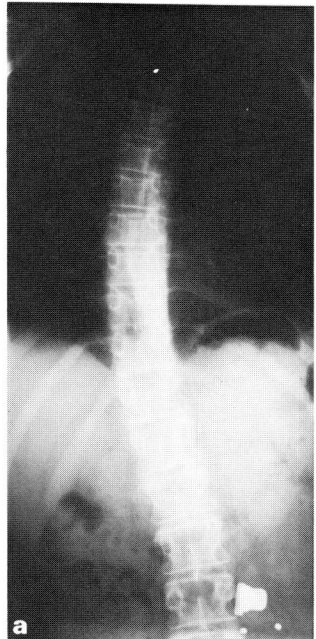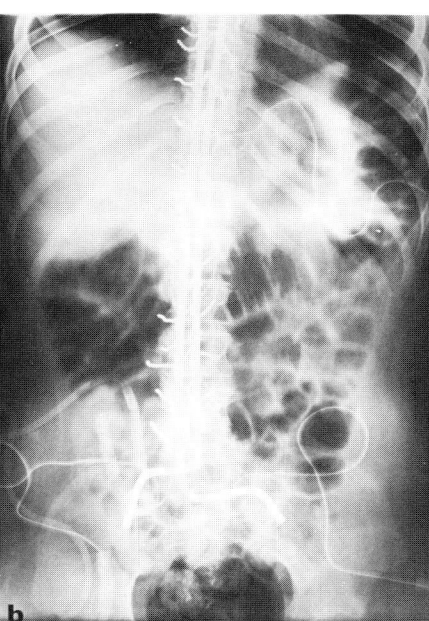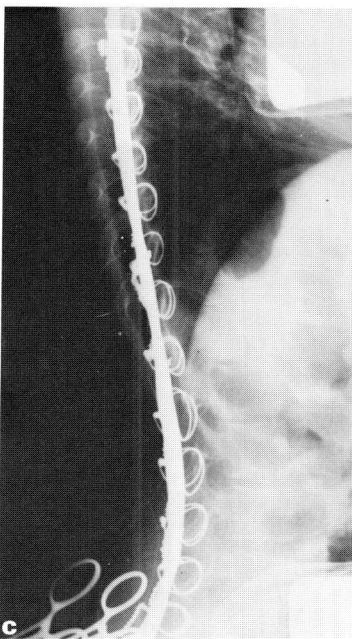

Fig. 6.12. Luque stabilization of the spine in a patient with Duchenne muscular dystrophy.
(a) Pre-operative X-ray.
(b) Immediate postoperative X-ray of the abdomen showing the large bowel ileus. The Luque rods are fixed from D3 or D4 to the pelvis or sacrum.
(c) Lateral view. The rods are moulded to maintain the lumbar lordosis.

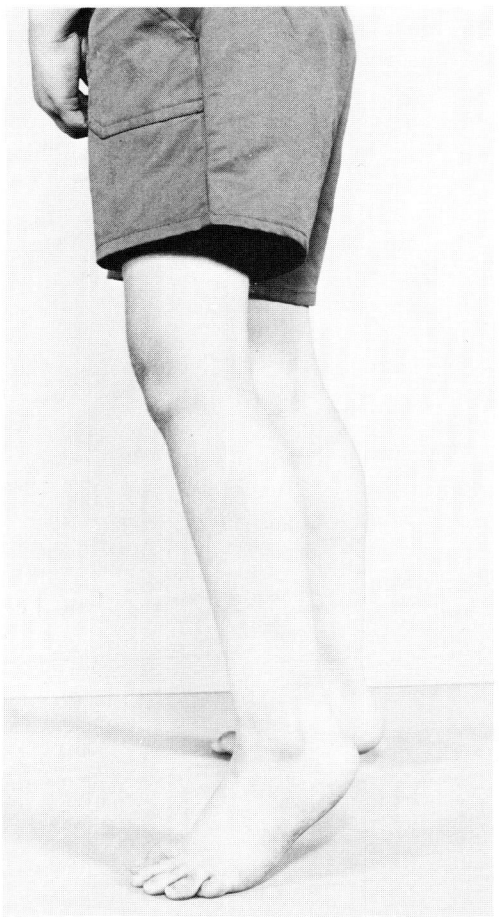

Fig. 6.13. Equinus deformity in an independently mobile patient with Duchenne muscular dystrophy.

talus and distal calcaneus in equinocavovarus.

Postoperatively the limb is immobilized in a below knee plaster cast until the wounds have healed, following which ankle–foot orthoses are worn.

Contractures of the knee and hip

Mobile patients

Contractures should be avoided or minimized by physiotherapy in the form of daily prone lying and stretching exercises. Contracture of the tensor fascia lata may affect the gait and require surgical release.

Mobile in calipers

Contractures must be corrected before calipers are fitted. This is occasionally required.

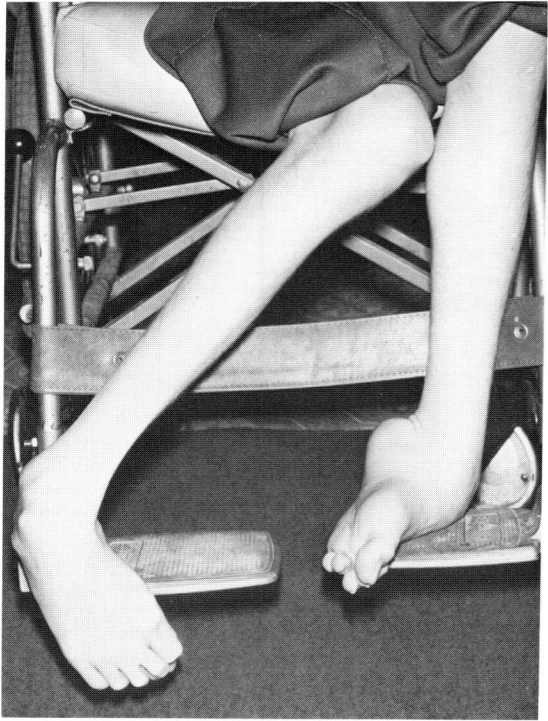

Fig. 6.14. Gross equinovarus deformities in a wheelchair bound patient with Duchenne muscular dystrophy.

rection is indicated. Elongation of the Achilles tendon alone is usually insufficient and elongation or transfer of the tibialis posterior tendon with tenotomy of the tendons of flexor hallucis and flexor digitorum longus and a posterior capsulotomy of the ankle joint may be required (Williams *et al.* 1984). Following surgical correction the deformity tends to recur, but at a slower rate than in unoperated patients (Williams *et al.* 1984). Transfer of the tibialis posterior tendon (Miller *et al.* 1982) may prevent the recurrence. Siegel (1980) advised curettage of part of the cancellous bone from the head of the

Wheelchair patients

Flexion contractures of the hips and knees always develop, but seem to be of little significance. Flexion of the hip is not associated with dislocation in Duchenne dystrophy and contractures of the hip or knees do not produce symptoms unless attempts are made to forcibly correct them. We have not found that surgical correction of these contractures was necessary in any of the 135 patients with Duchenne muscular dystrophy attending the author's Muscle Clinic.

Fractures

In our experience fractures are not a common complication of Duchenne muscular dystrophy although Matejczyk and Rang (1983) recorded an incidence of 18% during the course of the disease. Fractures of the long bones occur from falls out of a wheelchair as well as in ambulatory patients (Siegel 1977, Hsu 1979, Hsu & Garcia-Ariz 1981), the commonest site being the femoral supracondylar region (Matejczyk & Rang 1983). The wheelchair patient has very limited balance and his bones are very osteoporotic. Their fractures are frequently caused by very small force and are rarely displaced (Hsu 1979). Patients in wheelchairs should have safety belts applied for transport over rough outdoor terrain. When the braced child falls, the calipers tend to protect his lower limbs from direct trauma (Siegel 1977).

The fractures heal rapidly and should be immobilized in the lightest possible cast. In the mobile child fractures of the lower limb should be treated in a weightbearing cast. The patient may require admission so that intensive physiotherapy, including ambulation, can be supervised on a daily basis. Mobile patients should not be treated with traction or confined to bed as this may result in loss of their independent walking ability.

Anaesthesia

Problems relating to anaesthesia in children with Duchenne muscular dystrophy are well described and may include sudden death (Boba 1970, Ellis 1980), anaesthesia-related cardiac arrest (Seay *et al.* 1978), rhabdomyolysis (Miller *et al.* 1978, Boltshauser *et al.* 1980) and malignant hyperthermia (Brownell *et al.* 1983, Oka *et al.* 1982, Chapter 5). Hyperpyrexia has also been described in other types of neuromuscular disease, for example, central core disease (Denborough *et al.* 1973). Careful preoperative assessment of all patients is essential (*see* above). Suxamethonium, a neural blocking agent sometimes used in general anaesthesia, should be strictly avoided as reports suggest it may be responsible for hyperkalaemic cardiac arrest and sudden death (Genever 1971). In our series of patients undergoing correction of equinus deformity (Williams *et al.* 1984) the boys who were independently mobile, or mobile with calipers had an average lung function of over 75% of the predicted value, whereas those confined to a wheelchair had an average lung function of 60% of the predicted value.

In the later stages of the disease cardiomyopathy may occur resulting in a lowering of the cardiac reserve. This is not necessarily a contraindication to surgery, two of the author's patients undergoing foot surgery and three undergoing spinal stabilization having shown these changes. Conductive defects occur more commonly. Most of our patients with Duchenne dystrophy had a bundle branch block or some other form of conductive cardiac abnormality at the time of spinal stabilization. Congestive heart failure does not respond to conventional therapy and progresses rapidly (Mattioli & Melhorn 1982).

Table 6.5 shows the author's experience with cardiac and respiratory problems in patients with neuromuscular disease. Thirty-nine patients have been operated upon for scoliosis. One patient with minicore disease (a congenital myopathy) had a cardiac arrest. He was successfully resuscitated, but died four years later from cor pulmonale. One patient with Friedreich's ataxia died three weeks postoperatively from cardiac failure. One patient with Nemaline myopathy died whilst awaiting surgery. She had nocturnal apnoea and was on noctural cuirass ventilation. One patient with spinal muscular atrophy required serial bronchoscopies and suction postoperatively, as she was not able to cooperate with the physiotherapists.

Acute gastric dilation may occur postoperatively (Wislicki 1962) and all our patients with Duchenne dystrophy who underwent Luque spinal stabilization developed an ileus and required nasogastric suction and intravenous feeding for 2–5 days.

Table 6.5 Cardiac and pulmonary complications in patients with neuromuscular disease undergoing spinal stabilization.

	Number of patients	
Duchenne dystrophy	19	
Friedreich's ataxia	5	
Spinal muscular atrophy	5	
Congenital myopathy	3	
Misc. dystrophies, myopathies	7	
Total	39	

	Complications	
Peroperative deaths	0	
Cardiac arrest (resuscitated)	1	(Minicore disease)
Postoperative death	1	(Friedreich's ataxia, cardiac failure 3 weeks postoperatively)
Died whilst awaiting surgery	1	(Nemaline myopathy)
Required serial postoperative bronchoscopies	1	(Spinal muscular atrophy)

Other dystrophies

This section covers a number of conditions which require orthopaedic management but occur less frequently than Duchenne dystrophy (Chapter 5). The orthopaedic problems differ in the different disorders. For example, congenital dystrophy is associated with a high incidence of scoliosis, hip dislocation which often is present at birth, severe talipes equinovarus and contractures (Jones *et al.* 1979), whereas in the limb girdle dystrophies the main problem is abduction of the shoulders. The latter include a number of different syndromes, the primary condition often being spinal muscle atrophy. There is a slowly progressive weakness of the proximal upper and lower limb muscles, which is less rapid than in the muscular dystrophies and may become arrested (Walton 1983).

Scoliosis

The optimum form of treatment is surgical stabilization using Luque segmental stabilization. As in Duchenne dystrophy, the author prefers to stabilize the spine from D4 to the pelvis. The adult forms of muscular dystrophy seldom develop a significant scoliosis, presumably because their muscle weakness was mild during the growth period, for example, in limb girdle dystrophy (Siegel 1973).

Mobility

Where indicated, calipers should be used, but they are often unnecessary.

Foot deformities

Equinus and equinovarus deformities occur commonly in many of these conditions (Fig. 6.15). Contractures should be prevented by physiotherapy if possible. If the Achilles tendon is tight, regular gentle stretching exercises and night splints are indicated. Established equinus deformity usually requires surgical correction, the extent of surgery depending on the severity of the deformity. In many cases elongation of the Achilles tendon is sufficient, but as in Duchenne dystrophy it should not be overlengthened to avoid loss of standing stability. In more extensive contractures division of the tendons of flexor hallucis longus and flexor digitorum lon-

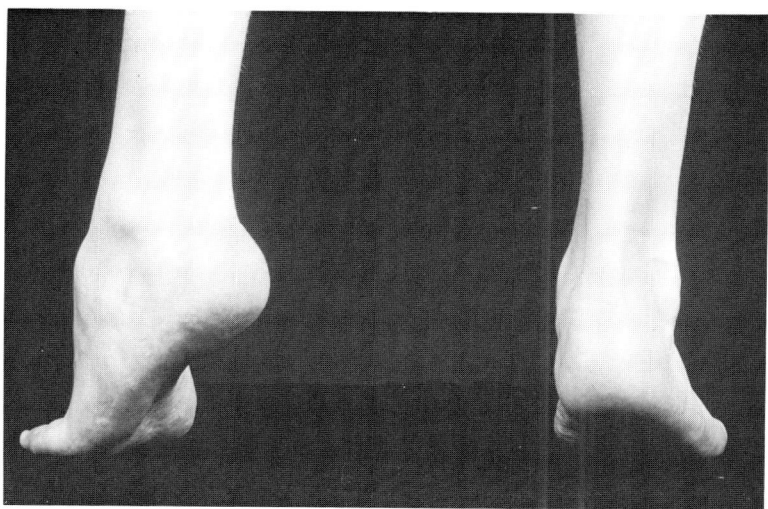

Fig. 6.15. Equinus deformity of the right, and equinovarus deformity of the left ankle and hind foot in a patient with congenital dystrophy.

gus, posterior capsulotomy of the ankle and sub-talar joints and either elongation or transfer of tibialis posterior may also be required.

Hip and/or knee contractures

If the contractures interfere with gait, surgical release is required. This may include release of the hip flexors, iliotibial band and hamstrings.

Dislocation of the hip

Treatment depends on the underlying condition, the development of the patient and their expected locomotor function (Chapter 8).

If the patient is grossly disabled (mentally and physically), will not be expected to stand or walk (with or without the use of aids) and has no pain, treatment is usually not indicated. However, if the hip is painful, or if the patient is likely to be able to stand or walk (with or without the pro-vision of aids) the hip should be stabilized. Treatment will depend on the age of the patient and the development of the acetabulum. The hip muscles must be balanced and the femoral head reduced into the acetabulum. If the dislocation

has been present from birth, acetabular development is poor, and the patient is older than 12–18 months, some form of pelvic osteotomy is frequently needed. An upper femoral varus oseotomy is usually required.

Loss of shoulder abduction

Many of these patients learn trick manoeuvres, but abduction of the shoulders can be helped by stabilizing their scapulae to the chest wall. This minimizes the winging of the scapula and allows the residual musculature optimum mechanical advantage. We usually fix the scapula to the chest wall with at least three ¼ inch nylon or mersilene tapes, passed through drill holes in the blade of the scapula and around adjacent ribs. Scapular stabilization is of little value if the deltoids are atrophied (Copeland & Howard 1978) and surgery should be postponed until growth is complete.

Congenital myopathy

This includes a variety of conditions (Chapter 5). Many are associated with a cardiomyopathy and preoperative cardiac investigations are essential. Anaesthesia carries the risk of hyperpyrexia.

Most of the patients with a congenital myopathy are mobile, their commonest deformity being scoliosis. The principles of treatment are similar to those of spinal muscle atrophy, but the risk of anaesthesia is greater (Table 6.5).

Spinal muscle atrophy

Orthopaedic management is usually required in the intermediate variety, but only rarely indicated in the mild (Kugelberg–Welander syndrome) where the children are ambulant and should be encouraged to remain so, or in the severe form (Werdnig–Hoffmann disease) when the patient usually dies within the first year of life. Cardiomyopathy is not a feature of spinal muscle atrophy.

Mobility

Most of the children with intermediate spinal muscle atrophy are unable to walk when first seen. It usually is not possible to provide calipers until the child is 3–4 years old and during this period active physiotherapy is encouraged, provided the child will cooperate. Most children will manage with cosmetic calipers, although occasionally a rollator is also needed. Unlike Duchenne dystrophy patients with spinal muscle atrophy can be mobilized even though they have been chairbound for some time.

Scoliosis

Like Duchenne dystrophy the most important deformity in these children is their scoliosis. A curve was already present in nearly half of the patients when first seen at the author's clinic. It is the author's policy to obtain an erect (sitting) anteroposterior X-ray of the spine at 6-monthly intervals. Progressive curves or curves more than

20° are braced until the patient is old enough for surgical stabilization. Aprin *et al.* (1982) found that bracing was ineffective in preventing the progression of the scoliosis. They recommended a longer posterior fusion with Harrington rod instrumentation but we now prefer Luque segmental spinal stabilization, as this avoids the necessity for a postoperative plaster of Paris cast or spinal orthosis. However, these patients can tolerate a postoperative jacket and a posterior fusion with Harrington instrumentation or combined posterior and anterior fusion (Riddick *et al.* 1982) is feasible.

The type of bracing depends on the age of the child. In the first 2–3 years of life a plastazote jacket may suffice. In older children a moulded underarm orthosis is usually used. A Boston brace should not be used in these patients although a Milwaukee brace may occasionally be required (Chapter 7). If bracing does not hold the curve, earlier surgery may be required (Chapter 7).

Hips

Unlike Duchenne dystrophy dislocation of the hip does occur in patients with spinal muscle atrophy, although much less frequently than in spina bifida or cerebral palsy (Chapter 8). The dislocation is secondary to muscle imbalance and is preceded by progressive subluxation. Serial X-rays will indicate which hips are at risk and dislocation can usually be prevented by balancing the musculature. This usually requires release of the adductors and flexors, and a proximal femoral varus osteotomy, sometimes supplemented by an iliopsoas transfer. Dislocated hips require open reduction and muscle balancing procedures. If there is an associated scoliosis with pelvic obliquity, these should be corrected first before the hip is reduced (Chapter 8).

Flexion contractures may be gross (Fig. 6.16), can interfere with mobility and if so require surgical correction. Regular prone lying should be encouraged in an attempt to prevent fixed flexion contractures.

Neuropathies and ataxias

This group includes a variety of conditions, but cardiomyopathy is not a feature of the peripheral neuropathies.

In hypertrophic neuropathy (peroneal muscular atrophy, Charcot–Marie–Tooth syndrome), pes cavus is often noted in early childhood before the onset of symptoms. Later there is involvement of the hand with difficulty in fine manipulation. In the Dejerine–Sottos syndrome (hypertrophic neuropathy of infancy) the onset is usually in infancy with delay in early milestones and walking may only be achieved by the third or fourth year.

In the neuronal type of peroneal muscular atrophy there is marked atrophy of muscle and there may be an associated pes cavus. The commonest early symptom is difficulty with walking but the onset may not be until middle age and the patient may have excelled in sports in his youth.

Overall the commonest orthopaedic problem is foot deformity. This usually is in the form of pes cavus (Fig. 6.17), but equinus and equinovarus deformities also occur. The latter are treated by soft tissue releases, whereas a significant cavus deformity requires wedge tarsectomy or triple arthrodesis.

Scoliosis may also occur in these conditions and the management is similar to that for spinal muscle atrophy. Asymmetrical lower limb involvement may result in limb length inequality (Fig. 6.18) and if greater than 3 cm a limb lengthening procedure may be required to improve the gait and avoid the back pain frequently associated with significant limb length inequality.

Sensory neuropathies may present with trophic ulceration, osteomyelitis or septic arthritis (Fig. 6.19). These lesions can also occur with congenital insensitivity to pain (Greider 1983).

It may not be possible to use spinal cord monitoring in patients with a sensory neuropathy, because of the inability to stimulate a peripheral nerve.

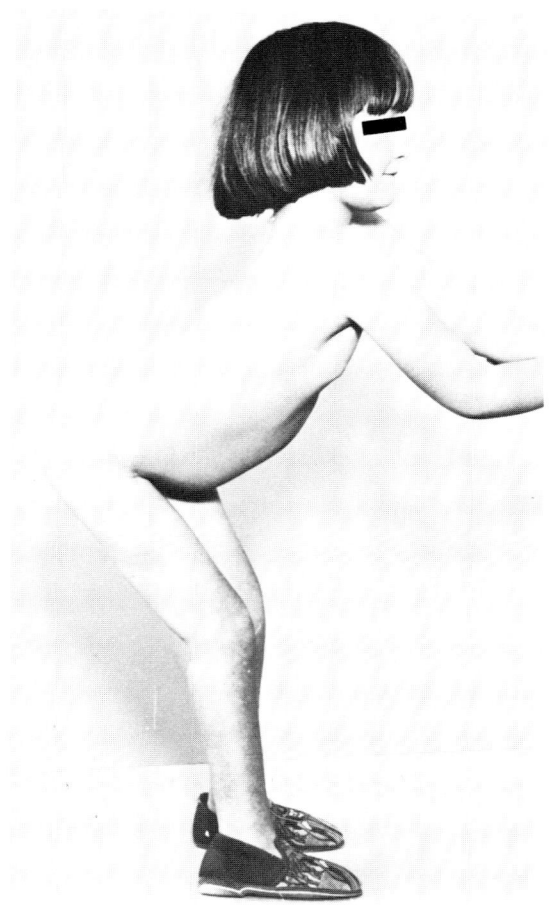

Fig. 6.16. Ninety degree fixed flexion deformity of the hips in a girl with spinal muscle atrophy. Following surgical release of the contracture she regained her independent mobility.

Knees and feet

The principles of management are similar to Duchenne dystrophy. Regular stretching exercises are encouraged. If the Achilles tendons are tight night splints are provided. Surgical release is required for those deformities which interfere with ambulation, prior to the fitting of calipers, and for symptomatic deformities.

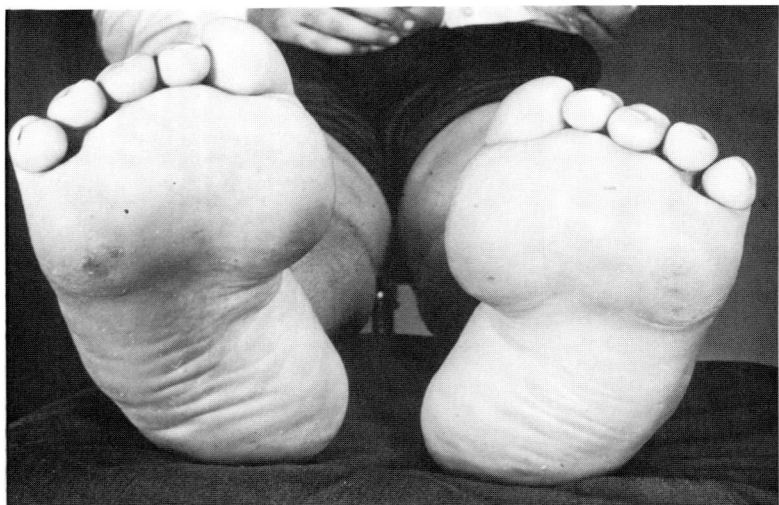

Fig. 6.17. Pes cavus deformity in a patient with peroneal muscular atrophy. He presented with pain under the prominent metatarsal heads and required triple arthrodeses to alleviate his symptoms.

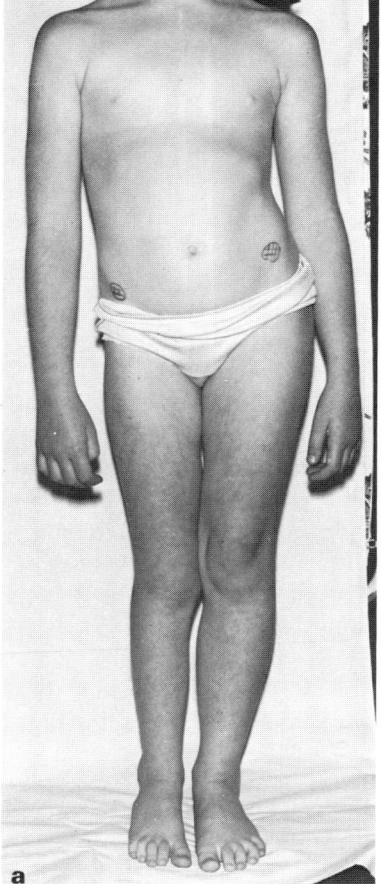
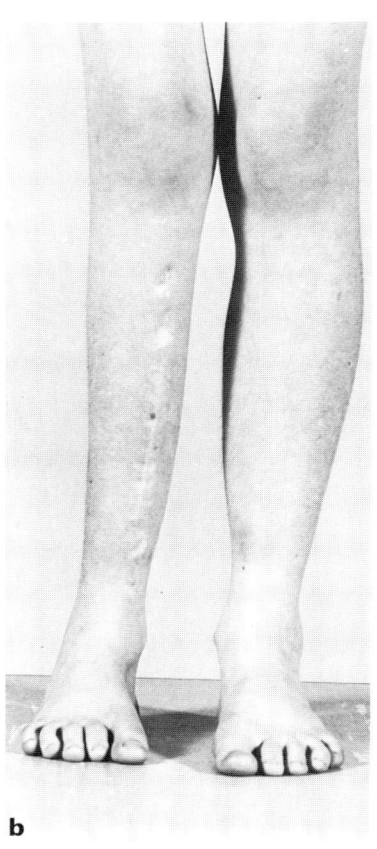

a

b

Fig. 6.18. Patient with polyneuropathy.
(a) Forty-two millimetre limb length discrepancy. The anterior superior iliac spines have been marked.
(b) Following tibial lengthening her discrepancy has been corrected.

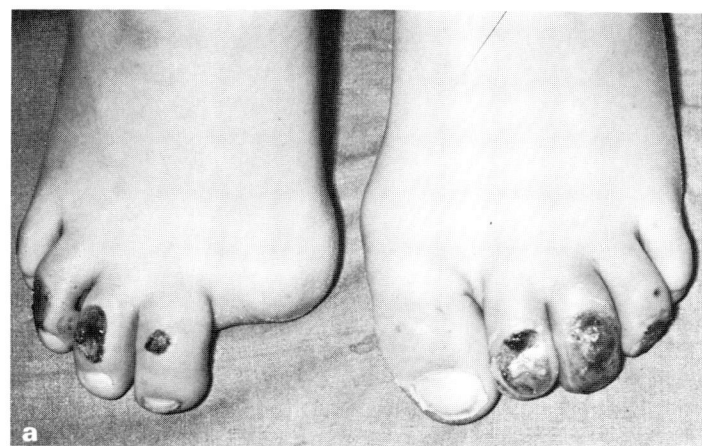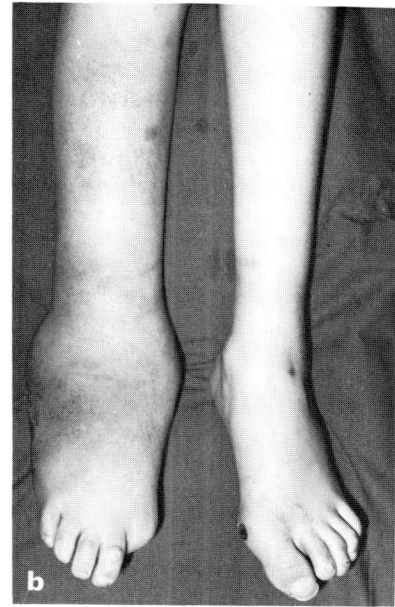

Fig. 6.19. (a) Patient with a sensory neuropathy who developed trophic ulceration affecting several of his toes. (b) Two years later he developed septic arthritis of his right ankle.

Friedreich's ataxia

This is commonly associated with scoliosis (Hensinger & MacEwen 1976, Cady & Bobechko 1984) and pes cavus. The scoliosis frequently requires surgical correction to allow comfortable sitting (Figs. 6.20 and 6.21). Cady and Bobechko (1984) suggested that bracing was of no value and recommended a long posterior spinal fusion as soon as the curve reached 40–50°. In an independently mobile patient, locomotion may be dependent on trunk movements and they may lose their mobility following an upper thoracic to pelvis stabilization. If the curve is still localized to the thoracic spine a localized stabilization should be carried out to preserve trunk mobility and allow for independent walking. If the curve subsequently involves the lumbar spine a second procedure may be required.

The cavus deformity may require treatment if the patient is ambulatory. A flexible deformity can be corrected by combining a Dwyer calcaneal osteotomy with a plantar release, but a triple arthrodesis is required if the cavus is rigid. Occasionally talectomy may be necessary if the deformity is extremely severe and rigid.

Friedreich's ataxia may be associated with cardiac abnormalities (Table 6.5) and a careful cardiac assessment is required prior to major reconstructive surgery. Taddonio (1982) analysed segmental spinal stabilization in 17 patients with a variety of neuromuscular disorders. The only death occurred postoperatively in 1 of the 2 patients with Friedreich's ataxia and who had cardiomyopathy. His series included 2 patients with Duchenne dystrophy, 2 with spinal muscle atrophy and 1 with congenital neuropathy.

Hereditary telangiectatic ataxia is frequently associated with a scoliosis, and which may require surgical correction for comfortable sitting.

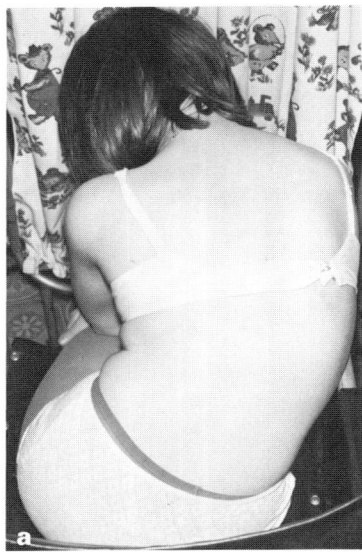 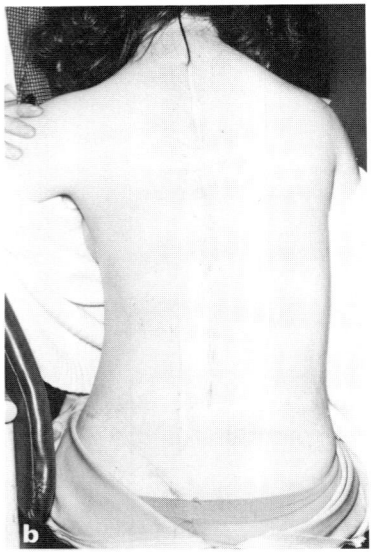

Fig. 6.20. (a) Seventeen year old, wheelchair bound girl with Friedreich's ataxia. She was unable to sit for more than an hour at a time because of pain under her right buttock.
(b) Following spinal fusion using Harrington instrumentation. Routine evaluation at six months post-operatively revealed a pseudarthrosis and she required a supplementary bone graft. Following the fusion, she was able to sit unsupported without pain.

Miscellaneous

There are a variety of miscellaneous neuromuscular conditions which may require orthopaedic management, which do not fit into any of the above categories. They include conditions such as rigid spine syndrome (Chapter 5); hereditary spastic paresis, where release of tight hip abductors for a scissoring gait or elongation of the Achilles tendon for an equinus deformity may be beneficial; inflammatory myopathies which may be associated with an equinus deformity or other contractures (Chapter 5); and myotonic syndromes, where the patient may present with a scoliosis or foot deformity (Chapter 5). Cardiac muscle is frequently affected in dystrophia myotonica and in these patients thiopentone must be avoided. Congenital talipes equinovarus occurs often in this condition.

Down's syndrome

Although this condition is not a neuromuscular condition by strict definition, nevertheless, it is associated with orthopaedic problems and, therefore, has been included in this chapter. Atlanto-axial subluxation has been reported on several occasions, Pueschel (1983) recording an incidence of 17% (40 of 236 patients). Thirty-four of the 40 patients with atlanto-axial instability (85%) were asymptomatic. These children should avoid contact sports, trampoline exercises or other injury which may lead to a cervical spine injury. If neurological symptoms occur, early surgical stabilization is advised (Pueschel 1983).

Another frequent complication of this condition is dislocation of the hips (Christofaro & Heskiaff 1981, Bennet et al. 1982). Bennet et al. (1982) found that the most effective treatment was pelvic and/or femoral osteotomy, combined with capsular plication and carried out in the phase of habitual dislocation. If left untreated subluxation and fixed dislocation followed. The results of surgery in the latter phases were poor and was not recommended. The patients remained mobile, even if untreated and pain was not a prominent feature.

Other orthopaedic problems include scoliosis, dislocation of the patella, genu valgum and pes planus.

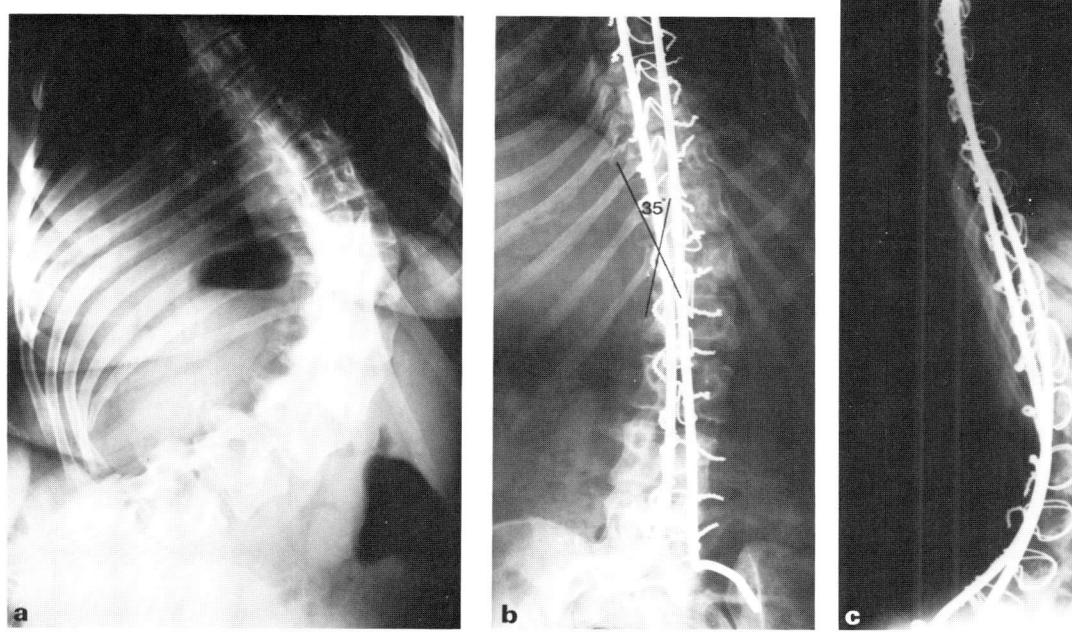

Fig. 6.21. (a) Thirty-two year old patient with Friedreich's ataxia. She has a 96° curve and associated pelvic obliquity. (b) Following the segmental spinal stabilization from D4 to the pelvis, she has a curve of 35° and her pelvis is horizontal. (c) Lateral view showing the lumbar lordosis, necessary for comfortable sitting.

Summary

Deformities occur commonly in the dystrophies, myopathies, atrophies, neuropathies and ataxias. They usually are secondary to muscle imbalance, and the incidence and type of deformity varies in the different conditions.

The most significant deformity is scoliosis. Progressive neuromuscular scoliosis produces increasing respiratory insufficiency and involves the pelvis, producing pelvic obliquity and difficulty with sitting. In Duchenne dystrophy it may be possible to control the scoliosis by prolonging standing with calipers, or a standing frame. If the curve is progressive, surgical stabilization is indicated. At the moment segmental stabilization appears to offer considerable advantages, in that a postoperative plaster jacket or spinal orthosis is avoided. Ideally, the operation should not be carried out under the age of 11–12 years. However, if the curve is progressive and cannot be adequately controlled, earlier stabilization may be necessary.

Contractures can occur in any joint. Contractures of the upper limb rarely require surgical correction in this group of patients. Contractures occur most often in the feet and ankles. The commonest are equinus and equinovarus deformities, but any type of deformity can occur. Surgical correction is required if the contracture interferes with gait or the fitting of calipers in a patient who requires the latter for walking or standing, and in a wheelchair-bound patient if the deformities are symptomatic. Equinus or equinovarus deformities can be corrected by a soft tissue release whereas a pes cavus deformity usually requires a wedge tarsectomy or triple arthrodesis.

Contractures of the hip and knees occur less frequently. They always develop in children confined to a wheelchair but under these circumstances rarely produce problems. Regular stretching exercises and prone lying may help prevent the deformity. If contractures do occur, do not respond to physiotherapy, and interfere with gait, surgical correction is indicated.

It must be emphasized that the orthopaedic management is part of the continuing treatment of these patients. Isolated orthopaedic surgery is of little value. It must be associated with a careful assessment, pre-operative physiotherapy programme and detailed postoperative rehabilitation. It forms part of the overall management of the child.

Orthopaedic surgery can do nothing to cure the underlying neurological disorder. It is aimed at preventing and correcting deformity. Major reconstructive surgery in these patients should not be undertaken purely for cosmetic reasons, but is indicated to aid mobility, alleviate discomfort and improve the quality of life.

References

APRIN H., BOWEN J.R., MACEWEN G.D. & HALL J.E. (1982) Spine fusion in patients with spinal muscular atrophy. *Journal of Bone and Joint Surgery*, **64A**, 1179–87.

BENNET G.C., RANG M., ROYE D.P. & APRIN H. (1982) Dislocation of the hip in trisomy 21. *Journal of Bone and Joint Surgery*, **64B**, 289–94.

BOBA A. (1970) Fatal postanaesthetic complications in two muscular dystrophic patients. *Journal of Pediatric Surgery*, **5**, 71–5.

BOLTSHAUSER E., STEINMANN B., MEYER A. & JERUSALEM F. (1980) Anesthesia induced rhabdomyolysis in Duchenne muscular dystrophy. *British Journal of Anaesthesia*, **52**, 559.

BROWNELL A.K.W., PAASUKE R.T., ELASH A., FOWLOW S.B., SEAGRAM C.G.F., DIEWOLD R.J. & FRIESEN C. (1983) Malignant hyperthermia in Duchenne muscular dystrophy. *Anesthesiology*, **58**, 180–2.

BURKE S.S., GROVE N.M., HOUSER C.R. & JOHNSON D.M. (1971) Respiratory aspects of pseudohypertrophic muscular dystrophy. *American Journal of Diseases of Childhood*, **121**, 230–4.

CADY R.B. & BOBECHKO W.P. (1984) Incidence, natural history and treatment of scoliosis in Friedreich's ataxia. *Journal of Pediatric Orthopedics*, **4**, 673–6.

CHRISTOFARO R.L. & HESKIAFF D. (1981) Bilateral habitual hip dislocation in a child with Down's syndrome: a case report. *Clinical Orthopaedics and Related Research*, **155**, 41–2.

COPELAND S.A. & HOWARD R.C. (1978) Thoracoscapular fusion for facioscapulohumeral dystrophy. *Journal of Bone and Joint Surgery*, **60B**, 547–51.

CRISP D.E., ZITER F.A. & BRAY P.F. (1982) Diagnostic delay in Duchenne's muscular dystrophy. *Journal of the American Medical Association*, **347**, 478–80.

DENBOROUGH M.A., DENNETT L. & ANDERSON R.M. (1973) Central core and malignant hyperpyrexia. *British Journal Medicine*, **1**, 272–3.

DRENNAN J.C., RENSHAW T.S. & CURTIS B.H. (1979) The thoracic suspension orthosis. *Clinical Orthopaedics and Related Research*, **139**, 33–9.

EDWARDS R.H., ROUND J.M., JACKSON M.J., GRIFFITHS R.D. & LILBURN M.F. (1984) Weight reduction in boys with muscular dystrophy. *Developmental Medicine and Child Neurology*, **26**, 384–90.

ELLIS F.R. (1980) Inherited muscle disease. *British Journal of Anaesthesia*, **52**, 153–64.

FIRTH M.A. (1983) Diagnosis of Duchenne muscular dystrophy: experiences of parents of sufferers. *British Medical Journal*, **286**, 700–1.

GALASKO C.S.B. (1977) Incidence of orthopaedic problems in children with muscle disease. *Israel Journal of Medical Sciences*, **13**, 165–76.

GARDNER-MEDWIN D. (1979) Controversies about Duchenne muscular dystrophy: (1) Neonatal screening. *Developmental Medicine and Child Neurology*, **21**, 390–3.

GENEVER E.E. (1971) Suxamethonium-induced cardiac arrest in unsuspected pseudohypertrophic muscular dystrophy: a case report. *British Journal of Anaesthesia*, **43**, 984–6.

GIBSON D.A., ALBISSER A.M. & KORESKA J. (1975) Role of the wheelchair in the management of the muscular dystrophy patient. *Canadian Medical Association Journal*, **113**, 964–6.

GIBSON D.A. & WILKINS K.E. (1975) The management of spinal deformities in Duchenne muscular dystrophy. A new concept of spinal bracing. *Clinical Orthopaedics and Related Research*, **108**, 41–51.

GREIDER T.D. (1983) Orthopaedic aspects of congenital insensitivity to pain. *Clinical Orthopaedics and Related Research*, **172**, 177–85.

HENSINGER R.N. & MACEWEN G.D. (1976) Spinal deformity associated with heritable neurological conditions: spinal muscle atrophy, Friedreich's ataxia, familial dysautonomia and Charcot–Marie–Tooth disease. *Journal of Bone and Joint Surgery*, **58A**, 13–24.

HSU J.D. (1979) Extremity fractures in children with neuromuscular disease. *The John Hopkins Medical Journal*, **145**, 89–93.

HSU J.D. (1983) The natural history of spine curvature progression in the non-ambulatory Duchenne muscular dystrophy patient. *Spine*, **8**, 771–5.

HSU J.D. & GARCIA-ARIZ M. (1981) Fracture of the femur in the Duchenne muscular dystrophy patient. *Journal of Pediatric Orthopedics*, **1**, 203–7.

JOHNSON E.W. & YARNELL S.K. (1976) Hand dominance and scoliosis in Duchenne muscular dystrophy. *Archives of Physical Medicine and Rehabilitation*, **57**, 462–4.

JONES R., KHAN R., HUGHES S. & DUBOWITZ V. (1979) Congenital muscular dystrophy. The importance of early diagnosis and orthopaedic management in the long-term prognosis. *Journal of Bone and Joint Surgery*, **61B**, 13–7.

KURZ L.T., MUBARAK S.J., SCHULTZ P., PARK S.M. & LEACH J. (1983) Correlation of scoliosis and pulmonary function in Duchenne muscular dystrophy. *Journal of Pediatric Orthopedics*, **3**, 347–53.

MATEJCZYK M.B. & RANG M. (1983) Fractures in children with neuromuscular disorders. In HOUGHTON G.R. & THOMPSON G.H. (eds). *Problematic Musculo-Skeletal Injuries in Children*, pp. 178–92. Butterworths, London.

MATTIOLI L. & MELHORN M. (1982) Duchenne's muscular dystrophy. The diagnosis and management of cardiac involvement. *Journal of the Kansas Medical Society*, **83**, 115–21.

MILLER G. & DUNN N. (1982) An outline of the management and prognosis of Duchenne muscular dystrophy in Western Australia. *Australian Paediatric Journal*, **18**, 277–82.

MILLER G.M., HSU J.D., HOFFER M.M. & RENTFRO R. (1982) Posterior tibial tendon transfer: a review of the literature and analysis of 74 procedures. *Journal of Pediatric Orthopedics*, **2**, 363–70.

MILLER E.D., SANDERS D.B., ROWLINGSON J.C., BERRY F.A., SUSSMAN M.D. & EPSTEIN R.M. (1978) Anesthesia-induced rhabdomyolysis in a patient with Duchenne's muscular dystrophy. *Anesthesiology*, **48**, 146–8.

MOOSA A. (1982) Duchenne's muscular dystrophy in six siblings. The case for early diagnosis and neonatal screening. *South African Medical Journal*, **62**, 765–7.

NUZZO R.M. (1980) Dynamic bracing: elastics for patients with cerebral palsy, muscular dystrophy and myelodysplasia. *Clinical Orthopaedics and Related Research*, **148**, 263–73.

O'BRIEN T., SIBERT J.R. & HARPER P.S. (1983) Implications of diagnostic delay in Duchenne muscular dystrophy. *British Medical Journal*, **287**, 1106–7.

OKA S., IGARASHI Y., TAKAGI A., NISHIDA M., SATO K., NAKADA K. & IKEDA K. (1982) Malignant hyperpyrexia and Duchenne muscular dystrophy. A case report. *Canadian Anaesthetists' Society Journal*, **29**, 627–9.

PUESCHEL S.M. (1983) Atlanto-axial subluxation in Down syndrome. *Lancet*, **1**, 980.

RIDDICK M.F., WINTER R.B. & LUTTER L.D. (1982) Spinal deformities in patients with spinal muscle atrophy. A review of 36 patients. *Spine*, **7**, 476–83.

ROY L. & GIBSON D.A. (1970) Pseudohypertrophic muscular dystrophy and its surgical management: review of 30 patients. *Canadian Journal of Surgery*, **13**, 13–21.

SEAY A.R., ZITER F.A. & THOMPSON J.A. (1978) Cardiac arrest during induction of anaesthesia in Duchenne muscular dystrophy. *Journal of Pediatrics*, **93**, 88–90.

SHAPIRO F. & BRESNAN M.J. (1982) Current concepts review: Orthopaedic management of childhood neuromuscular diseases. Part III: diseases of muscle. *Journal of Bone and Joint Surgery*, **64A**, 1102–7.

SEEGER B.R., SUTHERLAND A.D'A. & CLARK M.S. (1984) Orthotic management of scoliosis in Duchenne muscular dystrophy. *Archives of Physical Medicine and Rehabilitation*, **65**, 83–6.

SIEGEL I.M. (1973) Scoliosis in muscular dystrophy. Some comments about diagnosis, observations on prognosis and suggestions for therapy. *Clinical Orthopaedics & Related Research*, **93**, 235–8.

SIEGEL I.M. (1977) Fractures of long bones in Duchenne muscular dystrophy. *Journal of Trauma*, **17**, 219–22.

SIEGEL I.M. (1980) Maintenance of ambulation in Duchenne muscular dystrophy. The role of the orthopaedic surgeon. *Clinical Pediatrics*, **19**, 383–8.

SPENCER G.E. & VIGNOS P.J. JR (1962) Bracing for ambulation in childhood progressive muscular dystrophy. *Journal of Bone and Joint Surgery*, **44A**, 234–42.

SWANK S.M., BROWN J.C. & PERRY R.E. (1982) Spinal fusion in Duchenne's muscular dystrophy. *Spine*, **7**, 484–91.

TADDONIO R.F. (1982) Segmental spinal instrumentation in the management of neuromuscular spinal deformity. *Spine*, **7**, 305–11.

WALTON J. (1983) Changing concepts of neuromuscular diseases. *Hospital update*, 949–58.

WEIMANN R.L., GIBSON D.A., MOSELEY C.F. & JONES D.C. (1983) Surgical stabilization of the spine in Duchenne muscular dystrophy. *Spine*, **8**, 776–80.

WILLIAMS E.A., READ L., ELLIS A., GALASKO C.S.B. & MORRIS P. (1984) The management of equinus deformity in Duchenne muscular dystrophy. *Journal of Bone and Joint Surgery*, **66B**, 546–50.

WISLICKI L. (1962) Anaesthesia and post-operative complications in progressive muscular dystrophy. Tachycardia and acute gastric dilation. *Anaesthesia*, **17**, 482–7.

Chapter 7
The Management of Spinal Deformity in Neuromuscular Disease

M. J. McMASTER

Spinal deformity occurring as a consequence of neuromuscular disease can present one of the greatest challenges to the orthopaedic surgeon. These patients are very different from those with idiopathic or congenital scoliosis and must be assessed differently to avoid serious errors in management. In neuromuscular disease the treatment of the spine is influenced by a number of factors, such as respiratory muscle paralysis, sensory disturbance and functional disability of the limbs, which are not present in other types of scoliosis. Once a neuromuscular spinal deformity develops, it usually progresses and frequently requires treatment. If left untreated, the spinal deformity often becomes very severe and this may further decrease the respiratory function and make sitting and walking even more difficult.

Any neuromuscular disease producing weakness or spasticity of the trunk musculature can cause a spinal deformity provided the patient is still growing. In the past, poliomyelitis was the major cause of neuromuscular spinal deformity. Immunization has now virtually eradicated this disease from developed countries but there are many Third World countries where the condition remains a serious problem. Myelomeningocele and cerebral palsy are the commonest causes of neuromuscular spinal deformity in developed countries. In the past, many children with myelomeningocele rarely survived infancy, or early childhood, but more recently with early closure of the spinal defect, reliable means of controlling the hydrocephalus and antibiotics to control infection, an increasing number are surviving to adulthood when a spinal deformity

becomes their major problem (Hall & Bobechko 1973; Piggott 1980). These children along with those who develop a deformity following spinal cord injury are the most difficult to treat because of their sensory impairment. Other less frequent causes of spinal deformity are Friedreich's ataxia, spinal muscular atrophy, syringomyelia, and Duchenne muscular dystrophy.

In order to formulate a plan of treatment, it is necessary to understand the problems associated with the different patterns of neuromuscular spinal deformity and their course if left untreated.

Patterns of spinal deformity

In general there are two main groups of spinal deformities depending on the severity and distribution of muscle weakness affecting the spine. A third and much rarer type of spinal deformity occurs only in certain patients with myelomeningocele.

1 The commonest and most characteristic spinal deformity associated with neuromuscular disease develops in patients with either total paralysis or extensive symmetric weakness of their spinal musculature. Because of the lack of muscular support the spine 'collapses' under the influence of gravity when the patient is upright. Initially the spine remains flexible and the deformity can be easily corrected by passive means but with time it becomes fixed and increasingly more rigid.

The typical collapsing spinal deformity is a long smooth thoracolumbar scoliosis extending from the upper or mid thoracic regions to the sacrum and producing pelvic obliquity. In addition to the scoliosis, the spine is also frequently deformed in the sagittal plane with an increased lumbar lordosis and occasionally a thoracic kyphosis (Kilfoyle et al. 1965). When sitting the combination of a severe scoliosis and pelvic obliquity frequently causes the patient to list to one side and necessitates the use of one hand for support. This interferes with the use of the arm for normal activities and further increases the degree of disability. The pelvic obliquity causes the patient to sit with most of the body weight over one buttock and this can result in a pressure sore especially if there is sensory impairment. When standing the fixed pelvic obliquity produces an apparent leg length discrepancy and this makes fitting of long leg calipers and walking even more difficult. Because of the pelvic obliquity the hip on the high side of the pelvis is not fully covered by the acetabulum; this predisposes to subluxation or dislocation especially if there is a flexion adduction deformity of the hip as a result of muscle imbalance.

2 The second group is neuromuscular spinal deformities due to asymmetric weakness of the spinal musculature. This imbalance results in a wide variety of curve patterns depending on the distribution of the muscle weakness and can affect any part of the spine from the cervical to the lumbar regions. These curves which can resemble idiopathic scoliosis may be either single or double and are not necessarily associated with pelvic obliquity. Initially the spinal deformity is flexible, but with time it becomes fixed and there may also be decompensation of the trunk.

3 An uncommon, but very characteristic, angular kyphotic deformity can occur in some patients with myelomeningocele and is present although not always recognized at birth. These patients have a total paraplegia and the defect in their laminae which extends throughout the lumbar region is much wider than in the majority of patients with myelomeningocele (Hoppenfeld 1967). As a result the paraspinal muscles which normally extend the spine are carried forward and act at a mechanical disadvantage (Drennan 1970). Once the child begins to sit, the kyphus which usually has its apex at the second or third lumbar vertebrae deteriorates rapidly under the influence of gravity and becomes very severe at an early age (Sharrard & Drennan 1972). This progression is only stopped mechanically when the ribs come to rest on the pelvic brim. The child is thrown forward and forced to use both hands for support. Sitting or lying is difficult and the anaesthetic scarred skin over the apex of the kyphus easily develops pressure sores.

Prognosis

Neuromuscular spinal deformities frequently develop in early childhood and all deteriorate with growth; this deterioration becomes most rapid during the pubertal growth spurt. After skeletal maturity the rate of deterioration slows but unlike idiopathic scoliosis the spine does not stabilize and frequently progression continues until it is stopped mechanically when the ribs abut on the pelvis or the patient becomes so disabled that he cannot sit upright.

Thoracic curves distort the rib cage and if severe will decrease the vital capacity and further interfere with the respiratory function which may already be affected by paralysis of the intercostal muscles. In thoracolumbar curves, the diaphragm may be the only functioning respiratory muscle, and this can be hindered by the upward pressure of the abdominal contents as the spine collapses. Patients may die from respiratory failure precipitated by their increasing spinal deformity and not due to progression of their neuromuscular disease.

Factors affecting treatment

Progressive deterioration of the neuromuscular disease

The majority of neuromuscular diseases are static although the spinal deformity may progress. In a few conditions such as Friedreich's ataxia and Duchenne muscular dystrophy, the neuro-muscular disorder may also progress result-ing in increasing muscle weakness and finally death from cardiac or respiratory failure. Major surgical procedures on these patients neces-sitating bed rest and immobilization for more than a few days can result in a rapid increase in muscle weakness. As a result, patients who could walk prior to surgery, may no longer be able to do so afterwards. If spinal surgery is indicated it should be carried out at a relatively early stage before the patient is severely disabled and the period of bed rest should be as brief as possible.

Sensory impairment

In patients with myelomeningocele and spinal cord injury, the loss of sensation over their trunk and lower limbs will make them particularly liable to pressure sores. This is an important factor when deciding on the type of external support which may be necessary for conservative treatment or following surgery.

Respiratory function

The effect of a spinal deformity on respiratory function is very important when considering treatment. Many patients will already have an impaired respiratory function due to paralysis of their respiratory muscles and this cannot be altered by treatment. Further deterioration of the respiratory function can occur due to prog-ression of the spinal deformity but this can be prevented by treatment. Care should be taken that any external support for the spine should not impair respiratory function by constricting the chest or limiting the movement of the dia-phragm. Anterior spinal surgery may be hazard-ous because it involves a thoracotomy and tak-ing down the diaphragm which may be the only functioning respiratory muscle. A very careful assessment of the respiratory function and blood gases is necessary prior to surgery. Unfor-tunately there is no single test which indicates a

safe level for surgery. Postoperative com-plications are less likely if the vital capacity is greater than 40% of the predicted normal and there is an effective cough to get rid of secretion. If the vital capacity is less than 30% spinal surgery will be hazardous and postoperative assisted ventilation will be necessary (Nickel & Perry 1961; Makley et al. 1968; Bonnett et al. 1975).

Cardiac function

Duchenne muscular dystrophy is associated with cardiac myopathy and this may also occur but not so frequently in Friedreich's ataxia (Hen-singer & MacEwen 1976). These patients require careful pre-operative cardiac assessment and monitoring during surgery.

Hip deformities

A unilateral contracture of the iliotibial band may contribute to pelvic obliquity (Irwin 1949) and this should be released prior to treating the spinal deformity. Hip flexion contractures will produce lumbar lordosis whereas hip extensor contractures predispose to hyperflexion of the pelvis and a lumbar kyphosis.

Mental function

Patients with cerebral palsy or myelomenin-gocele may also suffer from mental deficiency and this may make it difficult for them to under-stand or comply with a complex treatment regi-men.

General condition

Many children with neuromuscular disease are unable to walk satisfactorily and as a result become obese. This makes it difficult to apply an external support to the spine and may also interfere with surgery. Patients with myelomeningocele and spinal cord injury frequently have bladder paralysis and their renal function must be carefully assessed and any infection treated prior to surgery.

Radiographic evaluation

A careful radiographic evaluation as well as a clinical examination is necessary before treatment. Radiographs showing the whole of the spine in both the anteroposterior and lateral planes are taken with the patient standing and sitting. These radiographs show not only the severity of the scoliosis but also any kyphosis or lordosis that might be present as well as pelvic obliquity and decompensation of the trunk. The sitting radiograph eliminates the effect of crutches, hip flexion contractures or leg length discrepancy. A radiograph taken with the patient suspended or in traction will show the flexibility of the curves and this is important when deciding on the type of surgical procedure necessary to correct the spine.

Treatment

The key to successful management of neuromuscular spinal deformities is to recognize their poor prognosis at an early stage and to start immediate treatment while the curve is still small and before it becomes rigid. The only satisfactory conservative means of treatment is to brace the spine, but unfortunately this is never sufficient as a definitive treatment. Even if the deformity were successfully controlled to skeletal maturity, the curvature would again deteriorate once the brace was removed and progress to a severe degree. Consequently a spinal fusion is usually necessary at the end of brace treatment.

Posterior spinal fusion is an established and successful method of preventing increasing spinal deformity, but unfortunately cannot be satisfactorily applied to very young children. Neuromuscular curves are often very long and

the extensive fusion that is necessary will stop all longitudinal growth in the posterior elements resulting in a severe degree of stunting of the spine as the child grows to maturity. Bonnett *et al.* (1975) also found that an increasing lordosis could develop in young patients due to the continued growth of the vertebral bodies anteriorly and lack of growth in the fused posterior elements. In order to minimize these difficulties it is best to delay spinal fusion until just before the onset of puberty when the growth spurt makes the curves increasingly more difficult to control in a brace. Because neuromuscular curves often start at an early age, a long period of conservative treatment may be necessary to prevent deterioration before they can be satisfactorily fused at the optimum age between 10 and 12 years. However, an earlier fusion will be necessary if the deformity cannot be controlled by other means.

Brace treatment

The object of treating neuromuscular curves in a brace is to minimize their otherwise relentless rate of progression and to maintain good alignment and sitting balance until an adequate amount of spinal growth has occurred and there is adequate bone stock for a spinal fusion. Unlike the treatment of idiopathic scoliosis these patients with weakness of their trunk muscles cannot perform corrective spinal exercises while in their brace. The brace is used therefore only as a holding device with the object of producing a stiff spine in a corrected position. No attempt is made to mobilize the spine out of the brace and no exercises are performed. Although the brace may provide an initial partial correction this is usually not maintained and the curve continues to deteriorate but at a much slower rate than before the brace was applied.

Indications

The brace must be applied before a fixed spinal deformity develops. There is no value in applying the brace after the patient has developed a large structural curve and especially if there is pelvic obliquity (Duval-Beaupere *et al.* 1975). Any patient with a curve of over 25 degrees which shows signs of progression is a candidate for spinal bracing.

Contraindications

There are no absolute contraindications to bracing a neuromuscular scoliosis although there are a number of factors which mitigate against a successful result. Curves of over 60 degrees and especially those with pelvic obliquity are very difficult to control in a brace. The holding pressure of the brace against the skin is often uncomfortable and can result in pressure sores especially if the skin is anaesthetic. Extreme obesity and lack of maternal care makes brace therapy much more difficult and the likelihood of pressure sores much greater. There are also certain types of neuromuscular disease which do not respond well to brace therapy. Patients with cerebral palsy, Friedreich's ataxia, and Duchenne muscular dystrophy, may already have difficulty in walking and the application of a brace may totally immobilize them. If, however, these patients are already wheelchair bound, the application of a brace can be much more beneficial. In some patients, breathing may be difficult because of respiratory muscle paralysis and the constriction of a brace around their chest may further increase their difficulties by limiting chest expansion.

A brace should not be applied to myelomeningocele patients with an angular kyphotic deformity because this is totally unresponsive and the brace is a potent cause of pressure sores.

Types of spinal brace

1 The *Milwaukee brace* has been most frequently used in the conservative treatment of idiopathic scoliosis and has also been successfully applied to neuromuscular curves (Bunch 1975). The Milwaukee brace consists of a carefully moulded plastic pelvic girdle connected to an encircling neck piece by extendable rods which provide a distracting force. A second correcting force is provided by means of an adjustable pad applied over the rib hump. Because these patients are paralysed, and cannot perform exercises while in the brace, the constant pressure of the pad may deform the ribs and also cause skin breakdown. In order to overcome these problems, the rib pad should be larger than normal and carefully conform to the chest wall. The pelvic girdle may be extended proximally to support the torso. The most frequent cause of failure of Milwaukee brace treatment is its application to curves which are too large. This type of brace is best applied to thoracic curves of less than 40 degrees and in patients with normal sensation.

2 An *underarm 'total contact' brace* (Fig. 7.1)

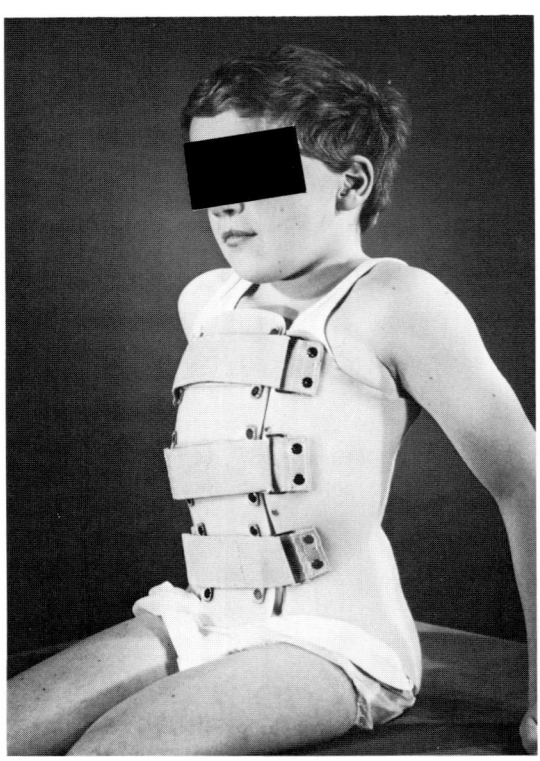

Fig. 7.1. A total contact underarm orthosis.

can be applied to the collapsing type of thoracolumbar scoliosis. This brace is not the same as that used in idiopathic scoliosis where a pressure pad within the brace provides part of a three point correcting system of forces. If this brace were applied to patients with reduced sensation it is likely to produce pressure sores. Patients with neuromuscular curves and reduced sensation are best treated in a total contact type of brace which spreads the pressure over a wide area so reducing the likelihood of skin breakdown. Care should be taken to make sure that these braces do not further compromise an already impaired respiratory system. Drennan *et al.* (1979) have produced a thoracic suspension orthosis which is a moulded body jacket suspended from a wheelchair by a swivel bracket. The thorax and subcostal margins act as weight-bearing structures and the effect of gravity on the suspended lower trunk corrects a collapsing scoliosis. The buttocks are kept just off the wheelchair and this prevents pressure sores.

Brace manufacture

Both the Milwaukee brace and the underarm jacket are made from a plaster mould of the patient held in the corrected position by applying traction to the head and pelvis. In Duchenne muscular dystrophy the underarm jacket is made in such a way as to extend the spine as this has been found to be the most stable position in preventing further deterioration (Wilkins & Gibson 1976). Patients with spinal muscular atrophy walk with a hyperlordotic thoracolumbar spine and the brace must be manufactured to maintain this position. If the brace were made with the lordosis corrected, as in idiopathic scoliosis, the patient would fall forward.

Both the Milwaukee brace and underarm jacket are made from strong but lightweight plastic materials and are lined with a nonabsorbent cushioning material to distribute the forces. The jacket is bivalved and secured with Velcro straps which allow easy removal for regular skin inspection.

Brace supervision

The patient is slowly weaned into the brace over a period of several weeks and this allows time for the skin to adapt to the pressure of the brace. The orthosis is worn only when upright and not at night when vertical support for a collapsing spine is unnecessary. If the patient were to wear the brace while asleep he is much more likely to develop pressure sores especially if there is anaesthetic skin. Good maternal care is essential and the brace should be removed several times each day to check for excessive pressure against the skin.

The satisfactory bracing of a neuromuscular spine deformity is difficult and requires meticulous attention. The best results are obtained when the spinal surgeon and the orthotist regularly see the patient together and the brace is made in close proximity to the clinic so that immediate alterations can be carried out as required.

Termination of brace treatment

Brace treatment may be terminated for several reasons. Firstly, if the curve cannot be controlled in the brace to an acceptable degree, it should not be allowed to progress and become fixed. Secondly, the brace may have to be removed if it produces intractable pressure sores. Thirdly, the patient may reach the optimum age for fusion, that is 10–12 years of age, and as fusion is always necessary one should not wait any longer. These curves are not like idiopathic scoliosis where if braced to skeletal maturity the spine becomes stable. Once the brace is removed from a neuromuscular scoliosis, the only option is to fuse the spine.

Operative treatment

Spinal fusion is frequently required to control neuromuscular spinal deformities. Before fusing the spine it is usual to correct the deformity as much as possible and then to hold the spine in the corrected position until the fusion is solid. A successful spinal fusion transforms the abnormally curved part of the spine into a solid bar of bone that is of sufficient strength to resist bending under the influence of gravity and the deforming forces of muscle imbalance. Correction may be lost due either to the development of a pseudarthrosis or to bending of a solid but weak fusion.

In the last 25 years there have been many major advances in the treatment of spinal deformities and there is now virtually no severity of curvature which cannot be significantly improved and stabilized by surgery. However, it is important to balance what is technically possible and what is practicable and safe for these patients, many of whom are severely disabled by their neuromuscular disease. Pre-operative evaluation is vitally important and the timing and indications for surgery require much more consideration than simply the presence of a spinal deformity. The spine must not be treated in isolation and the other problems due to the neuromuscular disease must be taken into consideration.

Indications for surgery

The surgery required for these patients is often the most difficult type of spinal surgery and should only be carried out in a specialized centre by a surgeon experienced in dealing with all types of spinal deformity. Any patient over the age of 10 years with a progressive structural curve should be considered a candidate for spinal fusion. If surgery is thought necessary it should be carried out early to prevent problems from developing, and fusion should not be delayed until after the adolescent growth spurt.

In deciding on surgery, a loss of function is more important than the size of the curvature. A progressive pelvic obliquity which becomes fixed may lead to progressive decompensation of the trunk, a loss of sitting balance and pressure sores. If the patient is less than 10 years old and being treated in a brace, the curve should not be

allowed to exceed 60 degrees and should never go beyond 100 degrees. The pulmonary function may already be impaired by respiratory muscle paralysis and the addition of a severe spinal deformity will only increase this problem. A severe curvature may also require anterior surgery via a thoracotomy and this may not be possible if there is a severe respiratory deficiency. It is important therefore to carry out any spinal surgery before the pulmonary function becomes affected by the deformity. Older patients can develop backache due to their curvature and this may be a relative indication for surgery. The cosmetic appearance is not a primary indication for surgery, but it is much better for the patient's morale to be able to sit upright rather than be bent and twisted.

Contraindications

The main contraindication to spinal surgery is a severe impairment of respiratory function which makes it likely that the patient would develop postoperative respiratory failure and this would not recover with assisted ventilation. Other relative contraindications are a short life expectancy due to cardiac or renal problems and severe mental retardation which would significantly interfere with the postoperative care.

Objectives of surgery

The objective of surgery is to correct the deformity and fuse the spine in its optimum position. The trunk should be supported in a balanced position over a stable and level pelvis. The torso should be vertical with the head centred over the thorax and pelvis. This will allow the patient to sit in a stable position and have independent use of the arms for activities other than supporting the trunk. In this position the weight is symmetrically distributed over the buttocks and there is less likelihood of pressure sores. In patients with total paraplegia the ability to walk in long leg calipers is frequently improved following a long spinal fusion to the sacrum. In these patients, the normal functioning muscles in the upper body are better able to control the pelvis and lower limbs through the long stable lever of the fused spine. A 'swing-to' gait with crutches and long leg calipers may be improved to a 'swing-through' gait which is more economical. However, in some patients with only partial paralysis of the lower limbs and trunk, the long fusion to the sacrum may interfere with gait. These patients often walk in calipers by alternately hitching up each side of their pelvis to get the foot off the ground and swinging the leg through. A lumbosacral fusion and rigid spine will prevent tilting the pelvis and interfere with this gait. A trial in a plaster jacket before surgery may be useful in evaluating any alteration in gait pattern that might occur after spinal fusion.

Selection and extent of the fusion area

The most common error in the surgical treatment of neuromuscular spinal deformity is to fuse too short a segment of the spine. The extent of the fusion is determined by examining the erect sitting and standing spinal radiographs in both the anteroposterior and lateral planes. This enables one to assess the whole spinal deformity which may be any combination of a scoliosis, kyphosis and lordosis. The fusion should extend over the entire length of these deformities as seen on both the anteroposterior and lateral radiographs. The upper level of the fusion is often well above that chosen for idiopathic curves and is usually one or two vertebra above the end vertebra as measured on the radiographs. The top of the fusion should lie directly above the centre of the sacrum and all rotated vertebrae should be included in the fusion. If the upper level of the fusion is not high enough, the curve will continue to progress above the fused area. In a collapsing spine with pelvic obliquity it is always necessary to extend the fusion distally to the sacrum. In curves due to asymmetric paralysis and without pelvic obliquity the spine should be fused to the lowest neutral vertebra and it is not necessary to

extend the fusion to the sacrum. The extent of the fusion area for any curve does not change whether the patient is operated on anteriorly or posteriorly.

Pre-operative correction

Methods of correcting the spinal deformity may be applied either before surgery or at the time of fusion. It is not possible to apply pre-operative corrective plaster jackets safely to patients with neuromuscular spinal deformities because of the high risk of pressure sores developing beneath the plaster especially if the skin is anaesthetic. The more successful means of correction are applied intraoperatively at the time of spinal fusion. The intraoperative techniques of correction can be applied either to the posterior bony elements or anteriorly to the vertebral bodies.

Halofemoral and halopelvic traction

Pre-operative halofemoral or halopelvic distraction has been recommended for the correction of large fixed curves (Bonnett et al. 1972; O'Brien et al. 1975) but the degree of correction is usually no more than can be obtained by intraoperative means alone (Lonstein & Akbarnia 1983).

There are a number of disadvantages of pre-operative traction. While in traction the patient is immobilized in bed during which time the vertebrae may become more porotic and this makes the application of metallic internal fixation devices to the bone less secure. Halo-traction applied to a patient with a meningomyelocele can be dangerous because the pins in the halo easily perforate the thin bone of a hydrocephalic skull. The presence of the pelvic pins passing through the wings of the ilium in pelvic hoop traction make it difficult to extend the fusion to the sacrum and also to obtain satisfactory bone grafting material from the iliac crest.

An advantage of halofemoral traction is that it can, on occasion, improve a limited vital capacity by reducing the intra-abdominal pressure so allowing the thoracic cavity to expand and making the patient a better operative risk. The traction may also be helpful in controlling an uncooperative patient and facilitating nursing care.

Posterior fusion and Harrington instrumentation

In the 1950s Harrington of Houston devised a technique of posterior spinal instrumentation which he first used to correct the scoliotic curves of patients with poliomyelitis (Harrington 1962). Since this time surgeons have used the technique in all types of neuromuscular spinal deformities with successful results.

Technique of Harrington instrumentation

Harrington instrumentation consists of two parts. A distraction system which jacks the curve out and supports the spine by means of a rigid stainless steel rod applied across the concavity and fixed to the spine by means of a hook at either end. These hooks can be applied to the spine anywhere from the first thoracic vertebra to the sacrum. A second and more flexible rod may be applied around the convexity and gains further correction by means of a system of hooks which apply compression to the spine. A transverse traction rod has also been devised to connect the distraction and compression rods and provides even greater stability. Harrington at first used his technique as a method of correcting the deformity without fusing the spine or applying external support. Unfortunately, the unrestricted movement caused the metallic hooks to cut out of the bone and it became obvious that a posterior spinal fusion with external immobilization was necessary if correction was to be maintained.

In neuromuscular collapsing curves, a long distraction rod is necessary and usually extends from the upper thoracic region to the ala of the sacrum on the high side of the pelvic obliquity. In severe curves a second distraction rod may also be applied in parallel nearer to the apex of the curve and this helps to distribute the distraction force and gains better correction (Fig. 7.2[a] and [b]). The distraction rod must also be prebent in the sagittal plane to correct and accommodate for a thoracic kyphosis and maintain a normal lumbar lordosis. Unfortunately, contouring the rod in the saggital plane significantly decreases the amount of distraction force that can be applied. In order to prevent the contoured rod from rotating out of its sagittal alignment a square ended rod is used and inserted into a lower hook with a square hole. To correct the pelvic obliquity it is necessary to apply a downward force on the high side of the pelvis and a specially adapted lower hook has been designed to fit over the ala of the sacrum. Unfortunately, as the distracting force corrects the scoliosis it may also cause a flattening of the normal lumbar lordosis. This is especially disadvantageous in a patient with hip flexion contractures who can walk independently, because it throws the body forward and makes it difficult to stand and walk without support. A lumbar lordosis may be maintained by bending the distraction rod to conform to the lumbar spine and by applying a compression system to the convexity of the curve before applying distraction. Osteoporotic bone is more easily fractured, and as a result displacement of the hooks is more frequent than in idiopathic scoliosis. In order to prevent displacement of the upper distraction hook, its fixation site may be reinforced with methyl methacrylate cement.

Posterior fusion

The incidence of pseudarthrosis following posterior spinal fusion in neuromuscular spinal deformity is higher than in idiopathic scoliosis. Bonnett *et al.* (1975) in a study of the evolution

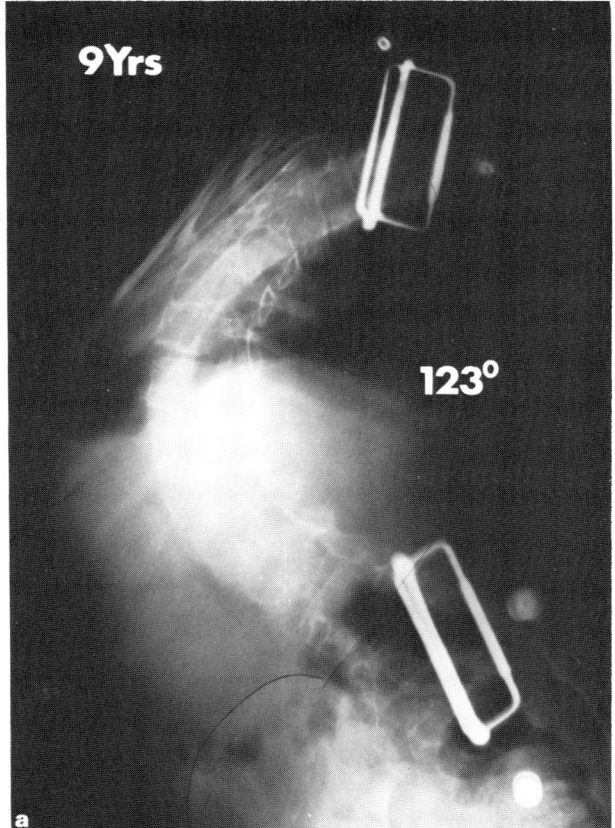
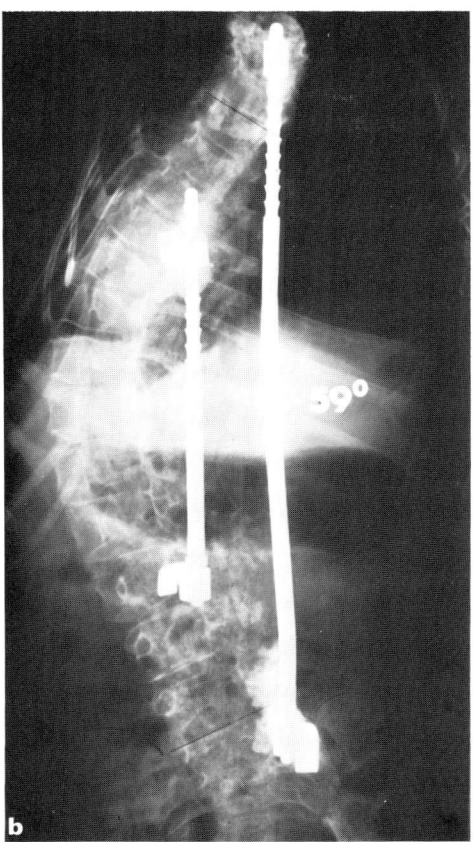

Fig. 7.2. (a) Anteroposterior erect spinal radiograph of a nine-year-old girl with spinal muscular atrophy. She has a collapsing thoracolumbar scoliosis measuring 123° and severe pelvic obliquity.
(b) Using two Harrington distraction rods, the curve has been corrected to 59° and the pelvis levelled.

of their treatment of paralytic scoliosis at Rancho Los Amigos Hospital, found that despite Harrington instrumentation and a careful fusion technique, the incidence of pseudarthrosis was 27%. This compares with a less than 1% incidence of pseudarthrosis in patients with idiopathic scoliosis (Erwin *et al.* 1976). Special care, therefore, is required in fusing the spines of patients with neuromuscular deformities.

If the patient has a myelomeningocele scoliosis, the skin overlying the spine will be scarred and adherent to the dura. Great care is necessary in dissecting the skin from the dura and some surgeons prefer two parallel incisions over the facet joints and strip the tissues laterally leaving intact the scarred and potentially infected tissues overlying the spinal defect (Mayfield 1981). The contents of the spinal canal are not excised. In paralytic scoliosis there is often more bleeding during the surgery because the muscles are weak and fibrotic and do not contract so aiding vasoconstriction. The venous canals in the osteoporotic bone are also larger and bleed more. In addition, the circulating blood volume is smaller in patients with a reduced muscle bulk and as a result they are less tolerant of excessive blood loss.

A very long fusion is usually necessary and there may be insufficient bone graft material from the iliac crests which are frequently hypoplastic and osteoporotic. Bone may be taken from both iliac crests and additional homologous bone may often be necessary. The author has found that deep frozen degenerate femoral heads removed during total hip replacements are a satisfactory source of homologous bone.

The spine is exposed by a meticulous subperiosteal dissection with removal of all remnants of soft tissue from the posterior bony elements. An interfacetal intertransverse fusion (Moe 1972) is performed followed by a deep and thorough decortication of all the posterior bony structures from the midline out to the tips of the transverse processes. This is followed by the application, throughout the fusion area, of large amounts of bone graft material cut into matchsticks. In myelomeningocele patients, the large

lumbar laminar defect and hypoplastic interfacetal joints make posterior fusion difficult and the incidence of pseudarthrosis may be as high as 46% (Osebold *et al.* 1982). In order to minimize this problem large amounts of graft material are laid bilaterally in the paraspinal gutters, on the sides of the defective laminae and on top of the vestigial transverse processes from the lower thoracic region to the sacrum.

Angular kyphotic curves in myelomeningocele patients are very rigid and it is necessary to first osteotomize the spine and resect a number of the vertebral bodies in order to gain correction. This is followed by instrumentation and posterior fusion (Fig. 7.3) from the thoracic region to the sacrum to prevent recurrence (Poitras & Hall 1974, Lindseth & Stelzer 1979).

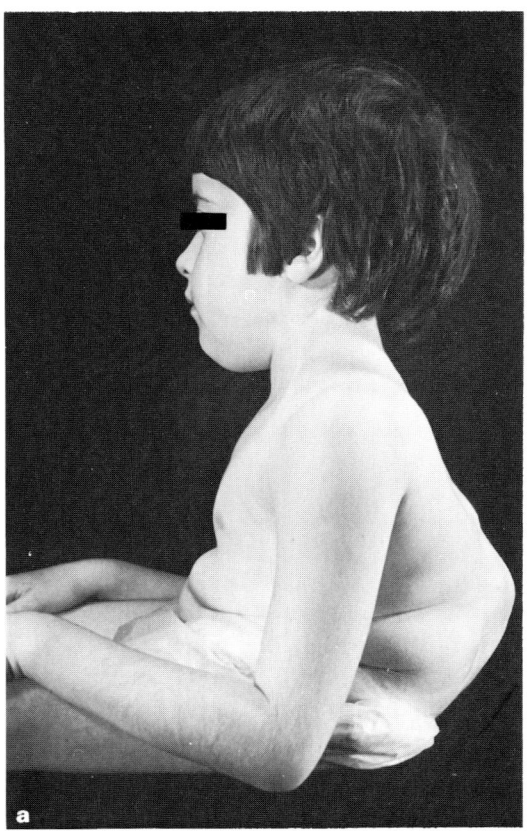 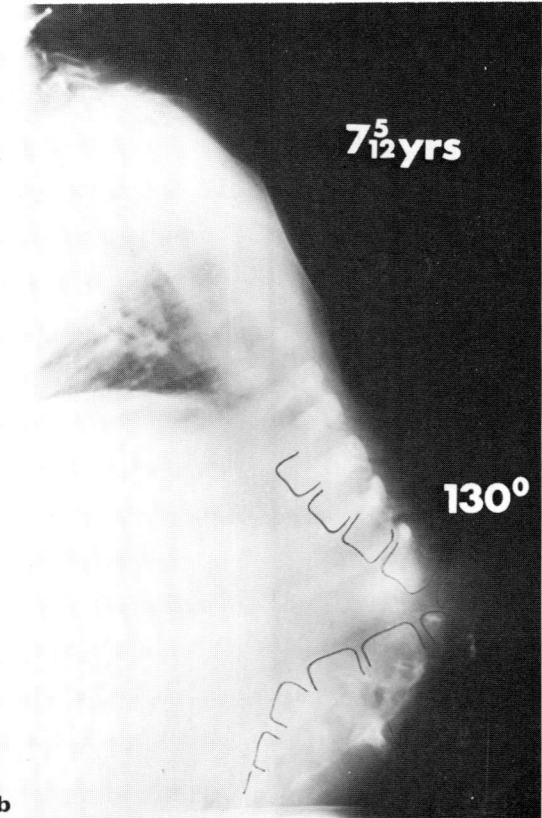

Fig. 7.3. (a) and (b) A seven-year-old girl with a myelomeningocele and a 130° angular kyphus in the lumbar region.

Indications

Most neuromuscular scoliotic curves remain fairly mobile until a late stage and a posterior spinal fusion with Harrington instrumentation is often sufficient providing the posterior elements are intact and there is not a very severe rigid curve extending to the sacrum. In myelomeningocele patients where there is a large laminar defect and insufficient posterior bony structures to fuse satisfactorily, it is usually necessary to supplement the posterior fusion by an anterior fusion with Dwyer instrumentation.

Contraindications

There are no contraindications to the use of Harrington instrumentation but the technique has certain disadvantages. The fixation of the hooks to the bone is not sufficiently secure to do without external immobilization. An underarm plaster jacket or brace is therefore necessary until the spine is solidly fused and this usually requires nine months. A plaster jacket can cause pressure sores if there is a sensory deficit and a removable type of plastic jacket is preferable.

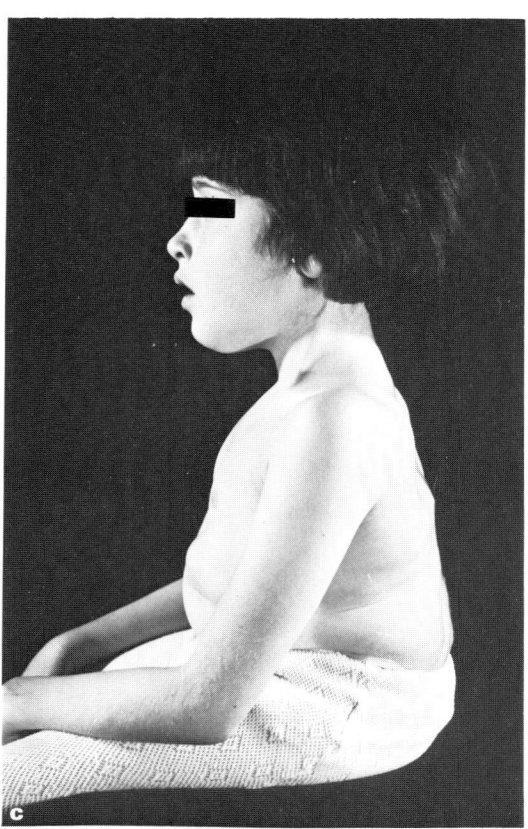
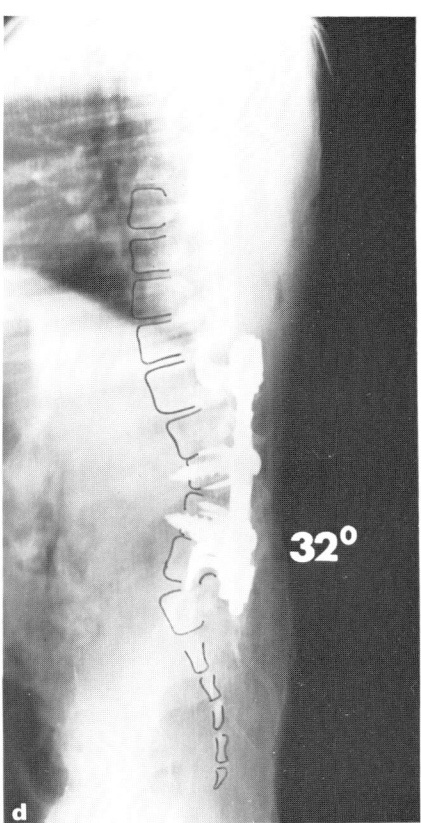

Fig. 7.3. (c) and (d) The deformity has been corrected to 32° by resecting the vertebrae at the apex of the kyphus. A posterior spinal fusion has been performed and correction maintained by a combination of Harrington and Dwyer instrumentation.

Anterior fusion with Dwyer instrumentation

In the late 1960s, Dwyer of Sydney, Australia, devised a completely different technique for spinal correction and internal fixation which was applied anteriorly to the vertebral bodies. Dwyer initially thought his technique was best applied to idiopathic scoliosis (Dwyer 1973), but the method is now mainly used in combination with a posterior fusion and Harrington instrumentation to correct severe neuropathic curves.

Technique

The convex side of the scoliosis is exposed through an extensive trans-thoracic and retroperitoneal approach in which the dia-

phragm is divided circumferentially. The intervertebral discs and vertebral end plates are excised throughout the length of the curve and the spaces packed with bone chips from an excised rib. Starting at one end of the curve, specially designed screw-and-staple units are inserted into each vertebral body and a flexible, braided titanium wire cable is passed through the holes in the heads of the screws. Adjacent vertebrae are compressed and the tension is maintained by crimping the screw heads into the cable. The process is repeated throughout the length of the curve which is gradually straightened (Fig. 7.4[a], [b] and [c]). Zielke et al. (1978) have modified the technique in an attempt to correct vertebral rotation as well as the lateral curvature. They replaced the Dwyer cable with a solid rod passed through the heads of the screws which are placed to derotate the

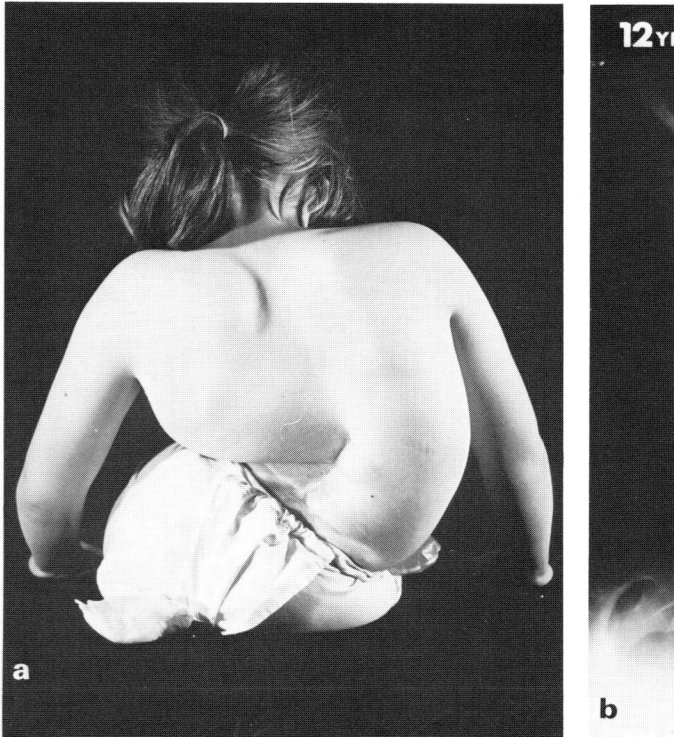 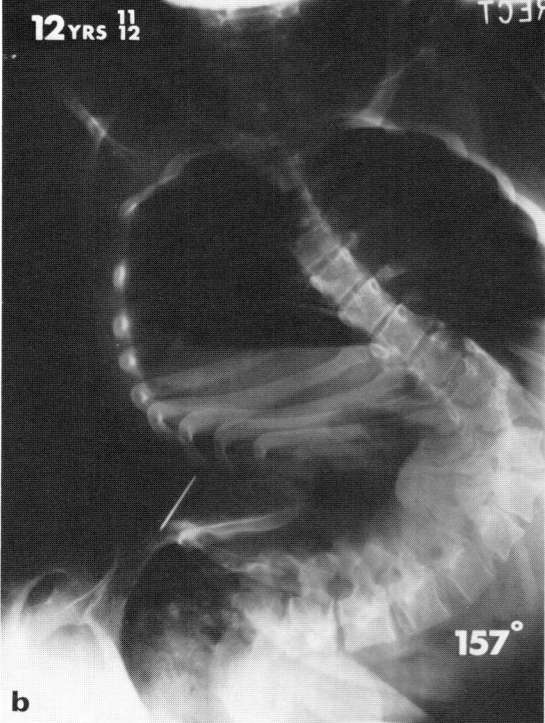

Fig. 7.4. (a) and (b) A twelve-year-old girl with a myelomeningocele and a very severe collapsing thoracolumbar lordoscoliosis measuring 157°. There is severe pelvic obliquity; she sits with all of her weight on one buttock and requires both arms for support.

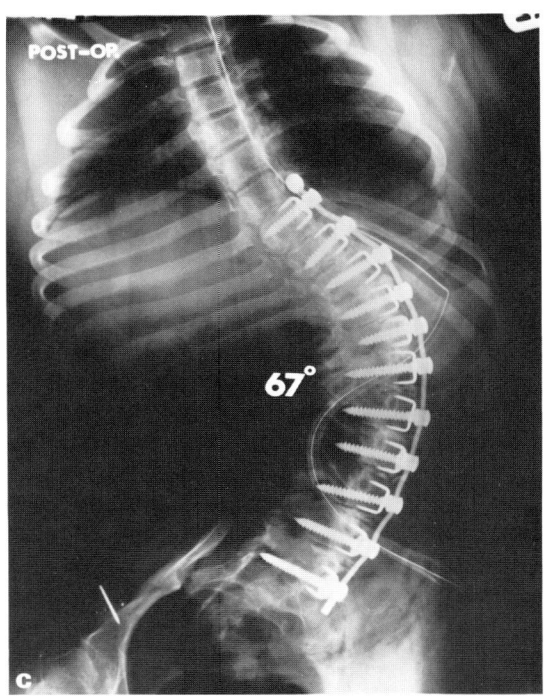

Fig. 7.4. (c) The curve has been corrected to 67° by Dwyer instrumentation and fused anteriorly.

vertebra to the fourth or fifth lumbar vertebra. A second disadvantage is that although the Dwyer technique provides good correction of the scoliosis, the incidence of pseudarthrosis is much higher than with Harrington instrumentation and posterior fusion alone. Bonnett *et al.* (1976) found that in patients with cerebral palsy the incidence of pseudarthrosis with Dwyer instrumentation alone was 72% compared with 40% with Harrington instrumentation alone. For these reasons, anterior instrumentation and fusion is never sufficient and always requires to be supplemented by a second stage posterior fusion with Harrington or Luque instrumentation usually carried out 10–14 days after the anterior surgery (Fig. 7.4[d] and [e]). This provides even greater correction because the spine

vertebral bodies as compression is applied (Moe *et al.* 1983).

Using these methods of anterior instrumentation an excellent degree of correction can be obtained and the segmental fixation is much more secure than with a Harrington distraction rod which grasps only the two end vertebrae. However, like Harrington instrumentation the internal fixation is not sufficiently secure to do without external immobilization until the fusion is solid. The major disadvantage of Dwyer instrumentation is that, for anatomical reasons, the screws cannot be easily inserted above the sixth thoracic vertebra or into the sacrum. Unfortunately neuromuscular collapsing curves are usually very long and, therefore, it is not always possible to correct and fuse the full extent of the deformity through an anterior approach. The typical thoracolumbar lordoscoliosis can only be satisfactorily fused and instrumented anteriorly from the tenth or eleventh thoracic

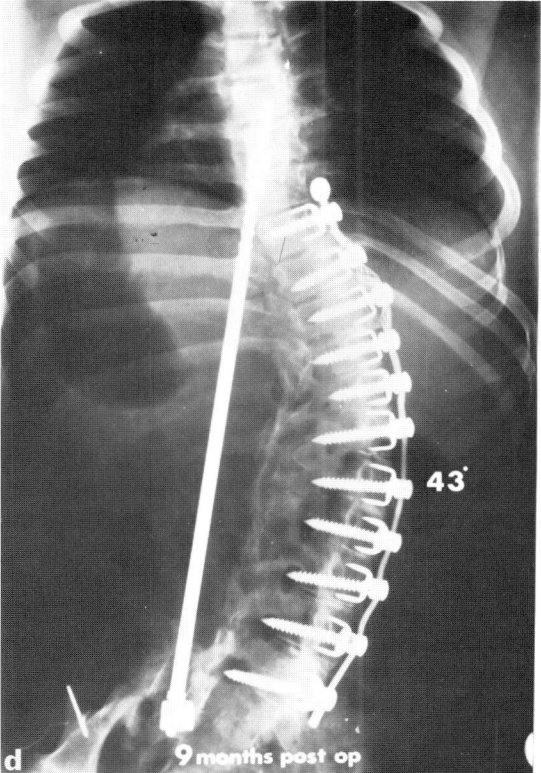

Fig. 7.4. (d) Using Harrington instrumentation, further correction to 43° has been obtained and the spine has been fused posteriorly from the upper thoracic region to the sacrum.

has been released both anteriorly and posteriorly. It also allows extension of the fusion, if necessary, to the upper thoracic region and distally to the sacrum to control the pelvic obliquity which is present in collapsing curves and must be included in the fusion (O'Brien *et al.* 1975).

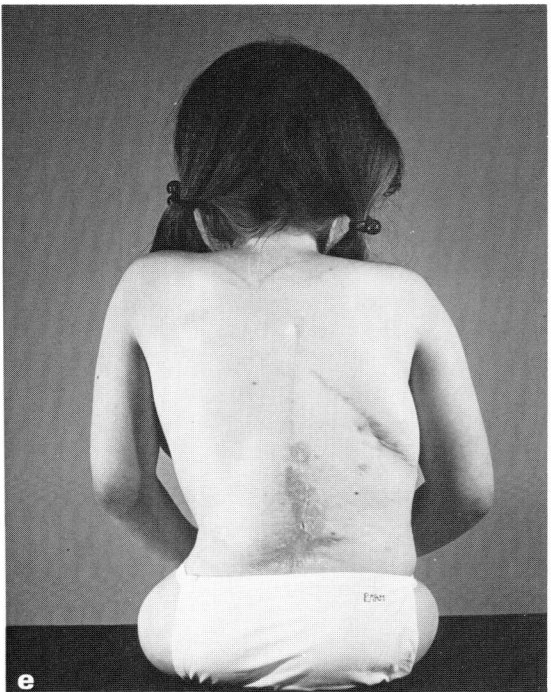

Fig. 7.4. (e) One year after the surgery, the patient has a balanced spine over a level pelvis and can sit without support.

The combination of an anterior spinal fusion with Dwyer instrumentation and a posterior fusion with Harrington instrumentation produces an excellent degree of correction with a very low incidence of pseudarthrosis and a stable spine (McMaster 1986). These results are much better than when Harrington instrumentation is used alone. Leong *et al.* (1981) found that in patients with poliomyelitis the combined procedure usually corrected collapsing thoracolumbar curves by over 60% whereas Harrington instrumentation alone usually achieved less than 40% correction. The incidence of pseudarthrosis was also reduced from 25% with

Harrington instrumentation alone to 12.5% with the combined procedure. Lonstein and Akbarnia (1983) found similar results in patients with cerebral palsy. The degree of correction was improved from 55% with Harrington instrumentation alone to 70% by the combined procedure and the incidence of pseudarthrosis lowered from 22% to 5.9%. Osebold *et al.* (1982) found that in patients with myelomeningocele the degree of correction was improved from 46% to 62% by the combined procedure and the incidence of pseudarthrosis lowered from 46% to 23%.

Indications

The main indication for an anterior spinal fusion with Dwyer instrumentation followed by a posterior spinal fusion and instrumentation is a severe rigid thoracolumbar or lumbar scoliosis with severe pelvic obliquity especially when combined with a lordosis. In these patients it is essential to level the pelvis and this can only be achieved by the combined procedure (O'Brien *et al.* 1975). The second indication is in patients with a myelomeningocele where there is a deficiency of the posterior elements and posterior fusion with Harrington instrumentation alone is likely to fail (Sriram *et al.* 1972).

Contraindications

The presence of a kyphosis is a contraindication to Dwyer instrumentation because the screws in the vertebral bodies lie anterior to the axis of flexion of the spine and when the cable is tightened it causes the kyphosis to increase. In some patients there is a severe rotation of the vertebrae in the scoliotic curve and this gives the appearance of an associated kyphosis (Stagnara *et al.* 1978). Correct placement of the screws during instrumentation will cause derotation of these vertebrae as the scoliosis is corrected with reduction in the rotatory kyphosis (Lonstein & Winter 1982). This type of kyphosing scoliosis is particularly suitable for the Zielke instrumentation.

Anterior fusion is usually contraindicated in patients with Duchenne muscular dystrophy and spinal muscular atrophy because they usually have severely impaired respiratory function, and the transthoracic approach necessitates dividing the diaphragm which is the main respiratory muscle and adds considerably to the operative risks.

It may not be possible to insert the Dwyer screws into the vertebrae of very young children because once the end plates have been removed, there is insufficient bone to hold the screws. In these young children it is possible to perform an anterior release and fusion without Dwyer instrumentation and follow this in the usual way with a second stage posterior spinal fusion with instrumentation.

Segmental spinal instrumentation (Luque technique)

Posterior spinal fusion with Harrington instrumentation when used alone or in combination with anterior fusion and Dwyer instrumentation has been used successfully in the treatment of neuromuscular spinal deformities but has proved to be less than ideal. The main disadvantage of these methods used either singly or in combination is that they do not provide sufficiently secure internal fixation and additional support is necessary in a plaster jacket or brace for at least nine months to allow the fusion to mature and the spine to become stable. This external support may further restrict an already impaired respiratory system and produce pressure sores in patients with anaesthetic skin. The ideal intraoperative method of correction and internal fixation for neuromuscular curves should be easily applied to a wide variety and combination of spinal deformities and provide sufficiently secure internal fixation to maintain correction without external support.

In 1973, Dr Eduardo Luque of Mexico City, began experimenting with wires passed beneath the laminae and around a Harrington distraction rod in an attempt to gain more rigid internal fixation of the spine in young patients with poliomyelitis. In 1975 after many modifications he finally introduced a totally different system of

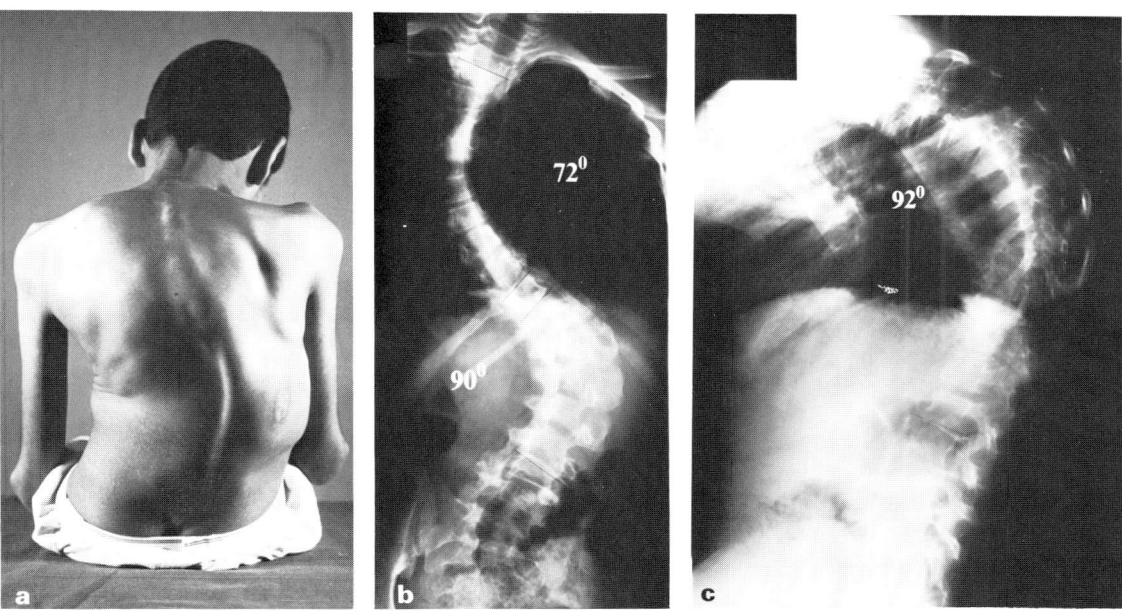

Fig. 7.5. (a), (b) and (c) A twelve-year-old boy with poliomyelitis and a severe collapsing thoracolumbar kyphoscoliosis.

spinal instrumentation in which the correcting forces are applied transversely to the spine at every level throughout the deformity rather than a distraction force across the concavity as in Harrington instrumentation or a compression force around the convexity as in Dwyer or Zielke instrumentation. The Luque method of segmental spine instrumentation also allows the deformity to be corrected in two planes as well as maintaining the normal physiological sagittal curves (Luque & Cardoso 1977, Luque 1982b). Because the technique provides an extremely rigid fixation, it eliminates the need for external support and is particularly applicable to all types of neuromuscular spinal deformities (Fig. 7.5). Initially the technique was used without fusion in an attempt to allow continued growth of the spine but eventually there was a high incidence of instrument failure and the method is now combined with a posterior fusion (Luque 1982a).

Technique

The spinal deformity is corrected and internally fixed by applying two prebent stainless steel rods, one on either side of the laminae, at every level throughout the length of the deformity. The two rods are bent to conform to the desired shape of the spine in both the sagittal and coronal planes as shown on the anteroposterior and lateral radiographs of the spine taken either with traction applied or the spine bent into a corrected position. These rods are attached to the spine at every level by means of wires passed beneath each side of the lamina and around each rod. The rods are bent at one end to an L shape to prevent migration up and down the spine. If pelvic fixation is required the short limb of the L is modified and driven into the transverse bar of the ilium on each side (Allen & Ferguson 1984). The spine is corrected as the contoured rigid rods are pushed into place and the wires are tightened

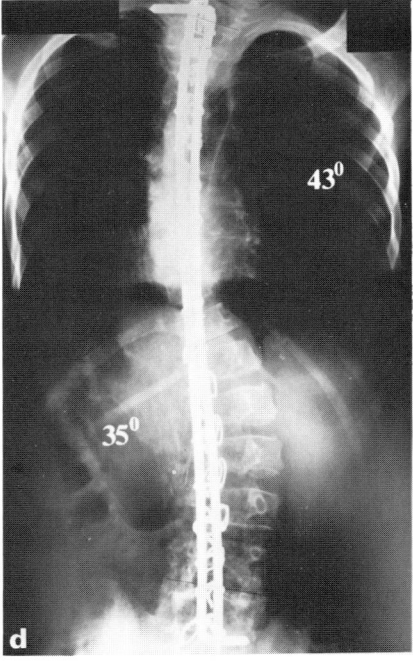
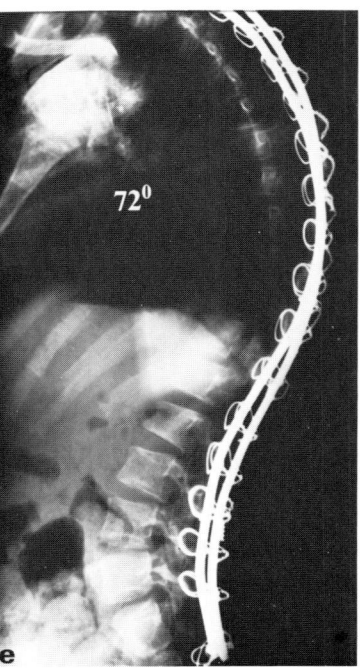

Fig. 7.5. (d) and (e) Using the Luque technique of posterior spinal segmental instrumentation, the spine has been well corrected and balanced over a level pelvis. The posterior spinal fusion extends from the cervicothoracic junction to the sacrum.

at each vertebral level by twisting. In this technique there is no distraction of the spine and correction is obtained in both the sagittal and coronal planes by a system of leverage and pushing and pulling the vertebrae into position. The system is further strengthened by wiring the rods together at several levels. A difficulty in this technique is predicting the amount of correction that can be obtained by prebending the rods. The primary objective is to balance the spine and it is important not to attempt over correction as this could be dangerous. At the end of the procedure the contoured rods should lie firmly against the laminae on either side of the base of the spinous processes. The two sites of attachment at each vertebral level provide an extremely rigid fixation and eliminates the need for external support (Fig. 7.5[f]). There is also the safeguard that if fixation is lost at any level it will not compromise the overall stability of the spine. In myelomeningocele patients there is difficulty in obtaining satisfactory fixation because of the

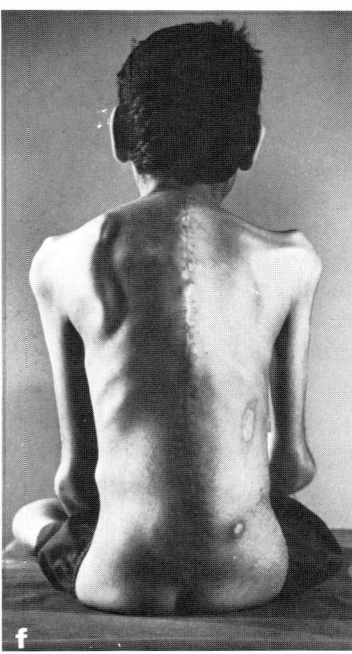

Fig. 7.5. (f) One week after the surgery, the patient is able to sit well balanced and without external immobilization.

laminar defect and the wires are passed around the pedicles and fastened over the rods which lie in the lateral paraspinal gutters.

As with Harrington instrumentation, the success of Luque instrumentation ultimately depends on producing a solid stable posterior fusion extending over all of the instrumented levels. There is no evidence that rigid internal fixation alone will result in fusion of the spine. The technique of posterior fusion used with Luque rods is slightly different to that described earlier with Harrington instrumentation. It is not possible to decorticate the laminae or to carry out a very extensive excision of the facet joints because this could weaken the laminae or allow the wires to cut through. Large amounts of autogenous bone grafts are therefore placed along the gutters lateral to the rods and this provides the best chance for a massive fusion.

Indications

The Luque technique can be applied to all types and combinations of spinal deformities providing they are still relatively flexible as shown on the bending or traction spinal radiographs. However, the technique does not always provide as good a correction of large curves or pelvic obliquity as with Harrington instrumentation (Taddonio 1982). The likely explanation of this is the lack of a distraction force and downward pressure on the high side of the pelvis. However, it has the advantage over Harrington instrumentation in that correction can be more easily obtained in two planes. Postoperatively the patient can be mobilized in a few days and because external support is unnecessary there is no restriction of respiratory function. This is particularly advantageous in patients with spinal muscular atrophy or Duchenne dystrophy who must be mobilized very rapidly after surgery to prevent an increase in their functional disability.

Contraindications

There are no specific contraindications to the use of Luque instrumentation in neuromuscular spinal deformities. However, in large rigid curves with severe pelvic obliquity, it may be necessary to first carry out an anterior spinal release with or without Dwyer instrumentation because Luque instrumentation alone would not gain sufficient correction (Fig. 7.6).

painful dysaesthesia which lasts for a few days. This is thought to be due to the movement of the wires against the nerve roots which occurs while the spine is being fused and before the wires are tightened.

The main disadvantage of the Luque techni-

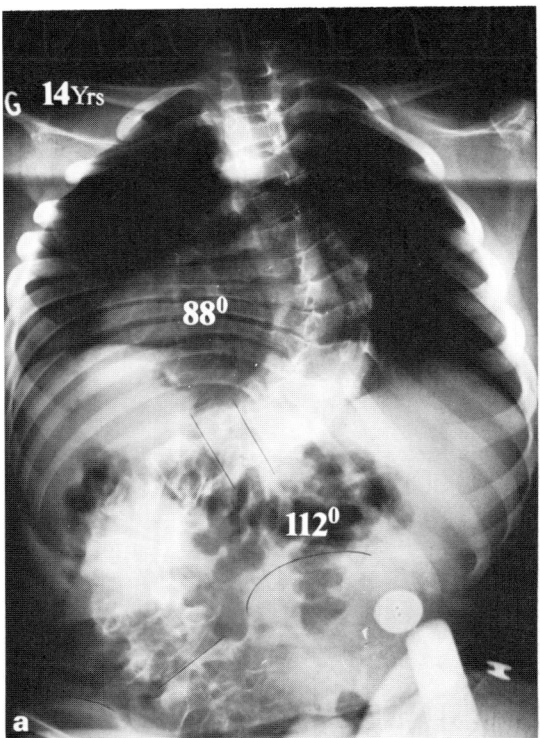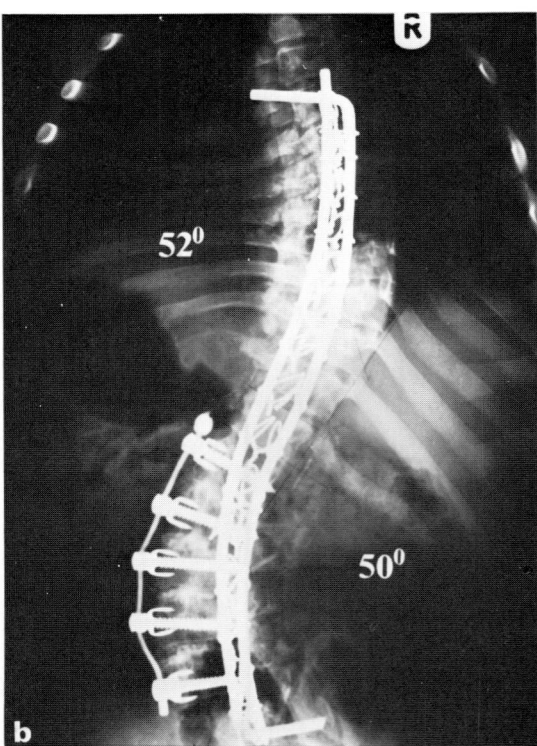

Fig. 7.6. (a) A fourteen-year-old boy with poliomyelitis and a very severe and rigid lumbar scoliosis with pelvic obliquity. (b) Because of the rigidity of the deformity, the lumbar scoliosis was corrected anteriorly by Dwyer instrumentation. Further correction was obtained ten days later using the Luque technique and the spine fused posteriorly from the upper thoracic region to the sacrum.

The Luque technique is a much more difficult and prolonged procedure than Harrington instrumentation and the desire to free the patient from external support must be weighed against the possible dangers of the technique. The main danger is that by passing the wire beneath the laminae the spinal cord could be damaged or an epidural haematoma could occur and press on the spinal cord. The most frequent complication is an isolated nerve root dysfunction producing

que is the large mass of metal that is applied to the posterior bony structures and decreases the area over which bone graft can be applied. This may interfere with the success of the posterior fusion and is particularly disadvantageous in the myelomeningocele patient who already has very little bone posteriorly. Radiographic assessment of the fusion is also difficult because of the overlying metal.

Postoperative management

Immediate care

Immediately after surgery the patient is nursed in a normal bed and log rolled from side to back to side. External support for the spine is unnecessary at this time provided internal fixation has been used. A Stryker turning frame is not used because many of these patients rely on diaphragmatic breathing and this is impaired when they are turned prone. Respiration may be helped by slightly elevating the end of the bed to prevent the abdominal contents from pressing on the diaphragm.

In the early stages, the most important aspects are to maintain respiratory function and to replace the blood loss. Care should be taken not to over transfuse these patients with fluids other than blood because it is possible to precipitate them into cardiorespiratory failure. If the preoperative respiratory function is poor it is possible that the patient will require supported ventilation in the postoperative period. Tracheostomy is rarely, if ever, required and an endotracheal tube with assisted positive pressure ventilation is nearly always sufficient. This is continued for a few days until the postoperative pain is gone and the patient has recovered sufficiently to breathe spontaneously.

Later care

After the immediate postoperative period, the aim should be to return these patients to their pre-operative status either walking or in a wheelchair by ten days. External support is unnecessary if Luque instrumentation has been used. However, if Harrington or Dwyer instrumentation has been used it will be necessary to apply some form of external support. The type of support will depend on the site of the curvature, skin sensation, pulmonary function and the reliability of the patient.

The most suitable form of postoperative external support is a bivalved total contact polypropylene body jacket similar to that worn in the conservative treatment of thoracolumbar and lumbar curves. This jacket is made from a mould of the patient taken after the surgical correction of the spinal deformity. The jacket which is light and comfortable allows regular inspection of the skin and this is particularly important in the myelomeningocele or spinal cord injured patient with impaired sensation. The jacket is only worn while the patient is upright and removed while in bed. A Milwaukee brace is used for upper thoracic curves as these would otherwise require a Risser–Cottrel type of plaster jacket. This type of brace is lighter than a cast and allows satisfactory chest expansion. The main disadvantage of both these types of brace is that they can be easily removed by the unreliable patient.

A plaster jacket of the lighter materials may only be used in the more mobile patients with normal sensation. An underarm jacket is sufficient for thoracolumbar and lumbar curves but a Risser–Cottrel jacket is necessary for higher curves. A plaster jacket should never be applied if there is anaesthetic skin or if it is likely to impair respiratory function. Some patients with weakness of their legs may find that the weight of the plaster makes walking more difficult and this is also a contraindication.

It is not necessary to include the hips in any form of postoperative spinal support as this will interfere with the mobility of the patient. The external support is worn for nine months to a year to allow the spinal fusion to mature and become stable.

Postoperative complications

The incidence of complications following the treatment of neuromuscular spinal deformities are much higher than for any other type of scoliosis. Death may occur in the postoperative period due to either cardiac or respiratory failure but the likelihood of this complication can be significantly reduced by careful pre-operative assessment and postoperative management. The problems of instrument failure and pseudarthrosis following surgery have already been discussed. Infection is always a problem and may affect either the chest or the wound. Failure to cough satisfactorily can result in postoperative atelectasis and bronchopneumonia. Wound infection is most frequent in the myelomeningocele patient with scarred skin and this can be reduced by plastic surgical procedures prior to the spinal fusion, avoiding entering the dura during surgery, and giving prophylactic antibiotics. Using prophylactic antibiotics, Osebold *et al.* (1982) reduced wound infection in myelomeningocele patients from 35 to 17%. Pressure sores can also be reduced by the use of removable jackets and regular inspection of the skin. Pathological fractures of the lower limbs due to osteoporosis can occur after prolonged postoperative bed rest and can be minimized by early mobilization.

Conclusion

We have now entered a new era in the surgical management of neuromuscular spinal deformities. The Luque method of posterior spinal segmental instrumentation promises to overcome many of the problems related to external immobilization and prolonged bed rest but longterm results are not yet available. Although this type of surgery is an arduous and complex task, it can be very rewarding to these severely disabled patients and even a relatively small gain in function can make a major difference to their lives. Many of these patients will spend most of their lives sitting and it is important that they should be able to do so with a balanced stable spine and have independent use of their hands for activities other than supporting themselves. The potential for disaster following surgery for neuromuscular spinal deformities is high, but satisfactory results can be achieved by expert surgical treatment in a specialized centre with adequate back-up facilities.

References

ALLEN B.L. & FERGUSON R.L. (1984) The Galveston technique of pelvic fixation with L-rod instrumentation of the spine. *Spine*, **9**, 388–94.

BONNETT C., PERRY J., BROWN J.C. & GREENBERG B.J. (1972) Halofemoral distraction and posterior spine fusion for paralytic scoliosis. *Journal of Bone and Joint Surgery*, **54A**, 202.

BONNETT C., BROWN J., PERRY J., NICKEL V., WALINSKI T., BROOKS L., HOFFER M., STILES C. & BROOKS R. (1975) Evolution of treatment of paralytic scoliosis at Rancho Los Amigos Hospital. *Journal of Bone and Joint Surgery*, **57A**, 206–15.

BONNETT C., BROWN J.C. & GROW T. (1976) Thoracolumbar scoliosis in cerebral palsy. Results of surgical treatment. *Journal of Bone and Joint Surgery*, **58A**, 328–36.

BUNCH W.H. (1975) The Milwaukee brace in paralytic scoliosis. *Clinical Orthopaedics and Related Research*, **110**, 63–8.

DRENNAN J.C. (1970) The role of muscles in the development of human lumbar kyphosis. *Developmental Medicine and Child Neurology*, **Suppl 22**, 33–8.

DRENNAN J.C., RENSHAW T.S. & CURTIS B.H. (1979) The thoracic suspension orthosis. *Clinical Orthopaedics and Related Research*, **139**, 33–9.

DUVAL-BEAUPERE G., POIFFAUT A., BOUVIER C.L., GARIBOL J.C. & ASSICOT J. (1975) Plexidur jackets for correction of paralytic scoliosis. Results after seven years of use. *Acta Orthopaedica Belgica*, **41**, 652–9.

DWYER A.F. (1973) Experience of anterior correction of scoliosis. *Clinical Orthopaedics and Related Research*, **93**, 191–214.

ERWIN W.D., DICKSON J.H. & HARRINGTON P.R. (1976) The postoperative management of scoliosis patients treated with Harrington instrumentation and fusion. *Journal of Bone and Joint Surgery*, **58A**, 479–82.

HALL J.E. & BOBECHKO W.P. (1973) Advances in the management of spinal deformities in myelodysplasia. *Clinical Neurosurgery*, **20**, 164–73.

HARRINGTON P.R. (1962) Treatment of scoliosis: correction and internal fixation by spine instrumentation. *Journal of Bone and Joint Surgery*, **44A**, 591–610.

HENSINGER R.N. & MACEWEN G.D. (1976) Spinal deformity associated with heritable neurological conditions: spinal muscular atrophy, Friedreich's ataxia, familial dysautonomia and Charcot–Marie–Tooth disease. *Journal of Bone and Joint Surgery*, **58A**, 13–24.

HOPPENFELD S. (1967) Congenital kyphosis in myelomeningocele. *Journal of Bone and Joint Surgery*, **49B**, 276–80.

IRWIN C.E. (1949) Iliotibial band: its role in producing deformity in poliomyelitis. *Journal of Bone and Joint Surgery*, **31A**, 141–6.

KILFOYLE R.M., FOLEY J.J. & NORTON P.L. (1965) Spine and pelvic deformity in childhood and adolescent paraplegia. A study of 104 cases. *Journal of Bone and Joint Surgery*, **47A**, 659–82.

LEONG J.C.Y., WILDING K., MOK C.K., MA A., CHOW S.P. & YAU A.C.M.C. (1981) Surgical treatment of scoliosis following poliomyelitis. A review of 110 cases. *Journal of Bone and Joint Surgery*, **63A**, 726–40.

LINDSETH R.E. & STELZER L. (1979) Vertebral excision for kyphosis in children with myelomeningocele. *Journal of Bone and Joint Surgery*, **61A**, 699–704.

LONSTEIN J.E. & WINTER R.B. (1982) Mechanics of the deformity and treatment in scoliosis, kyphosis and spine fractures. In GHISTA D.N. (ed.) *Osteoarthromechanics*, pp. 385–434. Hemisphere Publishing, Washington.

LONSTEIN J.E. & AKBARNIA B.A. (1983) Operative treatment of spinal deformities in patients with cerebral palsy or mental retardation: an analysis of 107 cases. *Journal of Bone and Joint Surgery*, **65A**, 43–55.

LUQUE E.R. (1982a) Paralytic scoliosis in growing children. *Clinical Orthopaedics and Related Research*, **163**, 202–9.

LUQUE E.R. (1982b) The anatomic basis and development of segmental spinal instrumentation. *Spine*, 7, 256–9.

LUQUE E.R. & CARDOSO A. (1977) Segmental correction of scoliosis with rigid internal fixation. *Orthopaedic Transactions*, 1, 136.

McMASTER M.J. (1986) Anterior and posterior spinal instrumentation and fusion of severe paralytic thorocolumbar scoliosis due to myelomeningocele. *Journal of Bone and Joint Surgery*, in press.

MAKLEY J.T., HERNDON C.H., INKLEY S., DOERSHUK C., MATTHEWS L.W., POST R.H. & LITTELL A.S. (1968) Pulmonary function in paralytic and nonparalytic scoliosis, before and after treatment. A study of 63 cases. *Journal of Bone and Joint Surgery*, **50A**, 1379–90.

MAYFIELD J.K. (1981) Severe spine deformity in myelodysplasia and sacral agenesis: an aggressive surgical approach. *Spine*, 6, 498–509.

MOE J.H. (1972) Methods of correction and surgical techniques in scoliosis. *Orthopedic Clinics of North America*, 3, 17–48.

MOE J.H., PURCELL G.A. & BRADFORD D.S. (1983) Zielke instrumentation (VDS) for the correction of spinal curvature. *Clinical Orthopaedics and Related Research*, **180**, 133–53.

NICKEL V. & PERRY J. (1961) Respiratory evaluation of patients for major surgery. In *American Academy of Orthopedic Surgeons Instructional Course Lectures*, **18**. C.V. Mosby Co., St Louis.

O'BRIEN J.P., DWYER A.P. & HODGSON A.R. (1975) Paralytic pelvic obliquity: its prognosis and management and the development of a technique for full correction of the deformity. *Journal of Bone and Joint Surgery*, **57A**, 626–31.

OSEBOLD W.R., MAYFIELD J.K., WINTER R.B. & MOE J.H. (1982) Surgical treatment of paralytic scoliosis associated with myelomeningocele. *Journal of Bone and Joint Surgery*, **64A**, 841–56.

PIGGOTT H. (1980) The natural history of scoliosis in myelodysplasia. *Journal of Bone and Joint Surgery*, **62B**, 54–8.

POITRAS B. & HALL J.E. (1974) Excision of kyphosis in myelomeningocele. Unpublished paper presented at the Scoliosis Research Society.

SRIRAM K., BOBECHKO W.P. & HALL J.E. (1972) Surgical management of spinal deformities in spina bifida. *Journal of Bone and Joint Surgery*, **54B**, 666–76.

SHARRARD W.J.W. & DRENNAN J.C. (1972) Osteotomy-excision of the spine for lumbar kyphosis in older children with myelomeningoceles. *Journal of Bone and Joint Surgery*, **54B**, 50–60.

STAGNARA P., DE MAUROY J.C., GONON G. & CAMPO-PAYSAA A. (1978) Scoliosis cyphosantes de l'adulte et greffes anterieures. *International Orthopaedics*, 2, 149–65.

TADDONIO R.F. (1982) Segmental spinal instrumentation in the management of neuromuscular spinal deformity. *Spine*, 7, 305–11.

WILKINS K.E. & GIBSON D.A. (1976) The patterns of spinal deformity in Duchenne muscular dystrophy. *Journal of Bone and Joint Surgery*, **58A**, 24–32.

ZIELKE K. (1978) Ventral derotation spondylodesis. The technique, results, indications. Preliminary report. In *Proceedings of the Fifth Meeting of the Scoliosis Research Group of the Yugoslav Association of Orthopaedic Surgery and Traumatology, Zagreb Medicinska Naklada*, 101–15.

Chapter 8
The Orthopaedic Management of Hip Problems

J. D. HSU, E. N. FEIWELL, M. KOFFMAN

Introduction

The growth and development of the hip in a child with neuromuscular diseases can be influenced by many factors. These changes may be predictable according to the nature and severity of the underlying condition. Some of these factors include: muscle tone (either present, absent or increased); positional sense; secondary changes from medication use; underlying congenital and/or developmental anomalies.

The bony abnormalities of the hip joint may include: the delay or failure to achieve full development of the femoral head and acetabulum; failure of coverage of the femoral head; failure of the seating of the femoral head; anteversion or retroversion of the femur; the development of degenerative changes of the hip joint.

Clinically, hip disorders involving incongruity and displacement of the femoral head in children with neuromuscular disease manifest as discomfort and pain. However, when the development of the abnormalities has been slow and longstanding, and when sensory input is disturbed, secondary factors such as difficulty in positioning and seating may become a common complaint.

The hip problems of the three major neuromuscular disorders: cerebral palsy, myelodysplasia and motor unit disease (neuromuscular disease) and their specific problems will be presented and discussed in this chapter.

Cerebral palsy

The clinical problem

All individuals with cerebral palsy have impairment of the voluntary control of some of their skeletal muscles due to nonprogressive encephalopathy acquired at an early age of development. The impaired motor control usually manifests itself peripherally in the form of spasticity, motion disorder, or a mixture of these two (Chapters 1 and 2).

The geographic distribution of this impaired motor control largely describes three separate groups of patients who have predominant spasticity: hemiplegic, diplegic, or total body involvement (TBI) (Chapter 2). One should recognize that there will be a rare patient who does not fit neatly into one or other of these three groups. Generally, all hemiplegic patients should be able to ambulate in the community, all diplegic patients should be either household or community ambulators, and almost all TBI predominantly spastic patients will never be able to progress beyond 'physiologic' ambulation (Chapter 2). Prognostic indicators elicited on physical examination of a young child with cerebral palsy may predict eventual ambulatory capability with considerable accuracy (Paine *et al.* 1964, Chapter 2).

The type of problems to be anticipated for the individual cerebral palsy patient in general, and for his/her hip in particular, bears some relationship to whether that patient has spastic hemiplegia, diplegia or TBI, or has a pure motion disorder. The patient who has a pure motion disorder without spasticity will not develop fixed contractures and will not be at risk for developing subluxation or dislocation of the hip.

The central nervous system disorder in these patients may adversely affect several important functions in addition to control of skeletal muscle. These may have a profound influence on the care of the 'whole person'. Examples are the presence of a seizure disorder or substantial deficits in cognition, communication, and/or one or more of the central nervous system sensory functions (Chapter 1).

The central nervous system functions (other than voluntary motor control) which have most impact upon the management of the hip in cerebral palsy are 'balance' and 'proprioception'. Assessment of balance about the trunk and hip is usually combined clinically. There are no effective means of evaluating proprioception about the hip joint in these patients. The influence that deficits in either of these two central nervous system functions have on the ability of a given individual with cerebral palsy to ambulate effectively is often difficult to estimate clinically.

The painful hip

What about the painful hip in cerebral palsy? Can it be predicted when a hip will become painful? Can it be prevented? Can it be treated? A severe neurologically involved nonverbal patient's pain may be difficult to interpret.

A subluxed or a dislocated hip may or may not be painful. The underlying cause of the pain from these hips is not completely understood. In our study, only one third of a group of cerebral palsy patients with dislocated hips were judged to be experiencing pain from those hips (Hoffer *et al.* 1981). Children rarely complain of a painful hip while it is subluxing or even when it is dislocated. A hip that is completely congruous is not likely to be painful except perhaps due to surrounding tendonitis or bursitis. A located hip that becomes incongruous due to premature degenerative changes may then become painful. The hips of the more severely involved adolescent or adult cerebral palsy patients are those which most frequently, but not exclusively, become painful.

The prospective development of pain in the hip of a patient with cerebral palsy cannot be predicted with any reasonable degree of certainty.

Successful management of the hip that has already become painful may not be possible, even in the hands of the most skilful surgeon. Some of the treatment options will be discussed later in this chapter.

Pathogenesis of deformities

Impairment of the voluntary control of the muscles about the hip when accompanied by spasticity results in 'muscle imbalance'. Grading of the strength or weakness of these muscles by conventional means is not appropriate; voluntary control is the issue. One is interested in determining to what extent an individual has selective control of the muscles about the hip and, therefore, is able to avoid stereotyped patterns of movement. The apparent activity of the individual muscles and muscle groups about the hip may vary with the position of the patient at the time of testing, for example, lying, sitting, or standing, as well as with the mix of reflex and voluntary stimuli acting upon the muscles at that time. The simultaneous activity of the antagonist group of muscles, if present, also influences the attitude that the hip joint will assume at that moment. When one position is favoured to the exclusion of others, contractures eventually develop. Persistent involuntary overactivity of the muscles due to spasticity may therefore result in limitation of motion of the hip joint and perhaps increased pressure between the opposing articular cartilage surfaces. The status of the articular cartilage is of primary importance in defining our treatment options. The position that the hip joint tends to assume in the unoperated spastic patient as a result of these muscle forces most often is one of flexion, adduction, and internal rotation. The exception is the hip that may have an abduction contracture in a TBI patient with 'windswept hips'. As the contractures progress in a skeletally immature patient, subluxation and eventual superolateral dislocation of the hip occurs. All dislocated and subluxed hips in cerebral palsy are acquired unless there is concomitant cogenital dislocation of the hip (which is rare). The more severe neurologically involved patients' hips are at greatest risk of dislocating at the earliest ages (Samilson *et al.* 1972).

A neurologically intact individual with a dislocated hip can still walk, but a cerebral palsied patient cannot. If a hip in a patient with cerebral palsy has not dislocated by the time skeletal maturity is achieved, it will not do so in the future in the absence of trauma or infection.

Another important factor in the genesis of hip subluxation and dislocation in these patients is the persistence of excessive femoral anteversion. This is thought to have some relationship to the continued presence of the newborn flexion contracture about the hip joint as well as to the patient's limited or non weightbearing status (Bleck 1980). Most, but not all, of the excessive valgus of the proximal femur seen on X-ray examination is just apparent and is due to the presence of excessive anteversion. The role that muscle activity plays in the development and in the correction of excessive femoral anteversion has never been proven. There is no good evidence that excessive femoral anteversion will improve solely in response to surgically correcting rotational muscle imbalance (Fig. 8.1).

Patient evaluation

Assessment of motor control

The function of the hip joint is important for sitting as well as for standing and walking. Reliable clinical information about the hip joint is obtained by observing the patient's attempt to perform the highest functional activity (sit, transfer, walk, run, hop) he/she is capable of doing with the least assistance necessary. In this manner, the clinical problem is formulated. The goal of treatment is to maximize function within the limitations imposed by the patient's neurologic deficits. In the authors' attempts to help the patient function better, they sometimes perform operative procedures which they reason ought to make the patient 'look' better. The

authors base this upon the empiric and biomechanical evidence that, within certain ranges of normal variation, the neurologically intact person automatically walks in the most energy-efficient manner available to them. A problem is the authors' limited ability to accurately depict and describe what should be the most energy-efficient manner of walking for the particular patient they are examining. They do not always know when the patient is doing the best he/she can with the neurologic equipment he/she possesses.

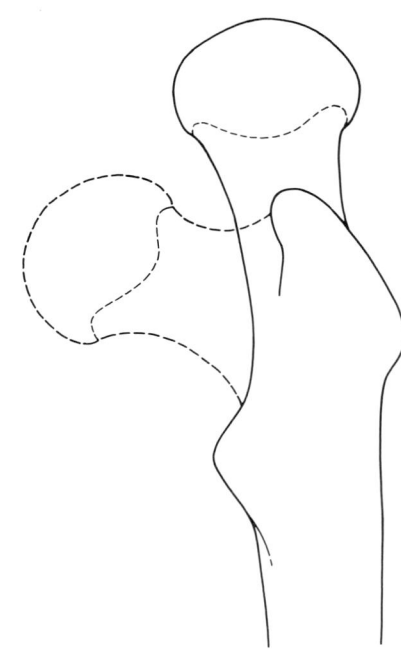

Fig. 8.1. Femoral anteversion–valgus. Both excessive valgus and anteversion of the proximal femur may be present; the anteversion predominates.

The brain lesion limits the selectivity of voluntary muscle control possible for the individual patient and this cannot be changed. The measurement of spasticity is quite inexact. The best assessment of spasticity is made when the patient is in the act of attempting the function under study, for example, standing or walking. A less accurate means is to perform passive stretch tests of muscle groups while the patient is recumbent. The limitations of interpreting the most commonly performed passive stretch tests have been shown (Perry *et al.* 1976).

To assess voluntary control of muscles requires the patient's participation and cooperation with the examination. Is the patient able voluntarily to isolate specific movements about the hip or can they only be made in association with certain other simultaneous movements at the knee and ankle? To deduce what specific muscles in a group are responsible for an abnormal position of the hip during the gait cycle by observation alone clearly has its limitations. The gait electromyogram (EMG) can record the activity of these muscles and may answer the question for us. The activity of the muscles may be 'normal phasic', prolonged, or entirely inappropriate. The gait EMG ordinarily does not tell us what portion of the activity of the muscle is under voluntary control and what portion is reflex ('spastic') in nature unless clonus is observed on the tracing. Likewise, the effective force that a given muscle is expressing during its period of contraction is not shown by the gait EMG.

The presumption is that whatever voluntary control the patient is capable of using can be used to best advantage if involuntary reflex activity and spasticity can be minimized.

Determining the presence or absence of abnormal and retained postural reflexes has its greatest value when one is looking for prognostic indicators in the young child (Chapter 1).

Bony deformity

Clinically, we are interested in having the thigh neither excessively internally nor externally rotated during gait. A number of means are available to measure femoral anteversion. Clinically, the patient can be placed in the prone position with the hip extended and the knee flexed. The thigh is rotated until the greater trochanter lies in the midlateral position. The degree of internal rotation of the hip at this point is taken to represent the angle of anteversion because the femoral neck is assumed to be parallel with the table. The roentgenographic method of determining femoral anteversion we have favoured in the past has been that of Reynolds and Herzer (1959). The neck shaft angle can be measured by placing the patient prone beneath an image intensifier and observing the position of rotation of the thigh at which the femoral neck appears to have its greatest length and taking an anteroposterior X-ray at that position. The true neck shaft angle is best measured on an X-ray taken when the femoral neck is parallel with the X-ray cassette.

The status of location and congruity of the hip is assessed first by observing the patient's functional activity and then by determining the range of motion of the hip. Next, plain X-rays of the hip in as close to neutral position as possible and in maximum abduction are taken. An arthrogram is rarely necessary to evaluate the congruity of the hip and the status of the articular cartilage surfaces. Computerized tomographic scanning of the hip may have a place in evaluating these patients.

Hemiplegia

Hemiplegic patients are all able to walk. Many have an internal rotation attitude of their thigh which may or may not also be associated with an adduction deformity. The patella will face medially during gait in these patients. The most common cause of this internally rotated thigh is excessive femoral anteversion. This is associated with subluxation of the hip in only a small percentage of hemiplegic patients.

A small number of young patients age six years or under may be found to have an internally rotated thigh during gait and may also have an adequate (20–30 degree) range of passive external rotation with the hip at rest and extended. If a gait EMG shows the semitendinosus to be continuously active only during the end of swing phase and early stance phase, as in a patient without neurologic involvement, transfer of this muscle-tendon unit laterally may be indicated.

Derotation osteotomy is indicated for excessive femoral anteversion which is responsible for an inefficient internally rotated gait. If there is an associated increase in the neck shaft angle of the proximal femur and/or subluxation of the hip, the osteotomy should be performed proximally. If neither of these two conditions exists, the derotation osteotomy may be performed in the supracondylar region (Hoffer *et al.* 1981). It is important to look for other rotational abnormalities of the limb which may be present below the knee. Additional surgery may be required to prevent the foot pointing in the direction of extreme external rotation following the femoral osteotomy.

A subluxing hemiplegic hip requires adductor release and a proximal femoral osteotomy with or without an iliopsoas lengthening.

Diplegia

These patients become household or community ambulators (Chapter 2). Many, but not all, use canes or crutches.

Their walking is delayed. Their hips are adducted, and frequently internally rotated and flexed. A 'hip action brace' which allows free abduction but which can be adjusted to block or stop any degree of adduction desired can be a useful training device to be worn while the patient is learning to walk. Unless a hip can be shown to be subluxing, surgery should not be performed while a young patient's ability to ambulate is improving functionally regardless of the 'appearance' of his gait. If the individual has reached a plateau, and the surgeon is convinced that the hip deformities are responsible for the patient's inability to walk more efficiently, then an analysis of what might reasonably be done surgically to improve ambulation is in order. Observational analysis with a sound knowledge of anatomy has traditionally formed the basis for decision-making. From observation of the position of the hip as well as of the pelvis and spine

above and the knee and ankle below, the inappropriate overactivity of certain groups of muscles is deduced. With respect to excessive adduction of the hip, this method is still helpful. Although the passive (static) muscle stretch tests have been shown to have limited specificity for a single muscle, if the passive abduction range of a hip is limited to less than 20 degrees when tested with the hips and knees each flexed 90 degrees, release of the pelvic origins of the adductor longus and gracilis and a portion of the adductor brevis without neurectomy of the anterior branch of the obturator nerve, may allow the diplegic child to progress further in his attempts to walk. Under these circumstances, the risk of adversely affecting gait by diminishing pelvic control due to excessive weakening of the adductors is negligible (Fig. 8.2).

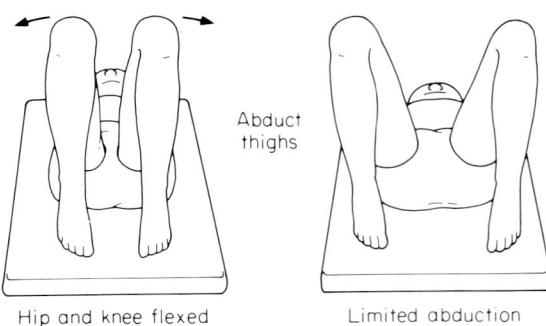

Fig. 8.2. True 'adductor' test. This is one of the most reliable of the passive stretch tests.

If the attitude at the hips during gait is a combination of excessive flexion, adduction and internal rotation in a child under six years of age, the surgical procedure on the adductors described above should probably be combined with an iliopsoas recession. When the diplegic child aged six years or older is 'scissoring' during gait with the hips in a position of adduction and internal rotation due to limited hip abduction and excessive femoral anteversion, femoral osteotomies may be performed at the time of the adductor and iliopsoas surgery.

Thus, a thoughtful approach to the young diplegic patient's hip problems will, of necessity, need to be based on a knowledge of the muscle overactivity and the bony abnormality usually responsible for a particular disabling deformity and whose correction carries with it the least risk of doing harm when one is treating these patients in a locale where gait analysis studies are not yet available.

Gait analysis with dynamic electromyography

Dynamic electromyography may help identify more precisely the particular muscle responsible for the unwanted and inefficient movement of the hip during gait. Improved predictability of the outcome of surgery is to be expected by combining the information from the dynamic EMG with that from observation alone. The dynamic EMG may help answer such questions as: is the iliopsoas or the medial hamstring contributing most to the internally rotated gait; is the iliopsoas or the rectus femoris contributing most to the hip flexion deformity; is there a great deal of overactivity of the quadriceps muscle group which could result in hyperextension at the knee if overzealous lengthening of the hamstrings is performed? A muscle whose activity on gait electromyography is 'normal phasic' is not primarily responsible for the patient's deformity. The decision whether or not to operate is determined by clinical criteria. The gait EMG may aid in deciding which operation is best for a particular patient. The information from the gait EMG complements, but in no way replaces, the need for thoughtful clinical observation. Gait analysis is becoming more computerized and electronically sophisticated. The positions of body segments relative to each other can be recorded and graphically displayed and correlated with a specific phase of the gait cycle within a brief period of time. Velocity, cadence and stride length can be rapidly calculated. Oxygen consumption studies can be used to analyze the energy efficiency of a patient's walking. These additional gait studies have expanded our understanding of the cerebral palsy patient's difficulties while walking (Sutherland 1978), and

may also contribute to improved management in the future.

Tendon transfers

Tendon transfers about the hip are rarely indicated in cerebral palsy in the authors' experience (they do not consider the iliopsoas recession as a 'transfer').

The so-called adductor posterior transfer may have a place in the diplegic patient who is independently mobile and who is not in need of additional surgery about the hip joint (Root & Spero 1981). We have no experience with iliopsoas transfer to the greater trochanter in patients with cerebral palsy.

Subluxation

The diplegic patient's hip may sublux superiorly and laterally due to the abnormal muscle forces imposed upon it by the spastic adductor group and perhaps by the iliopsoas as well. In the very earliest stages of subluxation, soft tissue surgery alone may correct the problem, but once any progression has occurred surgery must include proximal femoral osteotomy to be effective. The addition of an innominate osteotomy should not be necessary in the diplegic patient unless the subluxation has been of longstanding and is advanced. On occasion, an adolescent diplegic patient with a subluxing hip may require a Chiari osteotomy at the time of the soft tissue release and femoral osteotomy or as a second-stage procedure (Fig. 8.3). The progression to dislocation should be a rare event in a diplegic patient. This will result in loss of the patient's functional ambulation and treatment will be determined by the status of the articular cartilage.

Total body involvement

The total body involved (TBI) spastic cerebral

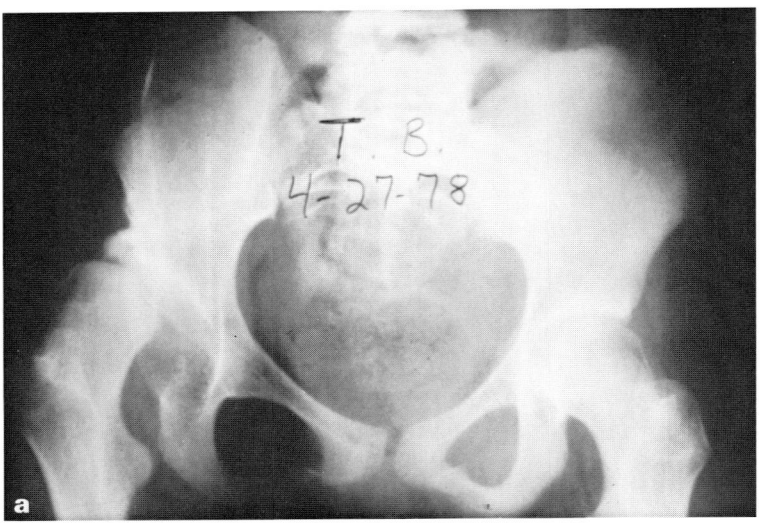

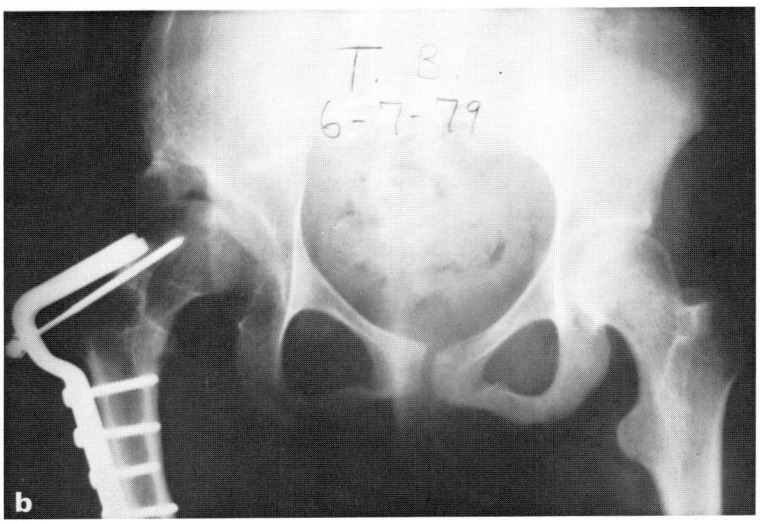

Fig. 8.3. (a) X-ray of an adolescent cerebral palsy patient with a painful subluxing right hip.
(b) X-rays after adductor release, proximal femoral osteotomy and Chiari osteotomy.

palsy patient is not a functional ambulator. Some of these patients may be able to walk a short distance in parallel bars or with a walker during a 'therapy' session or at home when someone is there to supervise them. Most of these patients are only able to transfer, to sit or to be propped up. A few will only be able to lie down due to the severity of their deformities. The TBI spastic cerebral palsy patient has a significantly greater risk of subluxation or dislocation of the hip than the hemiplegic or dip-

legic patient. Scoliosis and pelvic obliquity in the TBI patient potentiate the development of dislocation of the hip when they are present (Fig. 8.4).

The total body involved patient can be identified at an early age (Chapter 2). A poor prognosis of ambulation is not an excuse for inaction while a hip is subluxing. There are no satisfactory nonoperative means of preventing these hips from progressively subluxing and subsequently dislocating once this process is under-

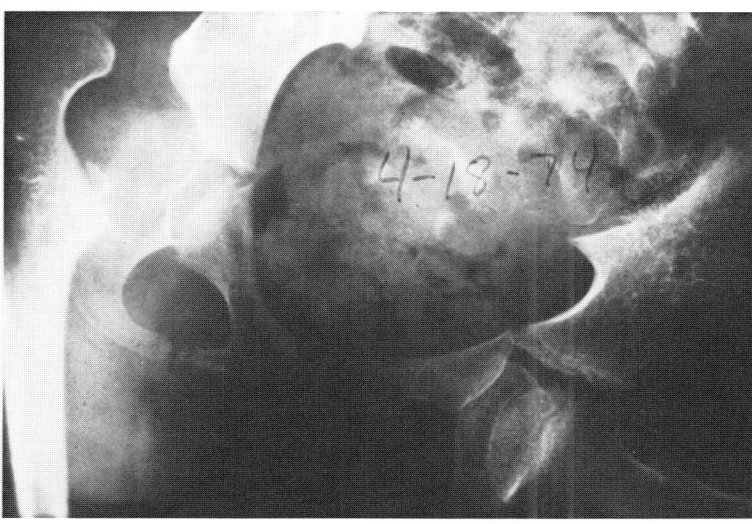

Fig. 8.4. Pelvic obliquity associated with a dislocated hip.

way. Surgical management should be aggressive, providing the anaesthetic risks are acceptable, as long as there is a possibility of restoring a congruous hip. For the majority of these patients, this means up to the age of 12 years. Release of the adductors alone is almost never enough. Iliopsoas and proximal hamstring lengthenings are frequently needed. There is no set age at which skeletal surgery should be added to the soft tissue releases for this problem; rather each patient must be treated as an individual. For example, a hip in a 4-year-old severely involved spastic TBI patient that is rapidly progressing toward dislocation should be treated with derotation-varus osteotomy of the proximal femur with or without skeletal shortening at the time of soft tissue release. The concept of performing an operation at one point in time on these hips which will take care of the problem forever should be laid aside. Some of these hips will require soft tissue releases at an early age only to have to be repeated again with bony surgery a few years later. Our goal is a mobile congruous hip because such a hip will allow the patient to sit or be propped and is less likely to become painful.

The results of intrapelvic obturator neurectomy are too unpredictable. This procedure is clearly ineffective in patients who already have fixed adduction contractures. In those who have overwhelming spasticity of the adductors without fixed contracture, there is the risk of abduction deformities occurring postoperatively; these are difficult to deal with.

The gait EMG has no place in the evaluation of a functionally nonambulatory patient.

The additional benefit of tendon transfer rather than simple release or lengthening in the management of the hip in the TBI patient has never been demonstrated.

Some of these patients will develop an extension attitude at their hips and/or their knees extreme enough to make sitting or propping impossible. Perhaps a prior iliopsoas lengthening has added to the development of this problem. In such a case, proximal hamstring release from the ischium and quadriceps tendon release at the knee may be necessary to gain hip and knee flexion (Bowen *et al.* 1981).

As the TBI spastic cerebral palsy patient approaches skeletal maturity, the risk of the hip subsequently dislocating diminishes, but the possibility of developing changes in the articular cartilage and pain increase. It is in the treatment of these patients that judgment is most difficult because usually we cannot predict which hips will become painful. Some pre-adolescent patients have hips which are dislocating or have dislocated with minimal or no apparent articular cartilage changes. Soft tissue releases, proximal femoral osteotomy with skeletal shortening, and an appropriate pelvic osteotomy may all be warranted in such a patient, particularly if the patient possesses relatively intact cognition and communication. A hip with advanced articular cartilage changes may be painful whether it is located, subluxed, or dislocated (Fig. 8.5). Once the hip becomes so painful as to preclude sitting or propping, the treatment options are very limited. The effects of proximal femoral resection are extremely unpredictable and result in

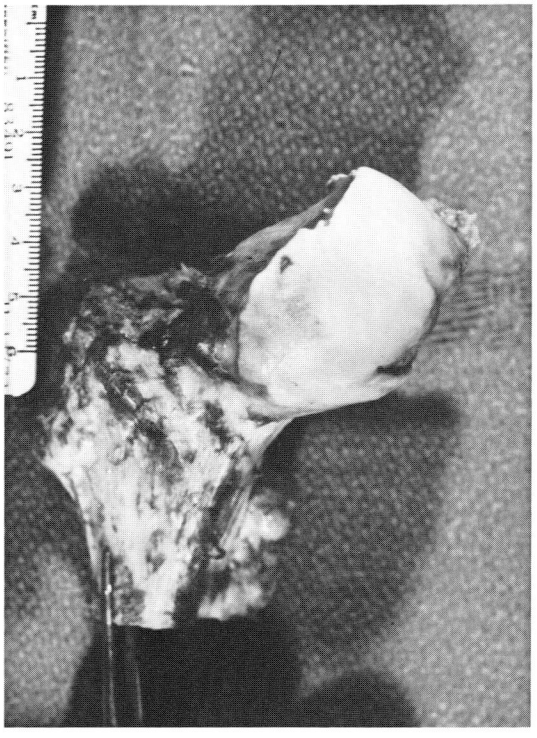

Fig. 8.5. The damage to the articular cartilage on the femoral head of this hip in an adolescent patient can be seen.

only a small percentage of operated hips that will allow sitting or propping for eight hours a day without some obvious pain. Total hip replacement has been unsuccessful for the authors in this group of nonambulatory patients. Hip fusion in a position of flexion and only slight abduction has been reported with some success;

we have no direct experience with this method of treatment. The painful hip remains largely an unsolved problem to date in the total body involved adolescent and adult cerebral palsy patient. Therefore, maintaining a congruous hip at a younger age should be a high priority.

As mentioned previously, some of these patients will have scoliosis with pelvic obliquity which complicates the treatment of the hip at risk. Orthoses have a very limited effect in slowing or halting the progression of these curves. Posterior spinal fusion to the sacrum with Harrington or Luque rods are necessary if one wishes to control the pelvic obliquity. The addition of anterior thoracolumbar fusion with the Dwyer of Zielke apparatus is an aid in improving the correction and in reducing the pseudarthrosis rate in some patients (Chapter 7).

Summary

The approach to the treatment of the hip in the cerebral palsy patient begins with an understanding of the types of problems likely to be encountered in each of the major subgroups; that is, spastic hemiplegic, diplegic, and total body involved patients; those with a pure motion disorder; and those patients who have some combination of spasticity and motion disorder.

There are occasions when patients with grossly similar hip deformities may be best treated by somewhat different operative procedures or no surgery at all. Obviously, the mere existence of a deformity about the hip is not, of itself, an indication for surgical correction of that deformity without regard to the type of cerebral palsy, the patient's age, and the patient's functional abilities, expectations and needs. Judgment requires at least as much of our attention as does technique.

For any given ambulatory cerebral palsy patient we cannot yet predict what should be the optimum and most efficient appearance of the gait. Refinements in gait analysis techniques probably offer the best hope of achieving this aim in the future.

The painful hip, particularly in the nonambulatory cerebral palsy patient, is still a largely unsolved problem. Prevention is the best approach.

It appears that the criteria for successful management are improving, and by being able to set realistic functional goals for these patients at an early age, resources are utilized more efficiently.

Myelodysplasia

General considerations

Problems related to the hip and myelomeningocele are primarily related to contractures and hip instability, the latter leading to adduction and flexion contractures. Treatment should be directed towards definite functional goals as compared to X-ray improvement. Hip reduction in the past has not been equated with ambulatory achievement (Barden *et al.* 1975, Feiwell *et al.* 1978). This includes ambulation, gait and bracing. The extended position of the hips would appear to be the most suitable goal for the ambulatory patient (Menelaus 1976) as it improves erect stability and decreases the energy expenditure.

Stillwell and Menelaus (1983) in their study of adult patients noted that hip flexion deformity, pelvic obliquity and scoliosis together precluded ambulation. Upper level patients who ambulate with knee–ankle–foot orthoses (KAFO) and crutches require flexion/extension ability and reduction is not important. Ascher and Olson (1983) believed that patients with L3 level lesions are more likely to ambulate with reduced hips than with unreduced hips. Above that level of neurologic deficit dislocation is not a factor. With lesions below the L3 level, the patients' capability of walking was less effected by one factor. Hip contractures were considered significant, but knee and ankle and spine deformities were much more significant in limiting ambulation. Prognosis for ambulatory ability and type of ambulation is a determining factor for the method of treatment of a hip deformity.

Ambulatory ability is primarily dependent on the level of neurologic lesion (Hoffer *et al.* 1973). Thoracic level patients rarely ambulate by the time they are teenagers or young adults; upper lumbar patients may ambulate in a small percentage of cases. These patients have voluntary hip flexion, and/or hip adduction and/or knee extension with sufficient power to move the joints (Table 8.1). The upper lumbar group includes neurologic levels from approximately L1 to just above the L4 level (some weakness of quadriceps is present). Patients with lesions between L3 and L4 have the greatest incidence of dislocated hips. The adductors are strong and the abductors are absent. The gross adductor–abductor imbalance encourages hip dislocation.

Table 8.1

Anatomic level	Functional level	Major lower extremity function
L1 L2 L3 L4	High lumbar	Hip flexors Hip adductors Knee extensors
L4 L5 S1	Low lumbar	Knee flexors Ankle dorsiflexors Hip abductor
S1 S2 S3	Sacral	Ankle plantarflexors Gluteus maximus

The lower lumbar patient has musculature which voluntarily flexes the knee and/or extends the ankle and/or abducts the hip. Patients who are approximately L4 level to the S1 level, have quadriceps that are almost completely innervated, their hip abductors have some function and the knee flexors bring further stability to the knee, as well as hip extension (Healey & Breed 1982).

Sacral level patients have plantar flexion of the ankle and toes and/or gluteus maximus function and their hamstrings should provide hip extension, as well as further knee stabilization. Good proprioception is present all the way down to the foot.

Other factors affect ambulation; in particular spasticity grossly changes the ambulatory potential (Hoffer *et al.* 1973, Mazur *et al.* 1986).

Ambulation in early childhood may be beneficial to the child's development and bring pride and satisfaction to the parents. If release of contractures at an early age allows appropriate bracing and ambulation then surgery should be performed. Menelaus (1976) advised that releases be performed between the ages of 7 and 18 months, depending on the child's stability and health. Repeat surgical releases in the older child or adult for short term goals of standing and walking in individuals unlikely to ambulate is not recommended. Wheelchair training is recommended for the older child with recurrent contractures and deformities and poor ambulatory potential. Major surgical procedures, prolonged therapy sessions and major bracing tend to inhibit development towards an independent individual. Individuals without voluntary knee control must wear KAFOs or higher bracing with pelvic control. It is these individuals whose energy costs become so great that continued ambulation at adulthood becomes impractical (Williams *et al.* 1983).

Hip flexion contractures

The normal newborn child has hip flexion contractures, that may be as great as 90° (Hoffer 1980). These rapidly stretch out, but are still present up to 30–40° prior to the time of ambulation. Following ambulation the hip flexion contractures reduce to 20°, and eventually to less than 0°. The child who has not had the opportunity to obtain the upright position will continue to have a hip flexion contracture. On this basis the individual who does not maintain an extended position of the hip is not expected to be able to avoid recurrent flexion contractures, even if multiple releases are performed. Either standing or ambulation in the extended position must follow hip release, and frequent or sustained periods of prone lying or bracing in the extended position must be continued through-

out childhood if hip flexion contractures are to be prevented. For the wheelchair patient, this is not as important, but it would be well to avoid hip flexion contractures of above 50° (into adulthood) which prohibit assumption of the prone position or as indicated in some adult males, an inconvenience with sexual contact.

In children with flexion contractures of under 40° soft tissue releases can be carried out anteriorly. The anterior hip release as described by Menelaus (1976, 1980) is carried out through an anterolateral approach as described by Salter (1961). The iliac apophysis is split, and the sartorius, rectus femoris and tensor fascia lata are released. The iliopsoas and even the anterior hip capsule may be sectioned as well. The iliotibial band should also be cut if tight. The prominence of the anterior superior spine area is removed. Suction drainage is utilized postoperatively. Menelaus (1976, 1980) maintained the patient in traction on a Bradford frame for six weeks postoperatively. The key to this procedure is to maintain hip extension by stretching and extended hip positioning. Scarring, which occurs with releases, will frequently produce significant recurrent hip flexion contracture that is even more difficult to treat if the extended position is not maintained.

In the older child, with hip flexion contracture of greater than 40°, extension osteotomy is necessary. Under the age of 10, additional bone deformation often occurs. The hip deformity may recur, particularly if the factors that originally caused the hip flexion contracture remain. These factors include persistence of the attachment of the iliopsoas; persistence of the other hip flexors in a patient who primarily sits and did not have hip stretching. Function is likely to deteriorate in a patient between the ages of 6 and 10 years who is a poor ambulator, with eventual inability to walk. If this is the case, extensive releases and osteotomies should not be performed. However, extension procedures would be reasonable in an older individual who is a community ambulator but has difficulties due to a marked hip flexion contracture.

Extension osteotomy is performed by removing a posterior based wedge from the sub-trochanteric region. If a lateral incision is curved anteriorly, in the manner of Watson-Jones, the anterior capsule can be freed of the iliopsoas and the tendon released at the osteotomy site. If the patient has a reducible hip, stability may be obtained by bringing the muscle laterally through a notch cut between the superior and inferior spines (Mustard 1952) and attached to the superior aspect of the greater trochanter. The osteotomy is maintained by heavy threaded Steinmann pins passed from the lateral cortex of the femur into the femoral neck and head. These pins may be left long and easily removed at a later date. The authors have avoided nail plate fixation because of the weak and small bone. The fixation has frequently loosened when the patients were left out of protective plaster post-operatively. Their preference is to pin the osteotomy and place the patient in a bilateral hip spica, allowing early weightbearing by standing the patient. If the bone is large enough and stout enough, and postoperative mobilization is anti-cipated, then more extensive internal fixation can be used.

Prior to the performance of an osteotomy, the patient must be able to flex the hip at least 30° beyond 90°. If the patient has limited hip flexion to 90° pre-operatively and an extension osteotomy of 30° is carried out, this will seri-ously inhibit sitting ability.

Adduction contractures

Muscle imbalance about the hip is greatest in patients with mid lumbar level lesions. In this group, hip adductor and flexor muscles are strong whereas abductor and extensor muscle function is absent. Patients with progressive subluxation develop further adduction con-tractures. Other sources of contracture are related to spasticity of the adductor muscles either due to abnormalities within the central nervous system from the beginning or abnormalities that subsequently develop due to cord tethering, hydromyelia or progressive hydrocephalus.

Adductor releases may be carried out at any age and as a part of other procedures. We recommend that the incision be transverse sev-eral fingerbreadths below the groin crease and centered over the adductor longus tendon. The adductor longus and brevis, gracilis and anterior portion of the magnus may be sectioned. The iliopsoas can be reached after the muscles have been divided and a one inch section removed. If transfer of the iliopsoas is anticipated then it may be cut from its insertion and dissected upward, tagged and left anteriorly for a subsequent anterolateral approach. The adductor muscles may be left after being transected as described and the patient then splinted in an abducted position or the adductor muscles may be sutured down to the posterior portion of the magnus at the ischial tuberosity. When this is performed a number 1 braided nylon is placed through the gracilis and anterior portion of the magnus and a second suture through the adductus longus and brevis. The magnus and gracilis are first sutured as far lateral and inferior as can be reached; then the adductor longus and brevis are sewn immediately adjacent to that. When posterior transfer is anticipated the skin incision can be placed slightly more posteriorly which facilitates transfer. If these muscles have all been removed adjacent to the bone, the obturator nerve and vessels which exit and split around the brevis are avoided. They do not have to be isolated during the dissection. The advantage of the adductor posterior transfer (Nickel et al. 1966) is that the adductors are permanently placed in a position in which they can still function to adduct the hip from abduction to neutral pos-ition, and may provide some extension power from the flexed position. This will result only if the femoral head is reduced in the acetabulum. The muscles have been lengthened as they have been passed from the more anterior superior position to the inferior posterior position (Figs. 8.6 and 8.7).

Thirty-two procedures were evaluated pre- and postoperatively in poliomyelitis and spina bifida patients. Adduction was successfully limited from the neutral position. No extension

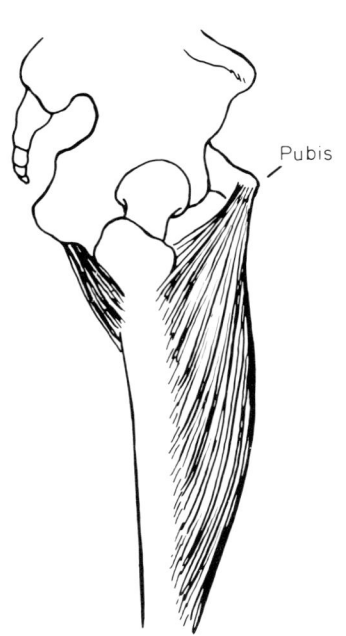

Pubis

Ischium

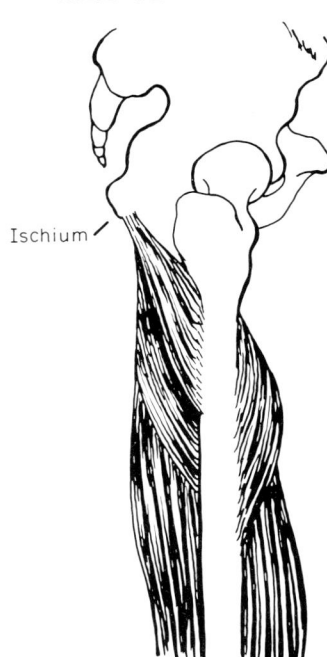

Fig. 8.6. Adductor posterior transfer. The adductors are removed from the adductor tubercle and the ischiopubic ramus, and attached posteriorly to the ischium. This includes the adductor longus, brevis, gracilis and anterior half of the adductor magnus. The muscles will lie posterior to the fulcrum of the hip joint.

power was obtained from 0° of extension. Some extensor function may have been present when the hip was in the flexed position. EMG studies (Griffin *et al.* 1977) have demonstrated function through stance phase providing some stabilizing function despite effectively reducing adductor power. The primary advantage is that the adductors have been permanently placed away from their origin and will not reattach as frequently happens during growth when simple sectioning is performed. London and Nichols (1975) advocated this procedure since they found that patients who had the most satisfactory hip reductions were those who had had adductor posterior transfer in conjunction with abduction transfers.

Older patients who have fixed adduction deformities that are not relieved by soft tissue release can be corrected by valgus osteotomies in the subtrochanteric region.

Abduction contractures

Bilateral abduction contractures are uncommon.

Frequently they are unilateral with the contralateral hip being adducted. The adducted hip will dislocate if no abductor power is present. This windswept deformity is difficult to treat. The resultant pelvic obliquity makes reduction of the adducted hip an impossibility as long as the other hip remains in the abducted position. Every time the patient's legs are placed together such as in sitting or lying, the pelvis is tilted and the contralateral hip adducted. The cause of this deformity is usually a contracted iliotibial band. Scarring in and about the joint may be another cause and is usually the result of prior surgical treatment. The Ober test will demonstrate the presence of an iliotibial band contracture. The patient is placed laterally on the opposite side, the hip is flexed and abducted with support placed under the distal femur. In that position the hip is then extended and while holding the ankle the knee is flexed and the distal femur support is released. In the hip extended position the extremity will remain abducted if the iliotibial band is tight.

Releases are carried out distally and proximally. The proximal release is performed

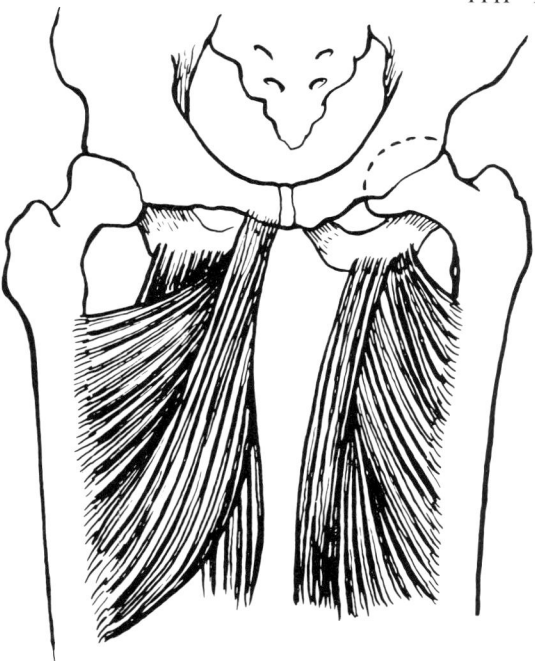

Fig. 8.7. Adductor posterior transfer. When the adductors are transferred from the pubis to the ischium it will be noted that the attachment on the ischium lies beneath the fulcrum of the hip. When the muscle pulls with the hip reduced it will only reach neutral position.

Fig. 8.8. Varus osteotomy.
(a) A heavy threaded pin is placed up the centre of the neck, the second pin is placed perpendicular to the shaft and X-rays are taken to be sure that the femoral neck pin is accurately placed in the anteroposterior and lateral views. The pin runs shy of the epiphyseal plate. The cut is made proximally in the inner trochanteric area. If some rotational correction is desired it is rotated at this time and then the angled wedge is removed. This will usually contain the iliopsoas tendon which may be simply divided or tagged for additional use.
(b) After the wedge is removed the osteotomy is closed and parallel threaded pins are placed across the osteotomy site but short of the epiphyseal plate. The femoral neck pin and the inferior shaft pin have been removed.

through a transverse incision below the iliac crest and placed anterolaterally. The Yount procedure is performed laterally several inches above the lateral condyle, with resection of 1–2 inches of the iliotibial band including the intramuscular septum (Yount 1926).

In all paralytic hips who lack an active abductor, release of the abduction contracture and stretching into adduction may lead to subsequent subluxation or dislocation. This complication must be weighed and a decision made as to which problem will cause the greatest difficulty. In hips that are scarred intra-articularly in abduction and not readily released by soft tissue releases, varus osteotomy is performed in the subtrochanteric area by a closing medial based wedge osteotomy. Fixation is similar to that described for the extension osteotomy (Fig. 8.8).

Windswept deformities

Patients may have asymmetrical musculature resulting in a flexed, externally rotated and abducted hip on one side with an adducted contralateral hip. Other sources are the deformities described above, namely a fixed abduction contracture on one side and a fixed adduction contracture secondary to dislocation, and contracted adductors on the opposite side. These

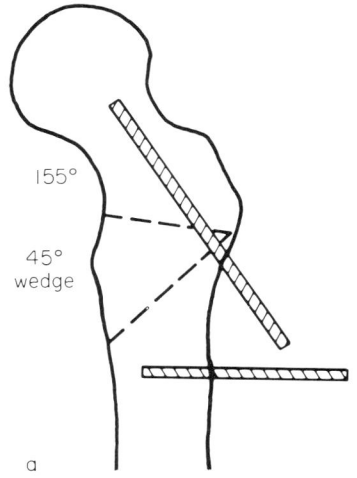

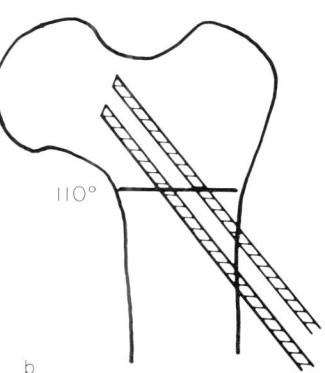

deformities are treated by the appropriate releases. It is important that bracing and positioning be continued postoperatively. A hip brace which allows flexion and extension, limited adduction with free abduction on the previously adducted side while maintaining the neutral position or slightly adducted position on the previously abducted side is used. If soft tissue releases are not adequate or are impractical then bilateral osteotomies may be performed (Weissman *et al.* 1961).

External rotation deformities

External rotation deformities occur at various neurologic levels due to passive contractures, imbalance of external rotators over internal rotators, or iatrogenic causes related to muscle transfers. Individuals with thoracic level paralysis have external rotation deformities secondary to positioning or spastic external rotators. Splinting in a more neutral position is performed, as well as frequent range of motion. Excessive force and an overcorrected position are avoided. Some external rotation is not of great significance in these children as long as they can be brought to within 30° of neutral for bracing and for sitting purposes. Those patients with greater external rotation contractures of the hip will require posterior release of the capsule and of the external rotators. The iliopsoas is released if internal rotation is obtainable when the hips are in flexion but not in extension. McKibbin (1968) has shown that the iliopsoas acts as an external rotator in the newborn infant and particularly in hips that are subluxed. When some improvement of external rotation is achieved by flexion, but it is obvious that the external rotators are also tight, both the external rotators and the iliopsoas are released.

Menelaus (1969) described treatment for external rotation contractures by placing the patient on the contralateral side and making a longitudinal lateral incision centered over the top of the greater trochanter. Both the posterior and anterior aspects of the hip can then be reached. The posterior hip is released by full medial rotation sectioning the external rotators and the posterior capsule. If a flexion and abduction contracture is present the fibrous tissue of the glutei are divided. The hip is externally rotated and tensor fascia lata, rectus, and psoas can be released if indicated. He also described reefing the anterior capsule. When the sartorius is tight it should be released by removing a section or by Z-lengthening. If the patient has thigh sensation care must be taken to avoid sectioning the lateral femoral cutaneous nerve.

Femoral derotation osteotomies are performed when bony deformity is present and the above procedures are not indicated. These are carried out either in conjunction with other osteotomies in the proximal femur or, if pure derotation osteotomy is indicated, distal osteotomy utilizing pin and plaster fixation may be the easiest. Sacral agenesis changes acetabular position, making it face laterally. This results in an external rotation deformity that may be treated by rotational osteotomy of the femur.

Hip dysplasia

Hip dysplasia in myelodysplasia is the result of an imbalance of forces about the hip creating greater adduction forces than abduction forces (Fig. 8.9). The prime prerequisite is a less than poor grade abductor strength. Evaluation of a series of patients with lower motor neuron lesions, primarily those with poliomyelitis, demonstrated that dislocation did not occur if abductor muscle power was better than poor grade (Nickel *et al.* 1966). That same study demonstrated that a combination of forces created dislocation of the hip. The most significant was the adductor muscles creating adduction positioning of the hip with the forceful direction pushing the hip laterally and superiorly. A study carried out by McKibbin (1968) demonstrated that, in the newborn, the iliopsoas caused flexion and external rotation and prevented medial rotation and improper seating of the femoral head in extension; this same action was seen in older

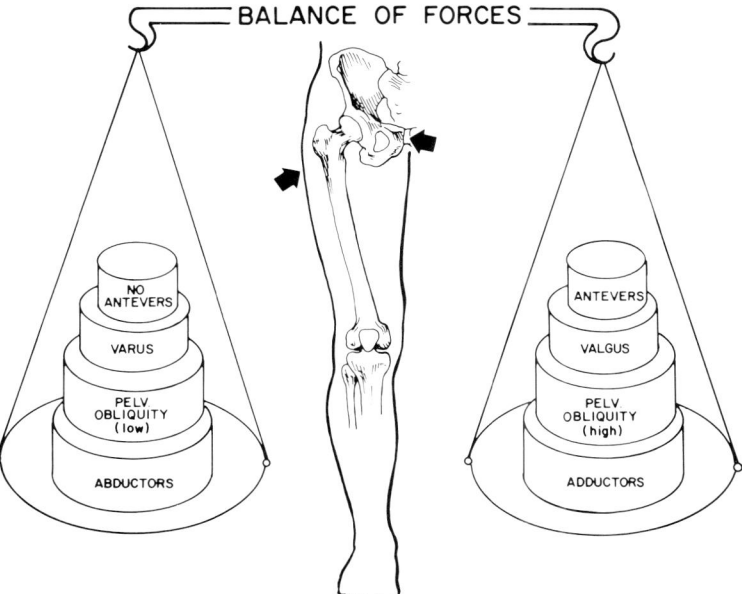

Fig. 8.9. Adduction forces tend to dislocate the hip. The strong adduction and no abduction creates the strong imbalance. Valgus deformity of the neck is the strongest and anteversion is the least forceful. The greater the imbalance the more rapid and likely the dislocation.

hips with increased anteversion or subluxation (Somerville 1959).

Increased valgus of the femoral neck causes an adducted position of the femoral head as related to the acetabulum (Fig. 8.10a). In the newborn child, hip valgus averages 20° more than the adult. Ordinarily the valgus will gradually decrease, but in the myelomeningocele child it may increase. Three factors appear to contribute towards this increase:

1 unbalanced muscle pull creating deformity about the proximal femur;

2 lack of stimulation of the greater trochanter due to an absent abductor and;

3 lack of weightbearing in the early years.

Brookes and Wardle (1962) demonstrated the effect of various muscles about the hip on decalcified femurs. They were able to demonstrate that valgus occurred with the pull of the iliopsoas, but the abductor muscles demonstrated an opposite force. They demonstrated the equilization of these forces on the femur when both were being applied at the same time in a ratio of five to three. In addition, they demonstrated that

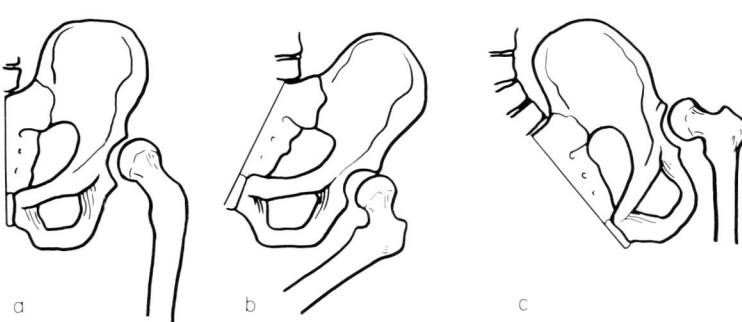

Fig. 8.10. (a) The neck is in valgus and the weightbearing pressures are on the outer aspect of the acetabulum.
(b) The neck is in normal or even varus position, but the adduction contracture places the weightbearing pressure on the outer aspect of the acetabulum.
(c) The femoral angle is normal. However, due to pelvic obliquity, the weightbearing pressure is again on the outer aspect of the acetabulum.

the extensor muscle decreased anteversion and flexor forces increased anterversion. It can be seen then that different combinations of muscle function will have different effects on the shape of the femoral neck. The iliopsoas may have a greater effect towards creating valgus in the high level lumbar patient of approximately L2–3 range where the adductors are still quite weak but the iliopsoas is full strength.

The effect of the greater trochanter on femoral neck position is readily seen. Increased valgus results after premature fusion of the trochanteric epiphysis. The lack of muscle pull on the greater trochanter decreases stimulation and growth.

Weightbearing has much less effect on the shape of the proximal femur, but probably contributes to it (Baker *et al.* 1962).

Additional causes of the adducted position are related to pelvic obliquity itself. This basically amounts to the relationship of the femur to the acetabulum. A short leg on the contralateral side will create an adducted position in weightbearing (Fig. 8.10b). An abduction contracture of the contralateral side creates the adducted position when the legs are lying parallel. Pelvic obliquity as a result of uneven musculature or scoliosis will create the adducted position on the upside and the abducted position in relationship to the hip on the down side (Fig. 8.10c). In these instances hips with inadequate acetabula or absent abductor muscles will readily dislocate. Somerville (1959) summarized the effect of the adducted position best, stating, 'the nearer the angle between the neck of the femur and the horizontal of the pelvis approaches 90° the more unstable the hip will become'.

The combinations of balancing factors about the hip effects the degree of severity as well as the rapidity of dislocation. The infant who has very strong adductors and flexors with no abductors will tend to dislocate early, even *in utero*. If the opposite hip is in relative abduction the tendency for the adducted hip will be to dislocate that much more rapidly. The individual with no hip muscle imbalance, that is full paralysis about the hip joint, will develop gradual dislocation if other factors are present which tend to place the hip in adduction. In the child who has some abductor power (low lumbar) the problem may be a very gradual, slow subluxation with no actual dislocation.

If hip dysplasia is to be treated, a balancing of forces must be carried out to obtain a stable hip. Concentric reduction must be obtained and the forces directed to maintain this reduction, by removing the deforming forces creating the adducted position and creating abduction forces. Various procedures have been described for changing these forces. If adductor function is present, sectioning of the adductors or posterior transfer as described earlier should be carried out. Release of the iliopsoas will alter the forces on the proximal femur. This will result in decreasing valgus creating stress in the proximal femur, reduce the tendency towards flexion contracture and hip reduction will be made easier. Varus osteotomy can be carried out if the child is over the age of two and has a significant valgus. Femoral osteotomy at 110° provides relative abduction of the hip and forces that are sufficient to resist recurrence of valgus. A closing wedge osteotomy is the most stable and parallel threaded pins across the osteotomy can be used to hold this. A wide variety of internal fixation devices have been described and may be used, but add to the complexity of the procedure. If the iliopsoas tendon has not been released from an adductor approach it can be readily reached and removed when the wedge of bone is taken.

Providing an abductor creates a positive force for maintenance of reduction. Abduction forces are provided by transfer of a muscle. In order for any force to be effective a satisfactory fulcrum as represented by a stable concentric reduction must be present. Any degree of instability will significantly decrease the force of a transferred muscle.

Two muscles have been used effectively as a lateral transfer, the iliopsoas and the external oblique. The iliopsoas has been the most popular since being reported by Mustard (1952) for poliomyelitic weakened hips. Garceau and Kinzel (1951) reported a midlateral transfer of the iliopsoas through a hole in the ilium. Mustard carried out his procedures through a notch in the anterior portion of the ilium and attached it to the greater trochanter. Fleming (1957) described combining the lateral psoas transfer with adductor tenotomy, femoral osteotomy and acetabular procedures. Sharrard (1964) reported the results of his posterolateral iliopsoas transfer. This transfer was designed to make up for the lack of extensor muscles as well as abductor muscle in myelomeningocele. By placing the muscle posteriorly it was reported to provide improvement of extension strength and therefore a better upright posture in addition to the abductor muscle benefits. There is a definite question as to the effectiveness of the muscle as an extensor both by clinical testing and by electromyography. The study by Buisson and Hamblen (1972) demonstrated that the iliopsoas functioned with the flexor muscles and did not give extension or change phase during gait.

The actual success of this transfer has been variable. Parker and Walker (1975) reported excellent success in lumbar level patients when performed early. Carroll and Sharrard (1972)

reported a long-term follow-up of Sharrard's initial group of patients and found a 60% success rate on a full gamut of neurologic deficit patients. Jackson *et al.* (1977) similarly described a poor result following posterior iliopsoas transfers and particularly indicated that it was exceedingly difficult to obtain a stable hip in older patients, that is above 5 years. In contrast Parsch and Goessens (1971) described excellent results in a group of patients with combined procedures that were performed between the ages of 3 and 7. There is a definite basis for posterolateral iliopsoas transfer in the myelodysplastic patient. In addition to the provision of lateral muscle power the iliopsoas has been removed from its deforming force anteriorly, which allows better hip extension from hamstring function and decreases the forces producing femoral neck valgus. The patient may lose the ability to flex the hip sufficiently to bring the foot on to a 12 inch step. A strong rectus femoris and sartorius muscle are needed to substitute for the iliopsoas strength. Very few patients evaluated in the authors' clinic can

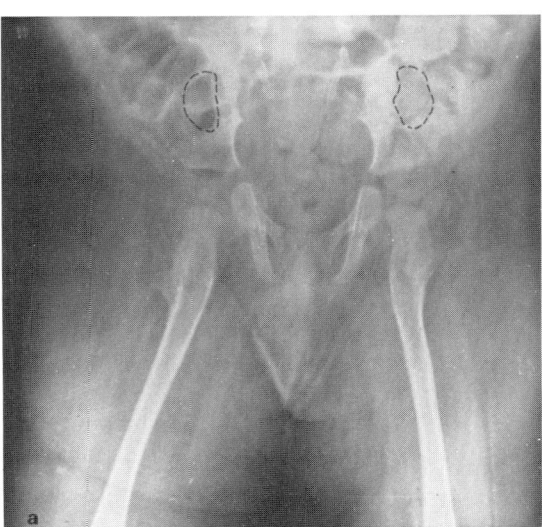 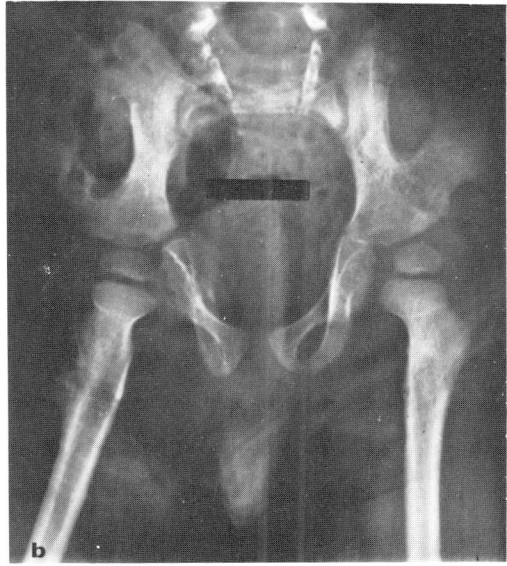

Fig. 8.11. (a) This child at nine months of age underwent iliopsoas transfers. Six months after the transfer the size of the holes in the ilium can be seen.
(b) X-ray taken a little over two years later. With increase in size and function of the iliopsoas transfers, the iliac holes have enlarged.

straight leg raise above 40° following an iliopsoas transfer.

The procedure as described by Sharrard (1964) may be altered by leaving the iliacus partially attached within the pelvis. The hole in the ilium should be large enough adequately to allow passage of tendon and muscle and may be made lateral to the described posterior position. If the transfer has functioned successfully, the holes will enlarge with growth of the child (Fig. 8.11). The authors avoid passing the tendon through a tunnel in the proximal femur by creating a perichondral or periosteal flap with some roughening of the bone, and anchor the tendon under tension by means of a drill hole and suture through the bone. This avoids the possibility of fracture in the small bones and facilitates the attachment of the tendon.

The external oblique is a muscle which does not have the bulk of the iliopsoas but does have a more advantageous position, its origin being far lateral on the trunk at the lower rib cage, and it extends straight down to the greater trochanter after transfer. Theoretically it may also reduce body sway or Trendelenburg lurch during ambulation. This transfer also spares the iliopsoas and allows its use as a flexor. This may be of advantage or disadvantage. The external oblique transfer is described by Thomas et al. (1950). The dissection and transfer itself is relatively easy. The primary consideration is to complete the dissection posteriorly and anteriorly to the rib cage and rotate the muscles sufficiently so that a tube is formed and appropriate tension is placed on all aspects of the muscle at time of attachment.

Acetabular procedures are performed when the acetabulum is deficient in patients over the age of two. Salter type procedures are not recommended as the posterior aspect of the acetabulum becomes defective and dislocation posteriorly may occur. In these cases posterior shelf operations have been carried out. A Pemberton type osteotomy has been effective in that it decreases the volume of the enlarged acetabulum and brings the normal cartilage down over the femoral head (Westin et al. 1985).

Capsulorrhaphy may be carried out simultaneously. The acetabular procedure should be performed at the time of the iliopsoas transplant since the area is exposed and the only additional requirement is cutting of bone about the acetabulum.

The Chiari osteotomy must also be considered. Good results have been reported by Canale et al. (1975) in providing stability for the hip, but Jackson et al. (1977), reported poor results in those patients who had combined iliopsoas transfers and Chiari procedures. Their conclusion was that the iliopsoas transfer acted as a tenodesis which actually pulled the femoral head out of the acetabulum. The Colonna arthroplasty can stabilize the hip, but frequently movement is significantly limited and this procedure should not be carried out. Madigan and Worrall (1977) evaluated 29 hips and demonstrated that 83% of the patients had loss of motion in the flexion extension arch. The most favourable results were in those patients whose level was above T12.

The combined procedures to eliminate the imbalance of forces are logical. Sharrard's series (Carroll & Sharrard 1972) included this type of combination procedure and indicated that some of his failures were probably the result of inadequate adductor releases and inadequate femoral acetabular relationships at the time of transfer. They strongly recommended capsulorrhaphy for the lax capsule after reduction and Menelaus (1980) agreed with this. Nickel et al. (1966) recommended multiple procedures which included adductor posterior transfer, femoral osteotomy, iliopsoas transfer to the mid lateral area and Pemberton osteotomy when indicated. Most of their patients had had poliomyelitis, but some myelodysplastics were included. London and Nichols (1975) used the same combination with posterolateral iliopsoas transfer. They felt their most successful patient group was those who had adductor posterior transfer as compared with simple adductor release. McKay (1977), described a similar group of procedures for stabilization, but utilized the external oblique muscle as an abductor. Bunch and Hakala

(1984) had excellent success in the low lumbar patient when varus osteotomy was combined with posterolateral iliopsoas transfer.

If an iliopsoas transfer is indicated, a varus osteotomy should be carried out either at the same time or prior to the iliopsoas transfer. Varus osteotomy after a transfer has been performed creates apparent lengthening of the transfer and, therefore, considerable weakening of it (Fig. 8.12). If an osteotomy is required after a transfer has been carried out, the transfer must

1 failure of procedure;
2 fractures;
3 postoperative stiffness and contracture
  (a) intra- and extra-articular fibrosis
  (b) heterotopic bone formation;
4 dislocation of the opposite hip secondary to unilateral procedures.

All the general surgical complications may occur and must be considered, including infection and anaesthestic complications.

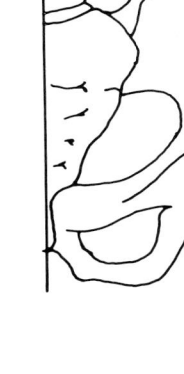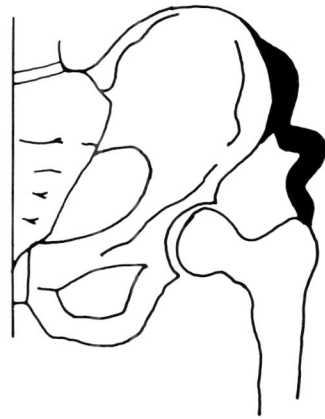

Fig. 8.12. If a varus osteotomy is performed after an iliopsoas transfer has been carried out the transfer becomes relatively lengthened and therefore markedly weakened. The transfer should be carried out after the osteotomy or it will have to be redone at the time of osteotomy.

be tightened at the time of surgery.

The final consideration of correction of hip position must be the position of the proximal femur relative to the acetabulum. Pelvic obliquity creates adduction of the hip on the high side and abduction on the lower side. The latter increases stability of the hip whereas the former creates increasing instability. It is impossible to reduce a hip that has inadequate superior coverage. This coverage cannot be provided in a hip with significant pelvic obliquity. In those instances pelvic obliquity must be corrected prior to attempting reduction of the hip (p. 149).

Complications of surgical reduction of the hip

Complications peculiar to myelodysplasia hip surgery include:

The general failure rate for reduction and surgery has been variable and dependent upon the selection of patients as well as the procedures performed. Sharrard's original series (Carroll & Sharrard 1972), demonstrated a 40% failure rate. A similar failure rate was encountered by Feiwell et al. (1978) and an even greater rate of failure of iliopsoas transfers was reported by Jackson et al. (1977). Parker and Walker (1975) selected a group of young patients (under 1 year), many of whom did not have a dislocation or subluxation, but were highly suspect for future occurrence, for iliopsoas transfer. They reported an extremely high success rate, but a significant number of complications occurred. Selection of the appropriate patient and the appropriate surgical procedures will lead to a higher rate of success. Operating on the older patient who has little musculature to provide stability will result in failure of maintenance of reduction.

Balancing hip musculature when bony deformity, that creates femoral acetabular instability, is present results in failure of reduction. The patient with little acetabular depth will not benefit from standard soft tissue procedures or even a femoral osteotomy. In this instance, an acetabular procedure will be required. The patient with pelvic obliquity greater than 10° will be unlikely to have a successful reduction.

Fractures of the lower extremity are extremely common following multiple hip operations. With immobilization sufficient bone is lost to weaken the extremity. Subsequent stiffness of the joints, particularly the hip joint, creates greater stress on the femur. Less frequently the tibia fractures as a result of tightness of the knee or rotation stresses in transferring. Patients in whom multiple operations have been carried out, which of necessity require more prolonged immobilization and increased stiffness about the hip postoperatively, have a significant incidence of fracture (Carroll & Sharrard 1972, Parker & Walker 1975, Feiwell et al. 1978). Methods of treatment to avoid this complication consist of early weightbearing in a cast, as early mobilization as possible, mobilizing with care and constant bracing whenever the patient is out of plaster. This includes getting in and out of bed and even bracing while in bed during the first few weeks after removal of the cast.

A major concern following surgical treatment has been the occurrence of contractures about the hip. A stable hip may result, but the patient may not be able to flex the hip to 90°. Twenty-seven per cent of the patients with unilateral or bilateral surgery in the series of Feiwell et al. (1978) and a similar percentage in Carroll and Sharrard's (1972) series had limitation of flexion. This grossly inhibits sitting ability and results in pressure problems on the sacrum and coccygeal area. Abduction contractures benefit reduction, but may lead to subluxation or dislocation on the contralateral side, due to the constant adducted position. Bilateral procedures are recommended to avoid unilateral abduction contractures in symmetrical neurologically involved patients.

Heterotopic ossification occurs in sporadic cases, and is disastrous since sitting becomes extremely difficult and limitation of motion is considerable. Treatment is difficult. Continued diligence in range of motion must be utilized over a prolonged period of time. Proximal femoral pseudarthrosis in nonambulators has been effective. Head–neck resections have been unsuccessful.

Selection of surgical candidates

The ideal patient for hip surgery is a two year old with a low lumbar lesion with subluxation of one hip. Since this child's prognosis as an ambulator is good and a unilateral hip dislocation would produce shortening of that extremity with some degree of contracture, surgical treatment is recommended. If the hip were in significant valgus, a varus osteotomy would be indicated. Adductor tightness should be relieved by sectioning or transfer, and if no significant flexion contracture was present, the iliopsoas would not be sectioned. An external oblique transfer would be preferable to an iliopsoas transfer. Transfer of the external oblique on the contralateral side is also recommended either at the same time or later. If the contralateral hip has a different neurologic picture with a greater degree of abduction strength than the side to be operated upon this will not be necessary.

The low lumbar patient below the age of 6 with bilateral subluxation may be treated in the same fashion. Acetabular procedures that increase anterolateral stability should be carried out if deficiency is present. Adequate varus osteotomy under the age of 6 will probably avoid acetabular procedure in most subluxations (Kasser et al. 1985).

The sacral patient will most likely not have a paralytic hip subluxation or dislocation since they should have an active abductor muscle.

However, if such were present, it is most likely to be congenital and should be treated as one would treat a congenital hip dysplasia.

Patients who have a high lumbar or thoracic level lesion should have their contractures released but reduction of the hips is not advocated. These patients will utilize KAFOs with a swing through gait and crutches if they ambulate in adulthood and are not likely to be affected by their hip dysplasia. Ascher & Olson (1983) believed that the L3 level may be benefited by reduction despite the use of crutches and KAFOs and the patient's decreased chance of adult ambulation. McKibbin (1973) described the early treatment of hip dysplasia in infants who had muscles crossing the hip joint with splinting in the abducted, slightly internally rotated, and extended position. Splinting of this type for 18 hours a day, up to the age of 24 months in patients with active muscles crossing the hip, produced improvement of acetabular depth and configuration and reduced contractures of the iliopsoas. His original series was small and there has been poor follow up since the original evaluation of the patients. Early adduction and iliopsoas release followed by splinting provided more successful subsequent surgical procedures compared with those children left to an older age before surgical intervention.

Splinting deters close holding and bonding, and inhibits the child's ability to achieve the normal milestones of development. Since hip reductions are questionable in the upper level myelodysplastic patient, such inhibition is more detrimental with this form of conservative treatment. Healey & Breed (1982) recommended release of the iliopsoas in the early months of life with transference to the anterolateral capsule in L3–4 level patients to reduce deformity and the risk of contracture and dislocation.

Pelvic obliquity

Obliquity of the pelvis is a seriously disabling problem for the myelodysplastic patient. It causes difficulty in the sitting patient by creating poor balance and easier development of pressure sores on the down side ischial prominence, as well as in the walking patient by leg length inequality and dislocation of the hip on the

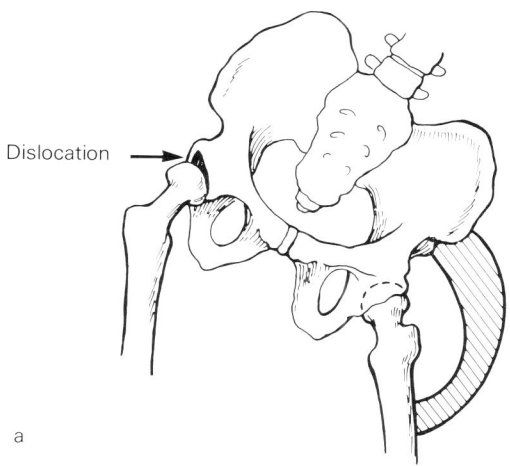

a

Fig. 8.13. (a) Abduction contracture is present. When the legs are brought together, as in standing or sitting, the contralateral hip is adducted because the pelvis is tilted. (b) When the hips are abducted and tension is released from the contracted area the pelvis becomes level.

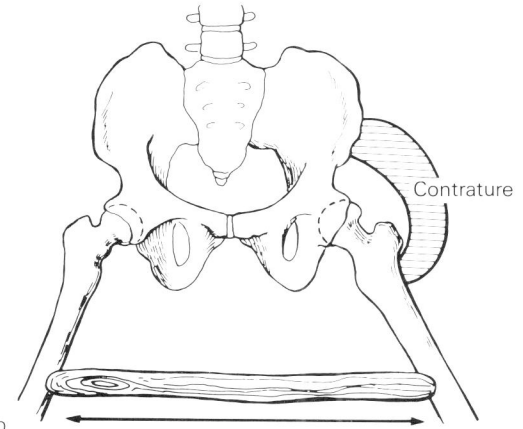

b

elevated side. Scoliosis is the primary cause of significant pelvic obliquity in the myelodysplastic patient, although contractures about the hip may also be a cause. In a fixed abduction contracture from a tight iliotibial band the pelvis is tilted when the legs are brought together because the contracted side cannot adduct any

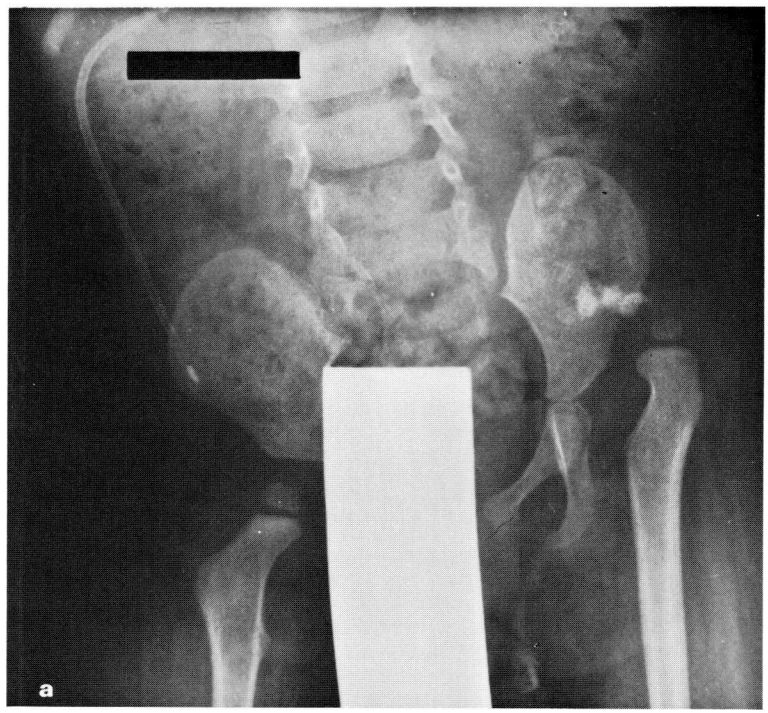

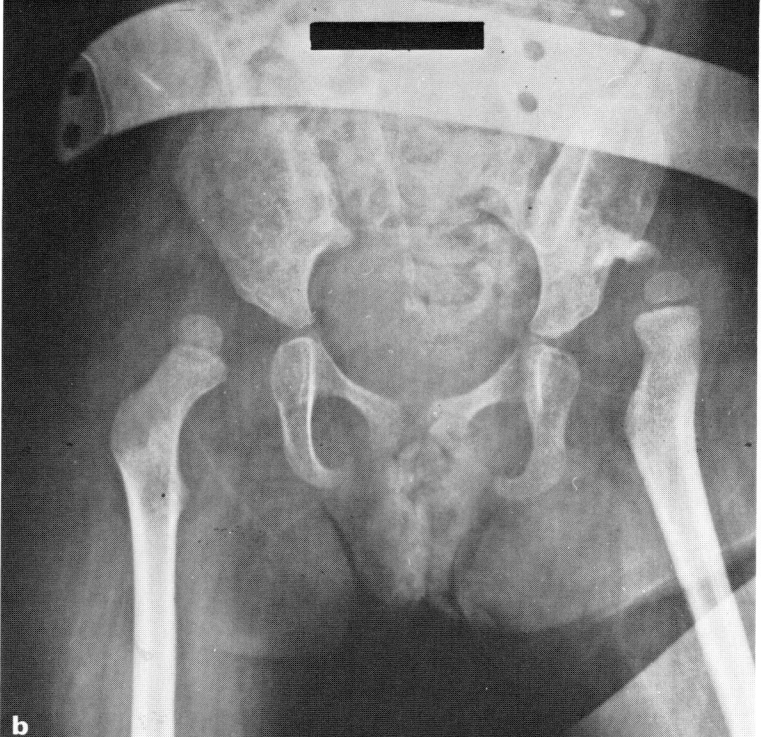

Fig. 8.14. (a) Attempted reduction of both hips will result in an iliotibial band contracture on the right. Pelvic obliquity results from the abduction contracture.
(b) When the iliotibial band contracture is released and the right hip is allowed to dislocate, the pelvis becomes level. Ambulation and sitting as an adult are effective.

further. In order to bring the legs parallel to the axis of the body, the pelvis must tilt and the opposite side must go into an increased adducted position (Fig. 8.13). When the hip is placed in abduction the pelvis becomes level. The contralateral side should be abducted if adduction contracture is considered the source

Correction of the contractures in the infrapelvic area will bring about correction of the pelvic obliquity (Fig. 8.14). If contractures are left long enough in the infrapelvic area, fixed contracture will develop in the spine (Irwin 1949).

In the case of pelvic obliquity caused by scoliosis the pelvis becomes part of the curve and is the last segment of an attempt to compensate for the curvature above. The pelvis rotates in the same direction and to a similar degree as the vertebra above it. Pelvic obliquity, in this situation, is fixed and the femur that is on the down side is in an abducted position in relationship to the acetabulum or the transverse line of the pelvis whereas the up side of the pelvis is creating an adducted position. The latter in a hip without any abductor musculature will leave it uncovered and, if the obliquity occurs sufficiently early in childhood, will result in dislocation. As a result of this obliquity significant leg length discrepancy occurs and affects ambulation. Not only does it affect the walking ability by requiring a significant lift under the short side but makes orthotic fitting more difficult in the high lumbar or thoracic patient who requires a lumbosacral hip–knee–ankle–foot orthosis (LSHKAFO) or an HKAFO. Often the increasing obliquity is manifested by the development of pressure areas from the orthosis.

The definition of pelvic obliquity and its measurement requires discussion. In many instances the apparent obliquity as related to the lumbar segments above it does not reflect the actual obliquity. A satisfactory definition of pelvic obliquity is difficult to find. Lindseth (1978) described the degree of pelvic obliquity as the relationship between the transverse axis of the pelvis and a line drawn across the end plate of the most proximal lumbar vertebra. This

method was not satisfactory in some of our patients. Kilfoyle *et al.* (1965) described scoliosis in paralytic patients whose centre of gravity fell lateral to the ischial tuberosities and indicated that these patients had difficulty in sitting as well as standing. These patients attempt to maintain their centre of gravity by trying to bring their weightbearing line back within the confines of the ischial tuberosity (Fig. 8.15).

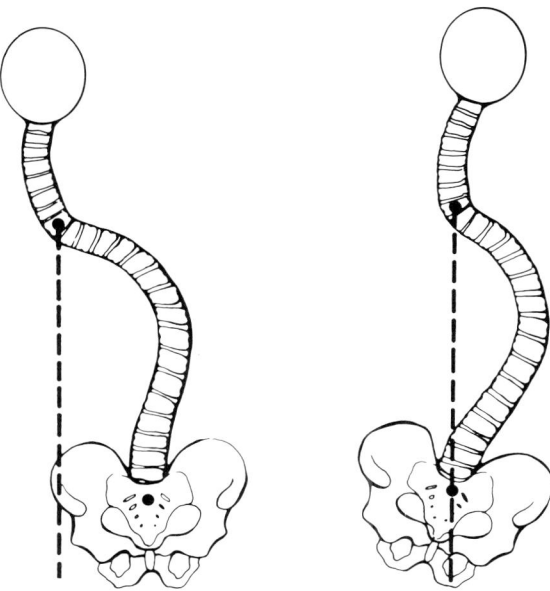

Fig. 8.15. The diagram on the left is of an individual with severe scoliosis placing the pelvis level on a surface. The weightbearing line would be far to the right and the individual would fall or be required to push with the right arm to keep from falling over to the right. The right hand figure demonstrates how the same individual would sit by directing the weightbearing line centrally over the S2 area. Balance would be maintained on one ischium. Unless a sitting X-ray was taken or the entire spine was X-rayed with the pelvis, functional pelvic obliquity would be difficult to determine.

The normal weightbearing line is evaluated by dropping a plumb line from the cervical/dorsal junction and having it end up in the mid portion of the sacrum. The weightbearing centre of gravity in the ambulatory patient has been determined to be about the S2 region. In an individual with a straight spine and level pelvis, the transverse axis of the pelvis is 90° to the weightbearing line. X-ray measurement of pelvic obliquity can be made by a sitting X-ray from D1 to the pelvis. Pelvic obliquity would be the angle that the transverse axis of the pelvis makes with the weight bearing line, as determined by a line through similar points on each side of the pelvis. The angle that the transverse axis of the pelvis makes with a perpendicular line to the vertical weightbearing line is the angle of functional pelvic obliquity.

Functionally the patient's activities of daily living are significantly affected. The simple act of putting on a shirt and buttoning it can be extremely difficult since the patient must lean on something in order to free both hands. Putting a shirt on overhead may result in the individual falling over. Pressure sores are exceedingly common since weightbearing is confined to a small area on the ischial tuberosity, rather than spread out over the buttocks and both posterior thighs. Various pressure cushions are used but do not completely solve the problem. Pressure areas appear and the patient continues with balance difficulties. The most satisfactory treatment would be to prevent fixed pelvic obliquity by surgically stabilizing the spine before it develops. Those patients who do have fixed obliquity are difficult to manage. Even straightening of the spine to a significant degree may fail to fully correct the pelvic obliquity. It is difficult in a fixed scoliosis to obtain full correction. O'Brien et al. (1975) used a combination of Dwyer instrumentation, Harrington instrumentation and at times halopelvic traction, but obtained complete correction of pelvic obliquity in only 40% of their patients. The average correction of pelvic obliquity was 78%. In those patients who had had fusions of their spine, Floman et al. (1982) described excellent success with spinal osteotomy. Complications following that procedure were high.

The posterior iliac osteotomy as described by Lindseth (1978) is a satisfactory method of correction. Derotation of the pelvis occurred by removing a wedge of bone from the down side posteriorly and opening the up side through a similar posterior osteotomy and inserting

the wedge of bone (Fig. 8.16). Lindseth (1978) closed the donor osteotomy and stabilized it by nonabsorbable sutures through drill holes in the ilium. The authors have found that the Knodt rod has been of benefit in closing the wedge (Fig. 8.17). Not only does it assist in the closure of the wedge, but it also maintains it with greater stability. One hook is placed into the sacroiliac joint and the second into a notch on the posterior ilium. A bilateral spica cast is used

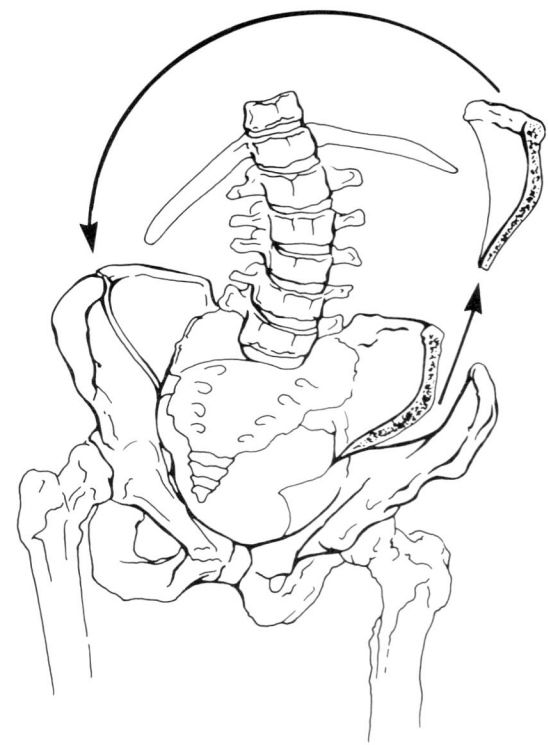

Fig. 8.16. A wedge of bone is removed adjacent to the sacroiliac joint on the downside of the oblique pelvis and placed in an osteotomy on the opposite side. The open wedge is closed while the osteotomy area is opened to allow insertion of the wedge. (Redrawn from Lindseth 1978.)

for six weeks. At the end of five weeks the cast is bivalved and range of motion exercises of the hips begun. The patient is started on a sitting programme at the end of six weeks, gradually building sitting tolerance. However this procedure should be carried out *only* when the spine has been stabilized or progressive changes are not anticipated. The procedure rotates the pelvis thereby swinging the up side downward. If the closing wedge is allowed to shift upwards, further correction is obtained of the tilt. The procedure not only changes the tilt, but also derotates the pelvis in an anterolateral direction, and shifts the pelvis laterally for improvement of the weightbearing line.

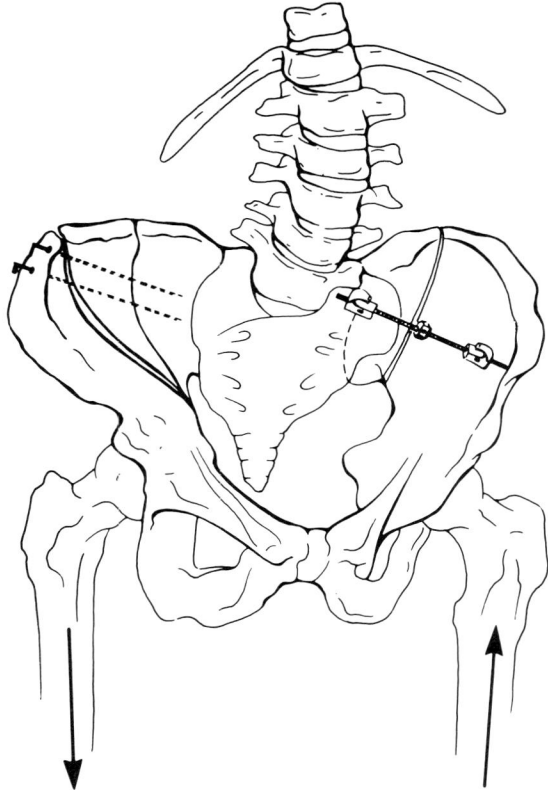

Fig. 8.17. Closure is facilitated by an assistant pushing up from below on the one leg and pulling down on the opposite leg to open the pelvic osteotomy. Parallel pins are placed through the wedge and a Knodt rod is used to close and help stabilize the osteotomy.

Duchenne muscular dystrophy (DMD)

Early, walking phase

Early growth and development of the DMD child is normal (Chapter 5). There is generally no delay in achieving the seated or standing position at the appropriate age. Hip development is expected to be normal. This does not preclude the possibility that a congenital dislocation or subluxation of the hip(s) may occur concomitantly and should it exist, be treated appropriately.

Lordosis is seen on standing at about the age of four to five years. Because of abdominal, gluteal and quadriceps muscle weakness, the child stands with a wider base and waddles when walking. As early as 24 months of age, the affected child demonstrates that he needs to climb up on himself to get up from the floor, evoking Gower's manoeuvre.

Late, walking phase

Although bony development in the hip joint continues normally, imbalance of the hip musculature can result in changes in upper femoral development (Fig. 8.18). Anteversion, generally not interfering with gait is frequently present. Walking and standing can continue until the child is 8–11 years of age when increasing generalized muscular weakness, increasing energy utilization for walking, and growth in height and weight causes the child to lose his balance and fall frequently (Sutherland *et al.* 1981). Bracing, surgical intervention to release contractures at the knees and ankles, appropriate tendon transfers in the foot to balance ankle control and motion may assist in prolonging ambulation and avoiding the secondary complications of immobility at an early age (Spencer 1973, Hsu 1976, Siegel 1978). The time that the DMD child ceases walking represents approximately half his expected lifespan (Hsu 1981).

Wheelchair dependent phase

The older DMD patient spends more than one half of his daily life seated, thus there is a natural prepondancy for hip flexion contractures to develop. Frequently, 60° of fixed hip flexion con-

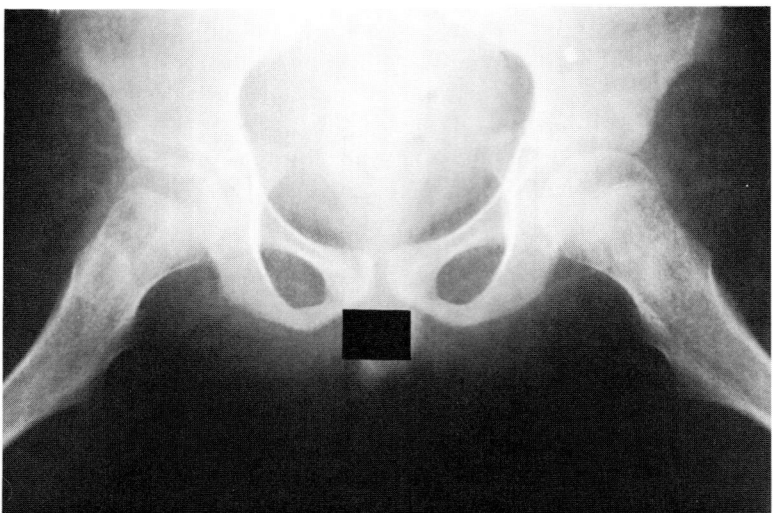

Fig. 8.18. Nine-year-old boy with Duchenne muscular dystrophy. Note well developed and well covered femoral heads. Femoral anteversion is present.

tractures occur. Treatment in the form of stretching and prone lying used in the younger, ambulatory patient is no longer effective. The hip flexion contractures generally do not cause pain or other symptoms, but unfortunately, they interfere with prone lying and when the DMD child sleeps, the legs either need to be supported or the affected children have to sleep on their sides and need to be turned by their parents or attendants periodically during the night.

Most of the older wheelchair dependent DMD children develop scoliosis with a curve greater than 35° (Hsu 1983, Sussman 1985). Associated with this is the development of a fixed pelvic obliquity, which can lead to changes in the hip that result in abnormal pressures and uncontrolled forces causing the femoral head to sublux. Degenerative changes can occur and are demonstrated in Fig. 8.19. Appropriate measures need to be taken utilizing position changes,

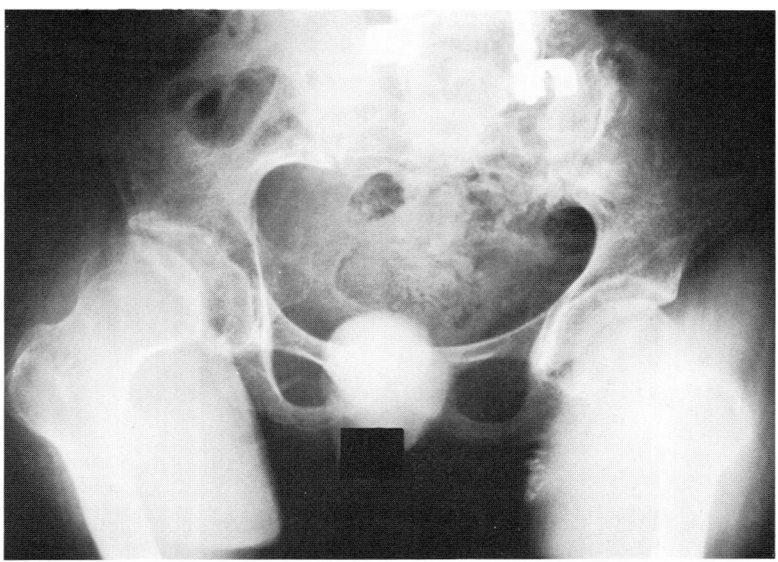

Fig. 8.19. Twenty-year-old male with Duchenne muscular dystrophy. Osteoporosis is seen in the femoral heads with some incongruity and lateral displacement.

seat adaptations, spinal fusion and release of the fixed soft tissue contractures. Localized pain may persist and anti-inflammatory medications can be used to increase the patient's comfort.

Surgical releases of hip flexion contractures, surgical resection of the femoral head, osteotomy of the acetabulum to provide improved femoral head cover is generally not indicated in these patients.

Spinal muscular atrophy (SMA)

Muscle weakness in the child with SMA can range from extreme hypotonia and total dependency (Werdnig–Hoffmann disease) to the minimally disabled, ambulating, thin young adult with near normal muscle strength and function (Kugelberg–Welander syndrome). The muscle weakness is not expected to progress significantly (Munsat *et al.* 1969). Approximately 80% of these patients are wheelchair dependent with activities of daily living (Hsu & Grollman 1979). Frequently, several members of the same family may be affected but the manifestation of muscle weakness differs. Some children are functionally more capable than others and achieve

ambulation, whereas their siblings are wheelchair dependent (Kessler 1968, Hsu & Grollman 1979).

Development of the hip in SMA children is dependent on the hip musculature, can vary considerably from patient to patient and needs to be individually assessed clinically and radiographically.

Radiographs of the young child show a shallow acetabulum and femoral head development may be delayed. As the child grows, the hips may develop further without pain, but, due to anteversion and the absence of hip abductors and external rotators, hip subluxation can occur easily, especially in nonstanding patients (Figs. 8.20 & 8.21).

Hip subluxation cannot be prevented. However, unilateral dislocation should be prevented and if it occurs, needs to be treated actively and aggressively. When the hip subluxes, the femoral head can undergo marked degenerative changes resulting in pain (Fig. 8.22).

Treatment for the incongruous head may be possible with the use of mild analgesic medication and improvement in spine position and

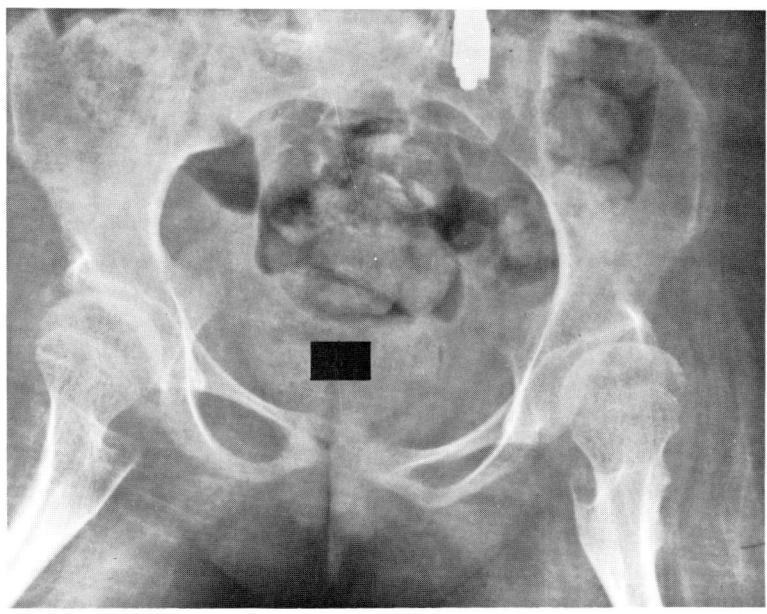

Fig. 8.20. Patient with spinal muscle atrophy. The left hip is partially subluxed at the age of 11 years.

seating. It is generally not necessary to use narcotic types of analgesic and femoral head resection is contraindicated as it could lead to further seating problems and the development of fixed pelvic obliquity.

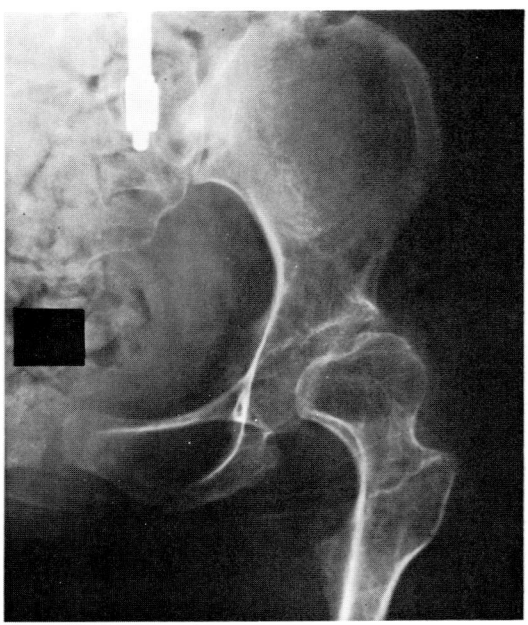

Fig. 8.21. Incongruity of the hip at the age of 21 years. (Same patient as in Fig. 8.20.)

Peroneal muscular atrophy

A recent report on the hips of patients with hereditary motor and sensory neuropathy (HMSN) Type I or II (Charcot–Marie–Tooth disease) showed the occurrence of hip dysplasia (Kumar *et al.* 1985). The hips may become symptomatic in early adolescence with weakness in the hip abductors, the development of a limp and a positive Trendelenburg test. Surgery is suggested for the severe cases to maintain function and to prevent the development of painful symptoms.

The hip in arthrogryposis

In contrast to the patient with spinal muscular atrophy, the arthrogrypotic child can have hips that are stiff in flexion, abduction and external rotation at birth. Dislocation is common and can be unilateral or bilateral.

Hip dislocation

Bilateral dislocations tend to be high and stable. They are generally symmetrical with a pelvis that

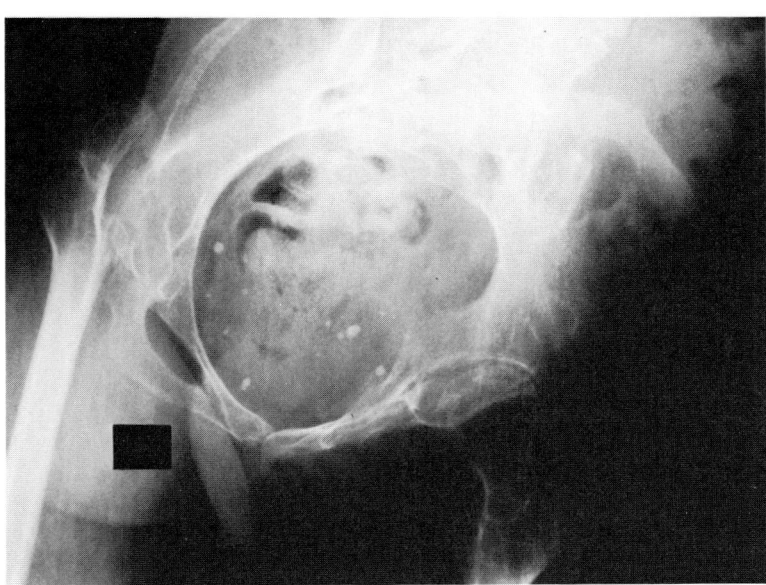

Fig. 8.22. Unilateral hip dislocation in a 31-year-old wheelchair dependent patient with spinal muscle atrophy.

is level and balanced. Gait is possible. Surgical treatment with open reduction and relocation is probably not necessary and can be very difficult to achieve. On the other hand, unilateral dislocation can bring about severe disability in sitting and in walking. Open reduction may be needed, as manipulative reduction and positioning is generally not possible, to minimize later pain and stiffness.

Polymyositis

The muscle weakness that occurs in polymyositis usually does not cause hip problems. However, hip pain and contractures may occur secondary to selective muscle weakness and intramuscular calcification. Physical therapy to maintain the range of motion is desirable (Shapiro & Bresnan 1982). When steroids are used in the treatment,

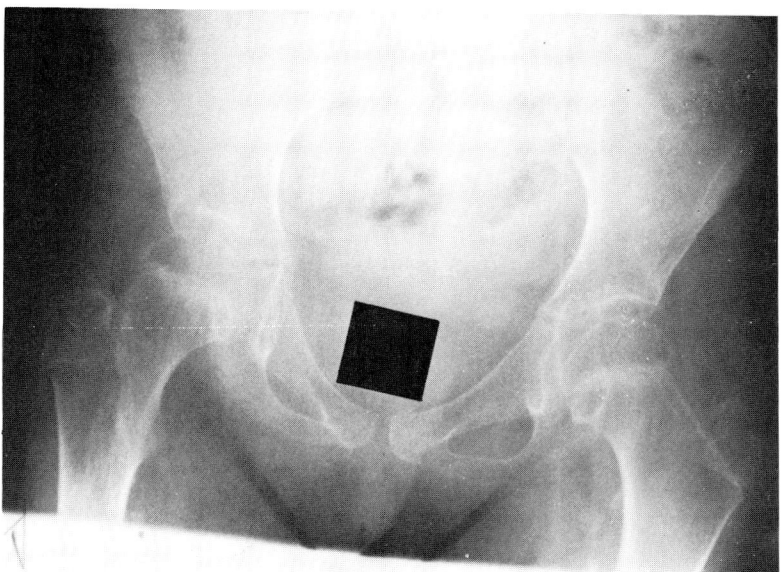

Fig. 8.23. Girl, eight years and ten months old, treated with steriods for polymyositis, showing marked osteoporosis of the femoral heads.

Hip flexion contractures

Hip flexion contractures can lead to decreased range of motion. There is associated lumbar lordosis and postural changes in the spine and pelvis as well as knee flexion contractures. Conservative measures are usually not helpful. Generally, recurrences are frequent following soft tissue releases especially in the non or minimally ambulatory child. If these are attempted, the knee flexion contractures should be corrected before an attempt is made to treat surgically the hip deformities. Subtrochanteric osteotomy at the end of the growth phase may be the most successful type of treatment and is recommended if the flexion deformity requires correction (Drummond *et al.* 1974).

secondary bony changes may occur. This needs to be recognized as increasing osteoporosis can lead to cortical atrophy, loss of bony architecture and collapse of the femoral head (Fig. 8.23).

References

ASCHER M. & OLSON J. (1983) Factors affecting the ambulatory status of patients with spina bifida cystica. *Journal of Bone and Joint Surgery,* **65A,** 350–6.
BAKER L.D., DODELIN R. & BASSETT F.H. (1962) Pathological changes in the hip in cerebral palsy. Incidence, pathogenesis and treatment. A preliminary report. *Journal of Bone and Joint Surgery,* **44A,** 1331–42.
BARDEN G.A., MEYER L.C. & STELLING F.H.C. (1975) Myelodysplastics — fate of those followed for more than twenty years or more. *Journal of Bone and Joint Surgery,* **57A,** 643–7.

BLECK E.E. (1980) The hip in cerebral palsy. *Orthopedic Clinics of North America*, **11**, 79–104.

BOWEN J.R., MACEWEN G.D. & MATHEWS P.A. (1981) Treatment of extension contracture of the hip in cerebral palsy. *Developmental Medicine and Child Neurology*, **23**, 23–9.

BROOKES M. & WARDLE E.N. (1962) Muscle action and the shape of the femur. *Journal of Bone and Joint Surgery*, **44B**, 398–411.

BUISSON J.S. & HAMBLEN D.L. (1972) Electromyographic assessment of the transplanted iliopsoas muscle in spina bifida cystica. *Developmental Medicine and Child Neurology*, **27**, 29–33.

BUNCH W.H. & HAKALA M.W. (1984) Iliopsoas transfers in children with myelomeningocele. *Journal of Bone and Joint Surgery*, **66A**, 224–7.

BYRNE R.R. & LARSON L.J. (1977) Hip instability in myelodysplasia. *Clinical Orthopaedics and Related Research*, **127**, 150–5.

CANALE S.T., HAMMOND N.L., COTLER J.M. & SNEDDON H.E. (1975) Pelvic displacement osteotomy for chronic hip dislocation in myelodysplasia. *Journal of Bone and Joint Surgery*, **57A**, 177–83.

CARROLL N.C. & SHARRARD W.J.W. (1972) Long-term follow-up of posterior iliopsoas transplantation for paralytic dislocation of the hip. *Journal of Bone and Joint Surgery*, **54A**, 551–60.

DRUMMOND D.S., SILLER T.N. & CREUSS R.L. (1974) Management of arthrogryposis multiplex congenita. *American Academy of Orthopedic Surgeons Instructional Course Lectures*, **23**, 79–95.

FEIWELL E.N., SAKAI D. & BLATT T. (1978) The effect of hip reduction on function in patients with myelomeningocele. Potential gains and hazards of surgical treatment. *Journal of Bone and Joint Surgery*, **60A**, 169–73.

FLEMING J.L. (1957) Iliopsoas transplant and femoral osteotomy for paralytic dislocation. *Journal of Bone and Joint Surgery*, **39A**, 697.

FLOMAN Y., PENNY J.N., MICHELI L.J., RISEBOROUGH E.J. & HALL J.E. (1982) Osteotomy of the fusion mass in scoliosis. *Journal of Bone and Joint Surgery*, **64A**, 1307–16.

GARCEAU G.J. & KINZEL R.J.W. (1951) Transplantation of the iliacus muscle for loss of hip abductor power. *Quarterly Bulletin of the Indiana Medical Center*, **13**, 27.

GRIFFIN P.P., WHEELHOUSE W.W. & SHIAVI R. (1977) Adductor transfer for adductor spasticity: clinical and electromyographic gait analysis. *Developmental Medicine and Child Neurology*, **19**, 783–89.

HEALEY P.M. & BREED A.L. (1982) The midlumbar myelomeningocele hip. Mechanics of dislocation and treatment. *Journal of Pediatric Orthopedics*, **2**, 15–23.

HOFFER M.M. (1980) Joint motion limitation in newborns. *Clinical Orthopaedics and Related Research*, **148**, 94–6.

HOFFER M.M., FEIWELL E.N., PERRY J., & BONNETT C. (1973) Functional ambulation in patients with myelomeningocele. *Journal of Bone and Joint Surgery*, **55A**, 137–48.

HOFFER M.M., PRIETTO C. & KOFFMAN M. (1981) Supracondylar derotational osteotomy of the femur for internal rotation of the thigh in the cerebral palsied child. *Journal of Bone and Joint Surgery*, **63A**, 389–93.

HSU J.D. (1976) Management of foot deformity in Duchenne's pseudohypertrophic muscular dystrophy. *Orthopedic Clinics of North America*, **7**, 979–84.

HSU J.D. (1981) Challenges in the care of the retarded child with Duchenne muscular dystrophy. *Orthopedic Clinics of North America*, **12**, 73–82.

HSU J.D. (1983) The natural history of spine curvature progression in the nonambulatory Duchenne muscular dystrophy patient. *Spine*, **8**, 771–5.

HSU J.D. & GROLLMAN T.B. (1979) Orthopaedic care of the spinal muscular atrophy child. *Journal of Neurology and Orthopaedic Surgery*, **1**, 47–50.

IRWIN C.E. (1949) The iliotibial band. Its role in producing deformity in poliomyelitis. *Journal of Bone and Joint Surgery*, **31A**, 141–6.

JACKSON R.D., PADGETT T.S. & DONOVAN M.M. (1977) Posterior iliopsoas muscle transfer in myelodysplasia. *Journal of Bone and Joint Surgery*, **61A**, 40–5.

KASSER J.R., BOWEN J.R. & MACEWEN G.D. (1985) Varus derotation osteotomy in the treatment of persistent dysplasia in congenital dislocation of the hip. *Journal of Bone and Joint Surgery*, **67A**, 195.

KESSLER G.B. (1968) Non-progressive proximal and generalized spinal muscular atrophy in siblings. *Bulletin of the Los Angeles Neurological Society*, **33**, 21–5.

KILFOYLE R.M., FOLEY J.J. & NORTON P.L. (1965) Spine and pelvic deformity in childhood and adolescent paraplegia. A study of 104 cases. *Journal of Bone and Joint Surgery*, **47A**, 659–82.

KUMAR S.J., MARKS H.G., BOWEN J.R. & MACEWEN G.D. (1985) Hip dysplasia associated with Charcot–Marie–Tooth disease in the older child and adolescent. *Journal of Paediatric Orthopaedics*, **5**, 511–4.

LINDSETH R.E. (1978) Posterior iliac osteotomy for fixed pelvic obliquity. *Journal of Bone and Joint Surgery*, **60A**, 17–22.

LONDON J.T. & NICHOLS O. (1975) Paralytic dislocation of the hip in myelodysplasia. The role of the adductor transfer. *Journal of Bone and Joint Surgery*, **57A**, 501–6.

MCKAY D.W. (1977) McKay hip stabilization in meningomyelocele. *Orthopaedic Transactions*, **1**, 87.

MCKIBBIN B. (1968) The action of the iliopsoas muscle in the newborn. *Journal of Bone and Joint Surgery*, **50B**, 161–5.

MCKIBBIN B. (1973) The use of splintage in the management of paralytic dislocation of the hip in spina bifida cystica. *Journal of Bone and Joint Surgery*, **55B**, 163–72.

MADIGAN R.R. & WORRALL V.T. (1977) Paralytic instability of the hip in myelomeningoceles. *Clinical Orthopaedics and Related Research*, **125**, 57–64.

MAZUR J.M., STILLWELL A. & MENELAUS M.B. (1986) The significance of spasticity in the upper and lower limbs in myelomeningocele. *Journal of Bone and Joint Surgery*, **68B**, 213-7.

MENELAUS M.B. (1969) Dislocation and deformity of the hip in children with spina bifida cystica. *Journal of Bone and Joint Surgery*, **51B**, 238–51.

MENELAUS M.B. (1976) The hip in myelomeningocele. Management directed towards a minimum number of operations and a minimum period of immobilization. *Journal of Bone and Joint Surgery*, **58B**, 448–52.

MENELAUS M.B. (1980) *The Orthopaedic Management of Spina Bifida Cystica*. Churchill Livingstone, Edinburgh.

MUNSAT T.L., WOODS R., FOWLER W. & PEARSON C.L. (1969) Neurogenic muscular atrophy of infancy with prolonged survival. The variable course of Werdnig–Hoffman disease. *Brain*, **92**, 9–24.

MUSTARD W.T. (1952) Iliopsoas transfer for weakness of the hip abductors: preliminary report. *Journal of Bone and Joint Surgery*, **34A**, 647–50.

NICKEL V., PERRY J., GARRETT A. & FEIWELL E. (1966) Paralytic dislocation of the hip. *Journal of Bone and Joint Surgery*, **48A**, 1021.

O'BRIEN J.P., DWYER A.P. & HODGSON A.R. (1975) Paralytic pelvic obliquity. Its prognosis and management and the development of a technique for full correction of the deformity. *Journal of Bone and Joint Surgery*, **57A**, 626–31.

PAINE R.S., BRAZELTON T.B. & DONOVAN D.E. (1964) Evolution of postural reflexes in normal infants and in the presence of chronic brain syndromes. *Neurology*, **14**, 1036–48.

PARKER B. & WALKER G. (1975) Posterior psoas transfer and hip instability in lumbar myelomeningocele. *Journal of Bone and Joint Surgery*, **57B**, 53–8.

PARSCH K. & GOESSENS H. (1971) Surgical treatment of spinal column and hip deformities in spina bifida. *Acta Orthopaedica Belgica*, **37**, 230–44.

PERRY J., HOFFER M.M., ANTONELLI D., PLUT J., LEWIS G. & GREENBERG R. (1976) Electromyography before and after surgery for hip deformity in children with cerebral palsy. *Journal of Bone and Joint Surgery*, **58A**, 201–8.

PERRY J. & HOFFER M.M. (1977) Preoperative and postoperative dynamic electromyography as an aid in planning tendon transfers in children with cerebral palsy. *Journal of Bone and Joint Surgery*, **59A**, 531–7.

REYNOLDS T.G. & HERZER F.E. (1959) Anteversion of the femoral neck. *Clinical Orthopaedics and Related Research*, **14**, 80–9.

ROOT L. & SPERO C.R. (1981) Hip adductor transfer compared with adductor tenotomy in cerebral palsy. *Journal of Bone and Joint Surgery*, **63A**, 767–72.

SALTER R.B. (1961) Innominate osteotomy in the treatment of congenital dislocation and subluxation of the hip. *Journal of Bone and Joint Surgery*, **43B**, 518–39.

SAMILSON R.M., TSOU P., AAMOTH G. & GREEN W.M. (1972) Dislocation and subluxation of the hip in cerebral palsy. Pathogenesis, natural history and management. *Journal of Bone and Joint Surgery*, **54A**, 863–72.

SHARRARD W.J.W. (1964) Posterior iliopsoas transplantation in the treatment of paralytic dislocation of the hip. *Journal of Bone and Joint Surgery*, **46B**, 426–44.

SHAPIRO F. & BRESNAN M.J. (1982) Orthopaedic management of childhood neuromuscular disease. Part III: diseases of muscle. *Journal of Bone and Joint Surgery*, **64A**, 1102–7.

SIEGEL I.M. (1978) The management of muscular dystrophy: a clinical review. *Muscle and Nerve*, **1**, 453–60.

SOMERVILLE E.W. (1959) Paralytic dislocation of the hip. *Journal of Bone and Joint Surgery*, **41B**, 279–88.

SPENCER G.E. JR. (1973) Orthopaedic consideration in the management of muscular dystrophy. *Current Practice in Orthopaedic Surgery*, **5**, 279–93.

STILLWELL A. & MENELAUS M.B. (1983) Walking ability in mature patients with spina bifida. *Journal of Paediatric Orthopaedics*, **3**, 184–90.

SUSSMAN M.D. (1985) Treatment of scoliosis in Duchenne muscular dystrophy. *Developmental Medicine and Child Neurology*, **27**, 522–4.

SUTHERLAND D.H. (1978) Gait analysis in cerebral palsy. *Developmental Medicine and Child Neurology*, **20**, 807–13.

SUTHERLAND D.H., OLSHEN R., COOPER L., WYATT M., LEACH J., MUBARAK S. & SCHULTZ P. (1981) The pathomechanics of gait in Duchenne muscular dystrophy. *Developmental Medicine and Child Neurology*, **23**, 3–22.

THOMAS L.I., THOMPSON T.C. & STRAUB L.R. (1950) Transplantation of the external obliquie muscle for abductor paralysis. *Journal of Bone and Joint Surgery*, **32A**, 207–17.

WATERS R.L. & LUNSFORD B.R. (1985) Energy cost in paraplegic locomotion. *Journal of Bone and Joint Surgery*, **67A**, 1245–9.

WEISSMAN S.L., TOROK G. & KERMOSH O.J. (1961) Intertrochanteric osteotomy in fixed paralytic obliquity of the pelvis. A preliminary report. *Journal of Bone and Joint Surgery*, **43A**, 1135–54.

WESTIN G., PERLIK P.C. & MARAFIOTI R.L. (1985) A combination pelvic osteotomy for acetabular dysplasia in children. *Journal of Bone and Joint Surgery*, **67A**, 842–50.

WILLIAMS L.O., ANDERSON A.D., CAMPBELL J., THOMAS L., FEIWELL E. & WALKER J.M. (1983) Energy cost of walking and wheelchair propulsion by children with myelodysplasia. Comparison with normal children. *Developmental Medicine and Child Neurology*, **25**, 617–24.

YOUNT C.C. (1926) The role of the tensor fascia femoris in certain deformities of the lower extremities. *Journal of Bone and Joint Surgery*, **8B**, 171.

Chapter 9
Surgery of the Knee
in Neurological Disease

P. AICHROTH

Introduction

Knee problems may occur in the following neurological states and will be considered in this chapter:
   flaccid paralysis;
   spastic paralysis;
   mixed neurological lesions of combined upper and lower motor neuron deficiency in spina bifida;
   arthrogryposis multiplex congenita.

Surgery of the knee which is affected by a flaccid paralysis

The flail knee may be produced by:

1   anterior poliomyelitis;
2   corda equina compression lesions;
3   some lower spina bifida lesions with neurological deficit;
4   other lower motor neuron lesions.

   The whole lower limb may be paralysed and

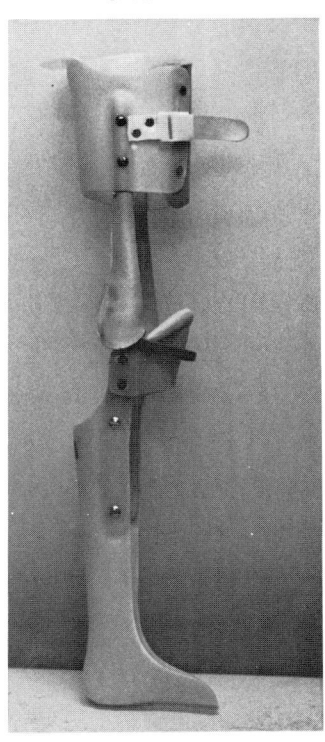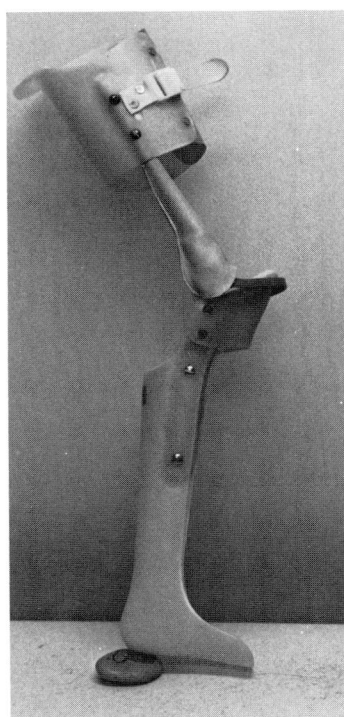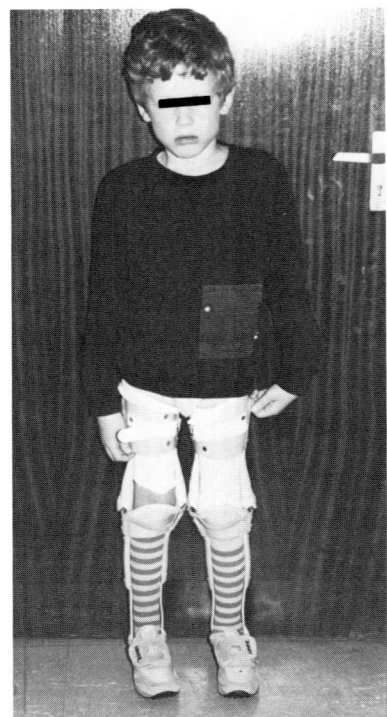

Fig. 9.1. Cosmetic type above knee caliper.

flaccid. The knee is only one minor part of this severe problem and usually requires bracing if the patient is to walk (Fig. 9.1). The hip innervation and strength must be carefully assessed. If the hip is also flail or very weak a full caliper system including a pelvic band is usually required (Fig. 9.2), whereas a flail knee with a good hip innervation and strength will usually require an above knee caliper for its control.

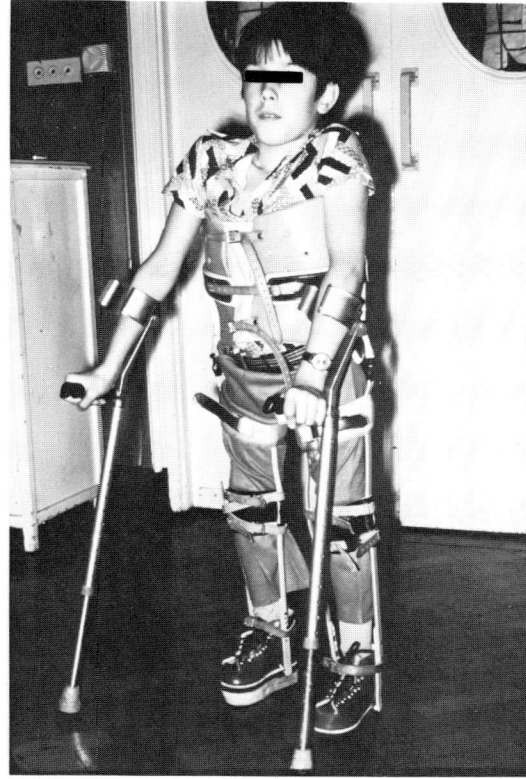

Fig. 9.2. Full caliper system including pelvic/thoracic band.

However, there are some situations where the flail knee fully extends, where hip extension is strong and where the ankle is in a satisfactory position and bracing may be avoided. In this situation the patient with a flail knee may walk without a caliper if the following criteria are present:

1 the hip extensors are strong, power 5 or at least power 4 on the MRC scale;

2 the knee fully extends or may even hyperextend a little;

3 the ankle is in equinus and fixed in this position when weightbearing.

The patient walks by strongly extending the lower limb at the hip as the foot strikes the ground (Fig. 9.3). The ankle is held in some equinus and as weight is put onto this lower limb the knee will be fully extended or hyperextended according to its laxity. Further powerful extension at the hip brings the body weight anterior to the hip and then the knee. The continued hip extension propels the body forwards and the first part of the step is completed. The surgeon therefore should make sure that the knee is able

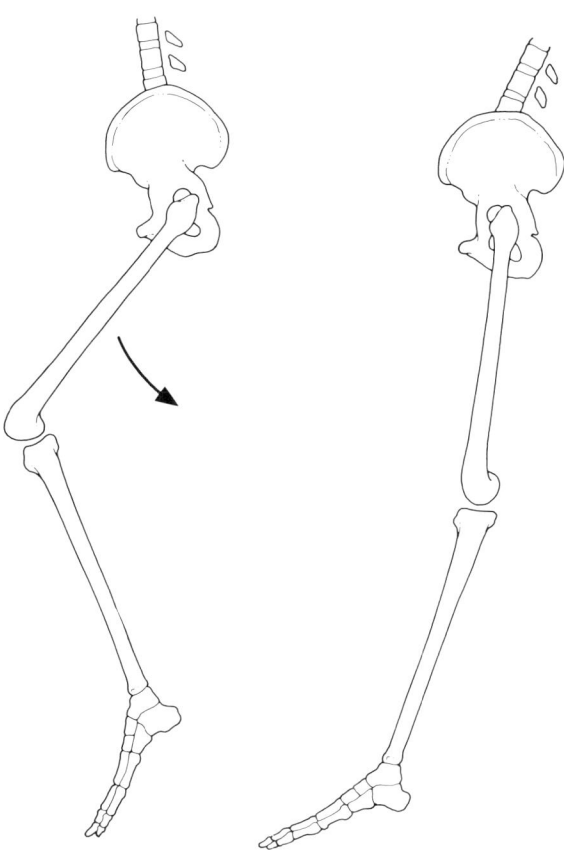

Fig. 9.3. The knee hyperextends when the equinus foot strikes the ground. The hip extensors are strong, the quadriceps paralysed.

to be fully extended or slightly hyperextended. If this is the position no operative knee procedure is required. However, if a knee flexion contracture is present the walking mechanism described in Fig. 9.3 becomes impossible and the limb collapses at the knee.

Surgical procedures which may be required to correct this flexion contracture are posterior knee capsule and tendon release, and/or supracondylar osteotomy.

Release of the posterior knee capsule and tendons

Indications

This procedure is indicated for a knee flexion contracture in the presence of a flaccid paralysis. The flexion contracture in a child is most amenable to this soft tissue release; up to 90° may be corrected in the small child, up to 60° in the adolescent, but no more than 30–40° in the adult.

Operative procedure

The operation is carried out under general anaesthesia with a bloodless field. The patient is placed prone with a sandbag beneath the anterior aspect of the thigh so that the posterior knee structures are placed on stretch. Two vertical incisions are recommended, medial and lateral, with their midpoint at the posterior joint line level (Fig. 9.4). The double vertical incision is preferable because a single vertical midline incision gives inadequate exposure, a transverse incision leaves substantial skin loss when the knee is extended, and an 'S' shaped incision leads to undue tension and some skin loss when the flexion contracture is relieved.

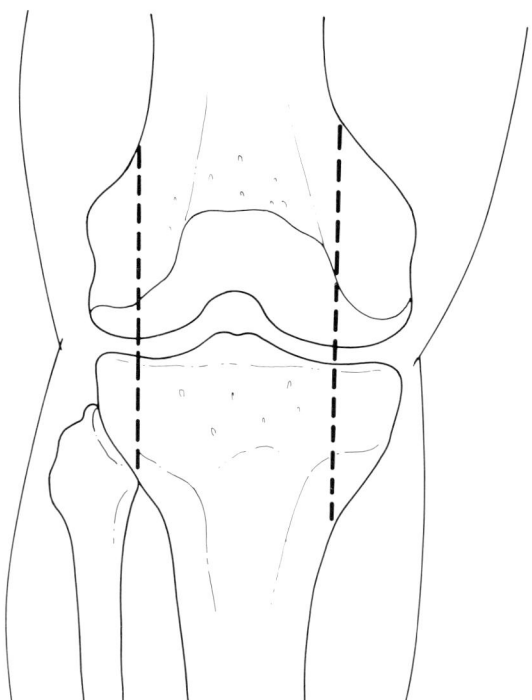

Fig. 9.4. Posterior knee release: *two* vertical skin incisions.

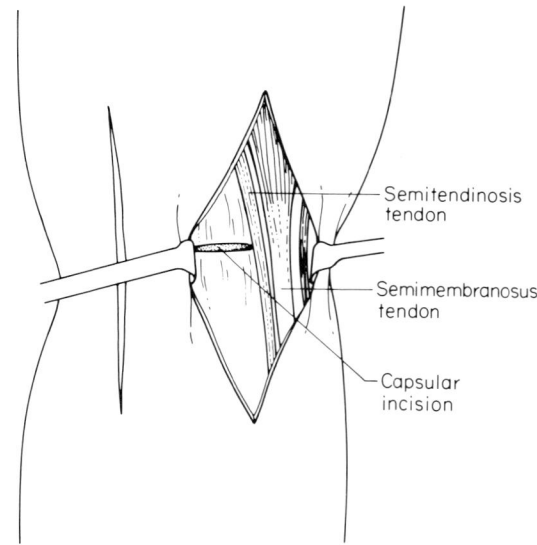

Fig. 9.5. Posterior knee release. The medial dissection.

Medial dissection The deep fascia is divided in the same line as the incision. At its midpoint the fascia is then divided transversely as far laterally as can be reached and medially to where the fascia blends with the medial tendons (Fig. 9.5).

The medial tendons and the neurovascular bundle are identified. The latter is found in the fat in the midline and is retracted laterally. The gracilis, semitendinosus and semimembranosus tendons are divided at the joint line. The gastrocnemius muscle or its fibrous equivalent is then seen overlying the posterior capsule. The knee capsule is opened transversely with a knife just above the joint line. The knee is then flexed a little allowing better lateral retraction of the neurovascular bundle. The transverse posterior capsule incision is extended medially to the posterior edge of the collateral ligament and laterally to the midline with the posterior capsular fibres intermingled with the posterior cruciate ligament and its tibial attachment.

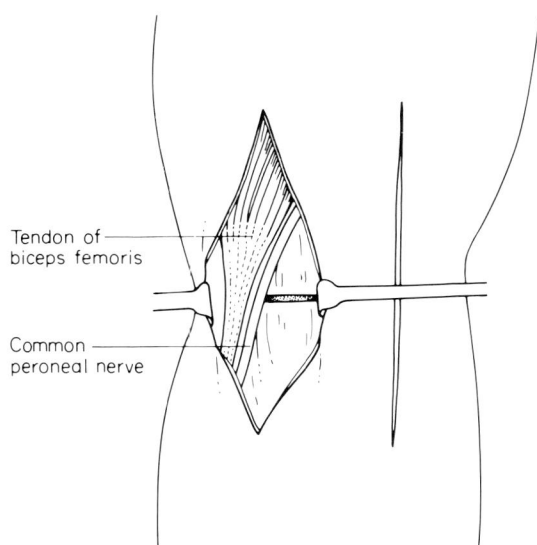

Tendon of
biceps femoris

Common
peroneal nerve

Fig. 9.6. Posterior knee release. The lateral dissection.

Lateral dissection The deep fascia is divided longitudinally in the line of the incision. The peroneal nerve (lateral popliteal nerve) is identified. If it is not immediately visible it will readily be found by gentle blunt dissection. The deep fascia is then divided transversely (Fig. 9.6). The large tendon of biceps is now found at the lateral side of the dissection and when positively identified it is divided transversely. The lateral gas-

trocnemius and the posterior capsule are divided just above the joint line in a similar fashion to that described on the medial side. With the knee flexed to relax the posterior structures the vascular bundle is retracted medially so that the posterior capsular division can be extended to the midline (Fig. 9.7). Any remaining tight bands of fascia are identified and divided as are any remaining tight capsular structures (including the tendon of popliteus).

Closure and after-care The neurovascular bundle is the only remaining tight structure and *must not* be overstretched. The wound is closed with a redivac drain and the limb is placed in a cylinder cast with the knee extended as far as possible without undue extension pressure. Forced extension may lead to incomplete return of vascular flow at the end of the operation, and the knee is best left in some flexion. The extension is increased at two-weekly intervals under general anaesthesia. An overstretched nerve will cause a foot-drop if the anterior tibial and peroneal muscles are innervated.

The cast should be retained for four weeks after full extension has been achieved.

Supracondylar osteotomy

Indications The adolescent or adult knee with a flexion contracture of more than 30° where full extension of the knee is required.

Osteotomy/osteoclasis operation

This procedure is ideal in the patient whose skeleton is still immature. It may be also applied to the *young* adult. The advantage of this procedure, which is undertaken in two stages, is the avoidance of an internal fixation device.

Operative procedure The patient is placed supine with a sandbag beneath the appropriate buttock. The limb is exsanguinated and a high pneumatic tourniquet is applied. A lateral inci-

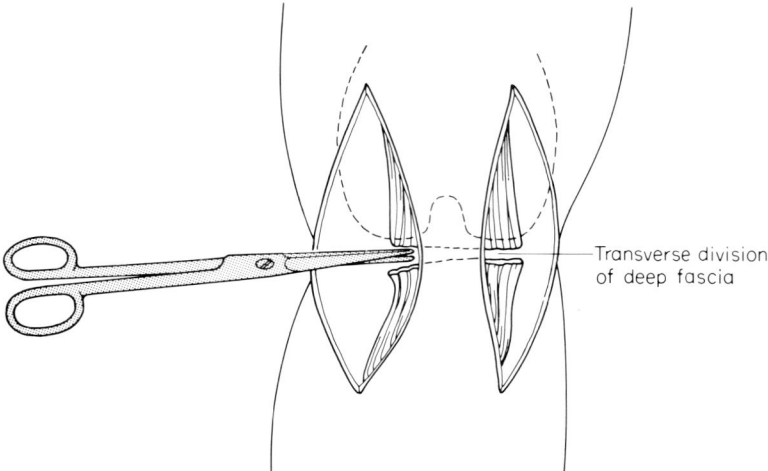

Fig. 9.7. Posterior knee release. The deep fascia requires transverse division.

sion is made from the joint line inferiorly to well above the supracondylar point (Fig. 9.8). The iliotibial tract is divided longitudinally and the supracondylar bone is exposed. The periosteum is incised longitudinally and elevated anteriorly and posteriorly, and the epiphyseal growth plate is identified in the immature patient. This is best undertaken by insertion of a marking needle into what appears to be the epiphyseal growth plate, the level being confirmed by an X-ray image intensifier or a radiograph.

angle of this wedge being equivalent to the flexion contracture. It is important that the surgeon ensures that the posterior cortex of the femur is not divided as this gives inherent stability. The cancellous bone of the excised wedge is divided into small portions and placed loosely back into the wedge deficit.

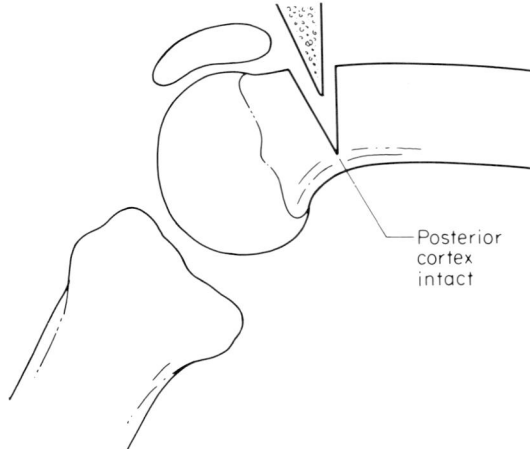

Fig. 9.9. Supracondylar osteotomy. Wedge excision based anteriorly.

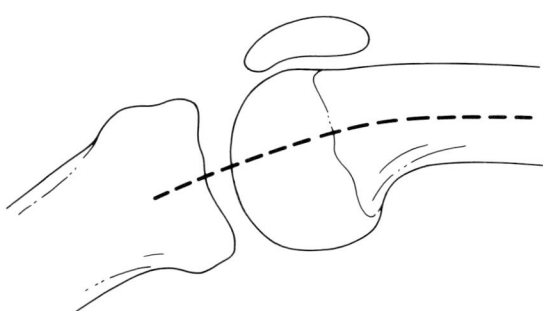

Fig. 9.8. Supracondylar osteotomy. The skin incision.

The femur is divided transversely 1.5–2 cm proximal to the line of the epiphyseal plate leaving the posterior cortex intact (Fig. 9.9). An anteriorly based wedge of bone is removed, the

The wound is closed in layers with drainage. A cast is applied in the *deformed* position maintaining the flexion contracture. Callus rapidly forms in and around the wedge.

Osteoclasis Two weeks after the osteotomy in the child, or three weeks in the adult, the cast is removed and the knee is fully extended by manipulation. The posterior cortex hinges, the early callus in the wedge compacts down and the femur maintains its position but allows the correction to be achieved at this supracondylar point. If the posterior cortex is divided at the time of the initial osteotomy this method will not succeed and internal fixation will be required to maintain the corrected position.

After the osteoclasis a further 4–6 weeks in an extended cast is required followed by physiotherapy.

Supracondylar osteotomy in the adult

If the adult is young and the flexion contracture to be corrected is not more than 30–40° the method of osteotomy/osteoclasis may be used. The alternative, however, is a corrective osteotomy in the supracondylar area with immediate internal fixation using a blade plate.

The osteotomy is marked out as shown in Fig. 9.10. The angle of the wedge, which is based anteriorly, is equivalent to the flexion angle of the knee. The blade-plate chisel is positioned in the condylar fragment with the chisel angle equivalent to the angle of correction. The chisel is passed across the condyle and its position and length checked radiographically with an image intensifier. The blade of the blade plate is inserted partly into the chisel tract. The wedge of bone is fully excised preferably leaving a minimum of posterior cortex. The blade plate is then driven home, the knee is extended and the plate is applied to the lateral femoral shaft with a bone holder. Appropriate apposition of the bone cuts is confirmed and full extension of the knee is checked. The plate is fixed with appropriate screws using a compression device if required.

Passive and active flexion of the knee may be started at an early stage but weightbearing is not allowed until the osteotomy has fully united at ten to twelve weeks.

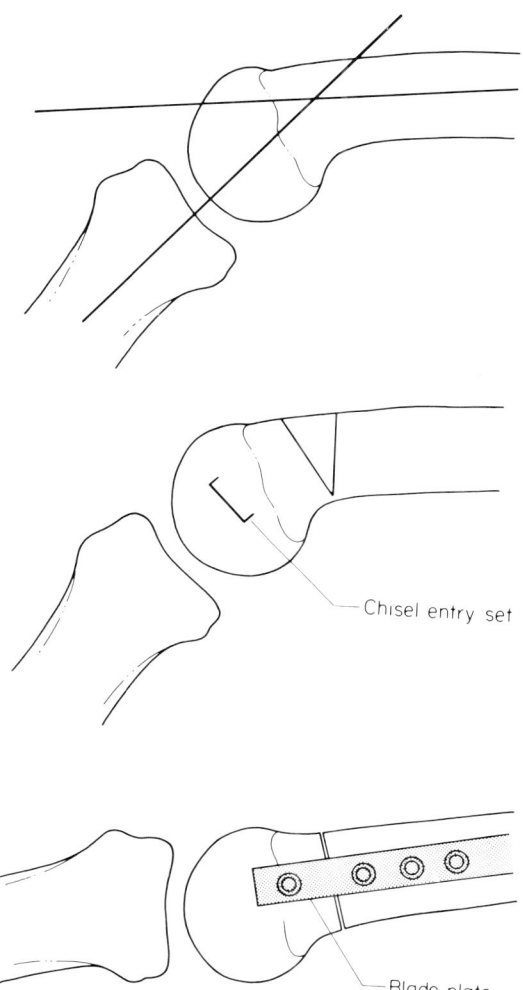

Fig. 9.10. Supracondylar osteotomy. Internal fixation.

Quadriceps femoris paralysis

Isolated quadriceps paralysis or severe weakness is most commonly due to poliomyelitis. If the hamstring muscles are normal in strength they may be transferred to the patella to provide some extension power to the knee thus improving its stability. The results, however, are variable and the surgeon must decide whether substantial surgical procedures of this type will be an advantage since the gait may be satisfactorily controlled by good hip extension power with the knee stabilized in walking by some fixed equinus at the ankle. Prior to this tendon transfer any flexion contractures of the knee must be fully corrected.

It is recommended that both biceps femoris and semitendinosus are transferred (Schwartzmann & Crego 1948).

tendinosus tendon is isolated and detached from its tibial insertion. A subcutaneous tunnel is again made from the anterior transverse knee incision and the tendon is delivered into the prepatellar region.

The prepatellar bursa is reflected and an incision is made through the quadriceps tendon and periosteum over the anterior surface of the patella. Drill holes are made obliquely through

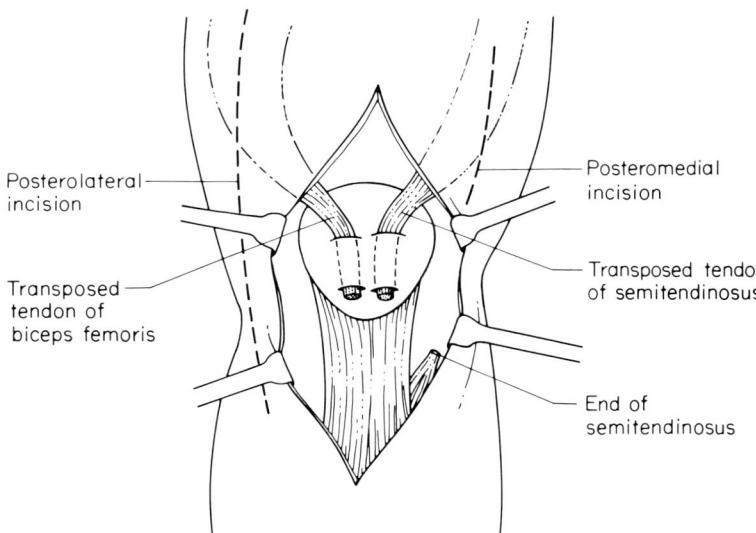

Posterolateral incision

Posteromedial incision

Transposed tendon of biceps femoris

Transposed tendon of semitendinosus

End of semitendinosus

Fig. 9.11. Hamstring tendon transplant.

Hamstring tendon transplantation to the patella (Fig. 9.11)

A longitudinal incision is made over the posterolateral aspect of the thigh from the junction of the proximal and middle thirds to the head of the fibula. The peroneal nerve is identified and retracted. The biceps tendon is isolated and is detached from its insertion at the head of the fibula. A transverse incision is made over the anterior aspect of the knee at the patellar level. The wound flaps are undermined and a subcutaneous tunnel is made. The intermuscular septum and iliotibial band may have to be excised to allow free passage of the transferred muscle belly.

A longitudinal incision is then made on the posteromedial aspect of the thigh and the semi-

the patella (Fig. 9.11). The biceps femoris and semitendinosus tendons are pulled through their respective tunnels and sutured to the patellar tendon under tension. The wound is closed with drainage. Tension on the transferred hamstring muscles is prevented by avoiding flexion of the hip. The patient is kept in bed for three weeks without hip flexion. A long leg cast is applied with the knee in the neutral position for five weeks followed by active and passive flexion of the knee under physiotherapy supervision.

The knee in spastic paralysis

The patient with spastic weakness of the lower limbs most commonly suffers from cerebral palsy. Other causes include:

1 hydrocephalus with cerebral damage;
2 spina bifida with a high myelomeningocele producing an upper motor neurone lesion;
3 other spinal dysraphisms may similarly affect the spinal cord producing a spastic paresis or paralysis.

The child with a spastic diplegia has a scissor-type gait with internal rotation, adduction and flexion of the hips, flexor spasm of the knees and equinus of the ankle (Chapter 2). To consider the knee alone is not possible, but if a decision has been made to attempt surgical correction of the lower limb deformities, the knee will certainly have to be treated.

The patient may not be able to walk at all, in which case a decision has to be made as to whether the patient should remain in a wheel-chair. In this event 90° of knee flexion will give a good lower limb position. If, however, the child is a potential walker an attempt should be made to reduce the flexion spasm of the knee, and if there is a flexion contracture this must be fully released.

Conservative treatment

Both reduction of knee flexion spasms and release of any *minor* flexion contracture may be undertaken by the physiotherapist. Serial splints may be used to increase the knee extension and other orthoses may be required to maintain the final position. The physiotherapist attempts to balance the flexion and extension muscle power. Increased power in the knee extensor apparatus may be attempted with quadriceps muscle drill and careful relaxation therapy.

Operative treatment

The surgeon must be prepared to supervise meticulously the pre-operative, operative and postoperative care in a child with a spastic paresis. Postoperative plasters and splints must be carefully inspected at frequent intervals as pressure problems may be severe. The rehabilitation of the child following any surgical procedure must be undertaken with full cooperation from the physical therapist and the parents as the rehabilitation course may be prolonged.

The main knee problems in spastic paralysis are:

1 flexion contracture;
2 extensor contracture due to quadriceps spasticity;
3 genu recurvatum.

It is considered essential to deal with hip and ankle problems before the knee is finally assessed and treated.

Flexion contractures may be released by posterior soft tissue dissection as described above. Eggers (1950) advocated transplantation of the hamstring tendons to the femoral condyles in order to improve hip extension and to decrease knee flexion in the cerebral palsy patient. If the flexion contractures are severe the release described above is preferable. Fractional lengthening of the hamstrings also has been advocated. The tendinous portion of the biceps femoris, semitendinosus and semimembranosus, are partially divided at two levels leaving the muscle fibres in continuity.

Extension contracture of the knee

This is a rare condition which is caused by excessive spasticity of the quadriceps femoris musculature. Treatment is usually conservative consisting of stretching and serial plasters. If severe, an anterior capsular release and quadriceps lengthening is required.

Genu recurvatum

Genu recurvatum may be excessive and an osteotomy of the upper tibia may be required. This may be undertaken by means of a wedge excision, an osteotomy/osteoclasis technique or the insertion of an anterior wedge graft in the upper tibia (Fig. 9.12).

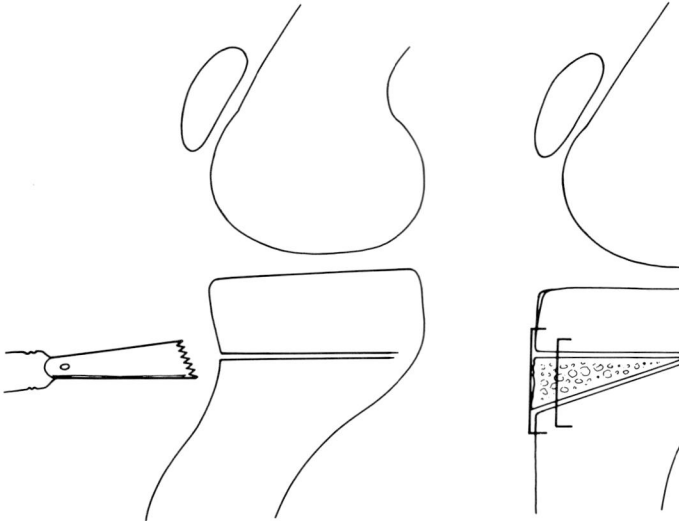

Fig. 9.12. Upper tibial osteotomy with wedge graft insert.

The knee in arthrogryposis multiplex congenita

This is a rare condition characterized by congenital constractures of multiple joints. Originally the aetiology was considered to be a primary disease of joints and Stern (1923) gave it the name 'arthrogryposis multiplex congenita'.

The child with these general congenital abnormalities of mesenchyme may present with very severe and multiple contractures of all limbs. The knees are usually flexed to a greater or lesser degree and a major release procedure may be required. The main points described in the posterior soft tissue release (*see* above) are followed, but the individual tendons are poorly defined and the posterior capsular structures are thick and poorly differentiated.

The knee joint may be held extended or hyperextended with no flexion possible. An anterior capsular release combined with a quadriceps tendon lengthening may be required. Conservative treatment is usually ineffective.

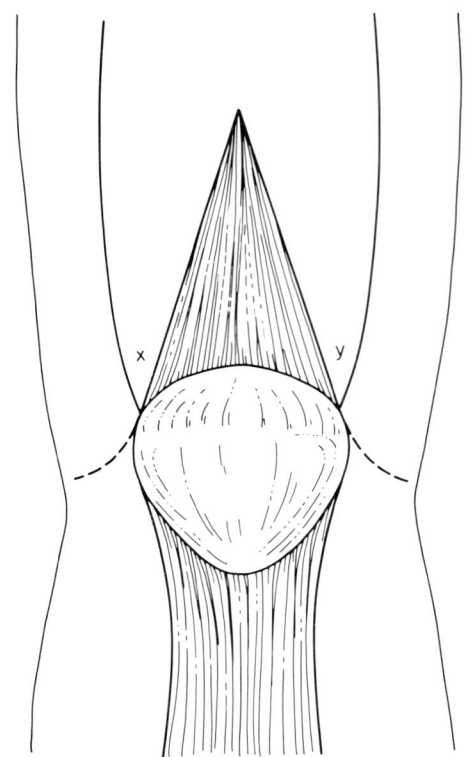

Fig. 9.13. Quadriceps lengthening. An inverted V shaped incision is made in the tendon.

Anterior capsule release and quadriceps lengthening

The knee is approached through a long lateral parapatellar incision after exsanguination and the application of a pneumatic tourniquet.

The quadriceps tendon and surrounding musculature is identified and cleared. An inverted 'V' shaped incision is made in the quadriceps tendon (Fig. 9.13). The quadriceps and patellar expansions are divided alongside the patella and the patellar ligament, the knee is flexed and any remaining tight structures are identified. The iliotibial band and any areas of the anterior capsule which are tight are divided. The tongue of the quadriceps is sutured to the quadriceps defect *with the knee in flexion* using a 'V-Y' plasty of the quadriceps tendon in its lengthening (Fig. 9.14). The wound is closed with drainage and the knee is maintained at 60° flexion in a well padded plaster of Paris cast.

After two to three weeks the wound is inspected and if it has healed passive flexion and extension is undertaken by the physiotherapist. Serial casts in 90° flexion and full extension are helpful in maintaining these positions.

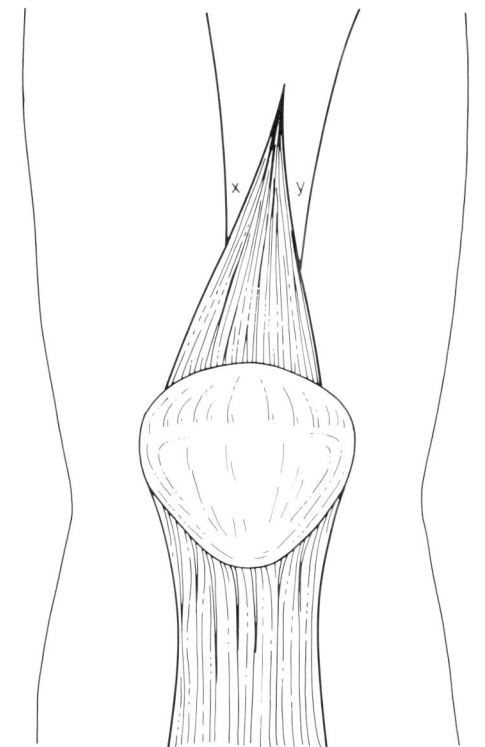

Fig. 9.14. Quadriceps lengthening. Points X and Y are sutured to the superior end of the inverted V.

References

EGGERS G.W.N. (1950) Transplantations of hamstring tendons to the femoral condyles in order to improve hip extension and to decrease knee flexion in cerebral spastic paralysis. *Journal of Bone and Joint Surgery*, **32A**, 80.

SCHWARTZMANN J.R. & CREGO C.H. (1948) Hamstring tendon transplantation for the relief of quadriceps femoris paralysis in residual poliomyelitis. *Journal of Bone and Joint Surgery*, **30A**, 545.

STERN W.G. (1923) Arthrogryposis multiplex congenita. *Journal of the American Medical Association*, **81**, 1507.

Chapter 10
The Orthopaedic Management of Foot Deformity

J. C. DRENNAN

Introduction

The single most important factor in planning the treatment of neuromuscular foot deformities is the establishment of a precise diagnosis. Evaluation must include careful personal and family history and physical examination complemented by appropriate enzyme, muscle biopsy, and electrical studies. The establishment of realistic treatment goals is based upon the orthopaedic surgeon's ability to define the distribution of muscle imbalance and associated neurologic deficiencies coupled with the patient's age, life expectancy, and functional potential. Patients with significant sensory deficit may not only lack pedal protective sensation and proprioception, but also may have very short feet which makes uniform plantar weightbearing distribution an essential objective of treatment. Associated upper extremity paresis may preclude the use of crutches and alter management.

The Heuter–Volkman law of cartilage growth has particular relevance to the skeletally immature foot. The short bones of the hindfoot are unique because the cartilage of the joint surface also provides the only growth plate for the entire bone. Both the articular and growth characteristics respond to compression or tension stresses and may be significantly altered by exceeding the physiologic limit of either form of stress.

The hindfoot has the dual responsibility for accepting body weight at the time of heel strike and serving as the keystone for the two longitudinal foot arches (Duckworth 1983). Hindfoot position is determined by the balance achieved by the four major extrinsic muscle groups. The triceps surae is the dominant muscle and its activity modifies the mechanical advantage of the other groups. This fact can be illustrated by comparing the foot deformities in patients with hereditary motor neuropathies Types I and II (Chapter 5). Type I patients retain triceps surae strength, and weakness in the peroneal and dorsiflexor groups leads to an equinocavovarus deformity. Type II patients combine paresis of the peronei and dorsiflexors with weakness of the triceps surae and a calcaneocavus deformity generally results.

The location of the peroneal tendons behind the lateral malleolus permits these muscles to maintain dynamically the distal fibula in proper alignment at the ankle. Peroneal weakness may result not only in the development of talipes varus but the fibula may also passively migrate posteriorly, thus giving the ankle joint a lateral plane of motion. Failure to recognize this secondary problem makes the joint vulnerable to early degenerative joint disease.

Orthopaedic objectives

Muscle imbalance leads to neuromuscular foot deformity. The orthopaedic goal is to achieve muscle balance and braceable plantigrade feet for both weightbearing and wheelchair activities. This responsibility includes prevention of unnecessary recurrent or iatrogenic deformities (Crego & McCarroll 1938).

Methods of correction

Manipulation and corrective casts

These methods are rarely definitive. Preliminary stretching of the soft tissues, including the neurovascular structures, may permit relaxed approximation of surgical incisions following extensive operative correction. The technique consists of prolonged gentle manipulation and application of well padded casts to retain the correction obtained by the manual stretching. This approach is particularly applicable to infants whose feet are too small for shoes and, therefore, orthoses cannot be used. Wedging casts are contraindicated in patients with insensate feet or dynamic muscle imbalance.

whose dynamic imbalance is limited to the hindfoot. Excessive varus–valgus forces may be managed by distributing pressure medially or laterally over a wide segment of the calf. This can be accomplished by adding a correction door to a plastic ankle–foot orthosis (Lin 1982, Fig. 10.1) or by using a metal upright brace with a wide, soft, leather T-strap.

Problems with orthoses

Shoes are an essential component of lower extremity orthoses. Deficiencies in current shoe design represent the single greatest worldwide problem in lower extremity bracing. Present day shoes are mass produced in one standard width

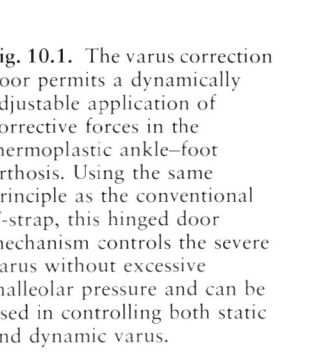
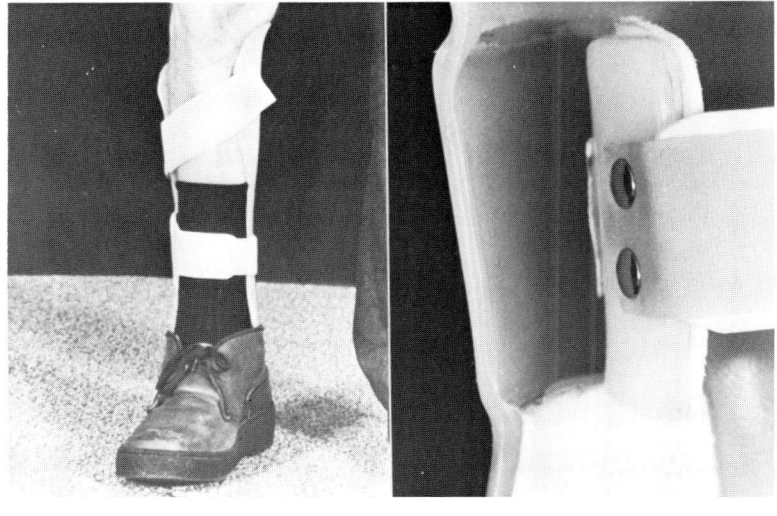

Fig. 10.1. The varus correction door permits a dynamically adjustable application of corrective forces in the thermoplastic ankle–foot orthosis. Using the same principle as the conventional T-strap, this hinged door mechanism controls the severe varus without excessive malleolar pressure and can be used in controlling both static and dynamic varus.

Orthoses

Braces are used to prevent deformity, maintain the corrected position, and permit balanced weight distribution. Paralytic feet require that the orthosis extend the entire length of the foot to prevent paretic forefoot equinus. Stopping the orthosis proximal to the metatarsal heads permits muscle activity during the second half of stance phase and is recommended for patients

per size and have a preform moulded synthetic heel–sole component. The limited shoe selection raises havoc with patients with uncommon feet, either because of increased pedal volume or excessive smallness. The problem is magnified when these patients need to use an ankle–foot orthosis. The functional compromise is selecting either excessively long shoes or athletic shoes. The former choice results in an awkward energy-inefficient gait pattern, while the latter selection is frequently impractical in temperate climates. Current plastic orthoses lack a functional ankle joint which will permit limited controlled ankle motion without the sacrifice of lateral force stability. Plastic orthoses may also fit too snugly to be practical when the patient has involuntary dynamic muscle imbalance.

Types of orthoses

UCBL orthosis   The University of California at Berkeley (UCBL) orthosis is designed to control flexible valgus instability of the subtalar joint and gives the foot architecture maximum passive support (Inman 1969). It is designed so that the combined orthosis and shoe cannot be rolled into a valgus orientation and thereby assures stabilization of the shoe on the walking surface. The orthosis exaggerates the posterior aspect of the longitudinal arch necessary to support the calcaneus in the area of the sustentaculum tali. The orthotic trimline passes beneath the medial malleolus and then rises to permit firm anchoring of the calcaneus. Forefoot pronation is controlled by extending the lateral trimline to the dorsal aspect of the fifth metatarsus. The orthosis stops proximal to the metatarsal heads and the medial trimline extends to the dorsal edge of the first metatarsus. Additional stabilization of hindfoot valgus can be gained by adding the medial Gillette extension modification (Colson 1979). This concept can be incorporated in the design of ankle–foot orthoses.

Ankle–foot orthosis (AFO)   Several clinical options can be included in the AFO design. The posterior leaf spring (PLS) controls paralytic foot drop, but still permits limited ankle motion while giving a dorsiflexion spring assist. This design permits sufficient dorsiflexion to allow a patient to climb stairs or rise from a chair. Combining the UCBL and PLS designs provides better control of the unstable subtalar joint than does the standard solid ankle–foot orthosis.

Greater mediolateral control is accomplished

by carrying the trimlines more anteriorly. The solid ankle AFO prevents excessive plantarflexion in both phases of gait and is of particular advantage to patients walking on a level surface. Forefoot equinus is prevented by extending the orthosis beyond the toes. The design includes a neutral 90° ankle position and is intended to be worn with shoes with a ¼-inch heel lift. The ankle–foot orthosis also partially substitutes for ankle dorsiflexors during the deceleration phase of gait immediately following heel strike to provide shock absorption for the ankle.

The Saltiel floor reaction ankle–foot orthosis   The Saltiel floor reaction AFO is only useful in spastic diplegic and myelomeningocele patients. The anterior shell AFO can be used to provide an extension moment to the knee in patients with a crouch gait (Saltiel 1969). The ground reaction forces are transmitted to the knee through the prepatellar pad (Fig. 10.2). The ankle component of the orthosis must be rigid to permit the extension moment to be applied to the knee during the stance phase of gait (Gage & Drennan 1983). The use of the Saltiel AFO is contraindicated in the presence of a fixed knee- or hip-flexion contracture which must be corrected to establish the prerequisites of full knee and hip extension.

Surgery

Surgical correction in the infant and young child is limited to soft tissue procedures. The joint capsules in rigid newborn foot deformities have never had the benefit of joint excursion and, therefore, can be expected to be contracted, whereas the joint capsules in acquired neuromuscular foot deformities frequently are lax. Surgery in patients under 3 years of age is limited to capsular and tendon surgery. Talectomy, which serves as a functional method of lengthening the tendons spanning the ankle joint, is included in this category. Older patients may require a combination of soft tissue and osseous surgical procedures. Feet that are already short should not undergo surgery that further shortens the bony column. Alternative procedures, such as calcaneal osteotomies and metatarsal osteotomies (Fig. 10.3), may be preferred. Patients with diminished proprioception

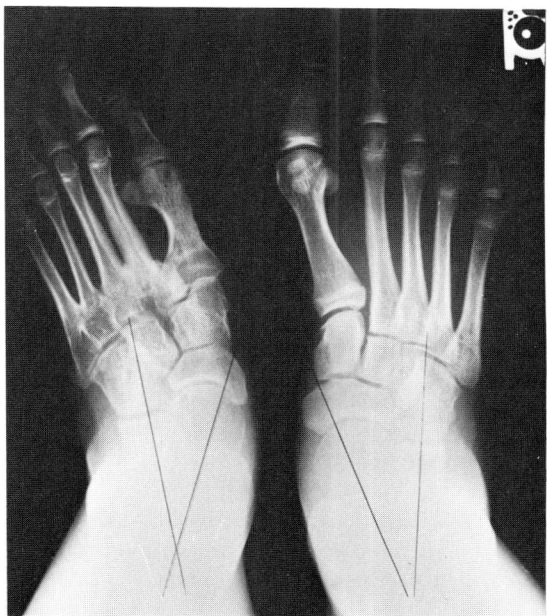

Fig. 10.3. An injudicious proximal first metatarsal osteotomy resulted in premature growth arrest. The metatarsal shortening precluded the toe-off segment of stance phase in this 12-year-old hemiplegic patient who also has developed a secondary bunion.

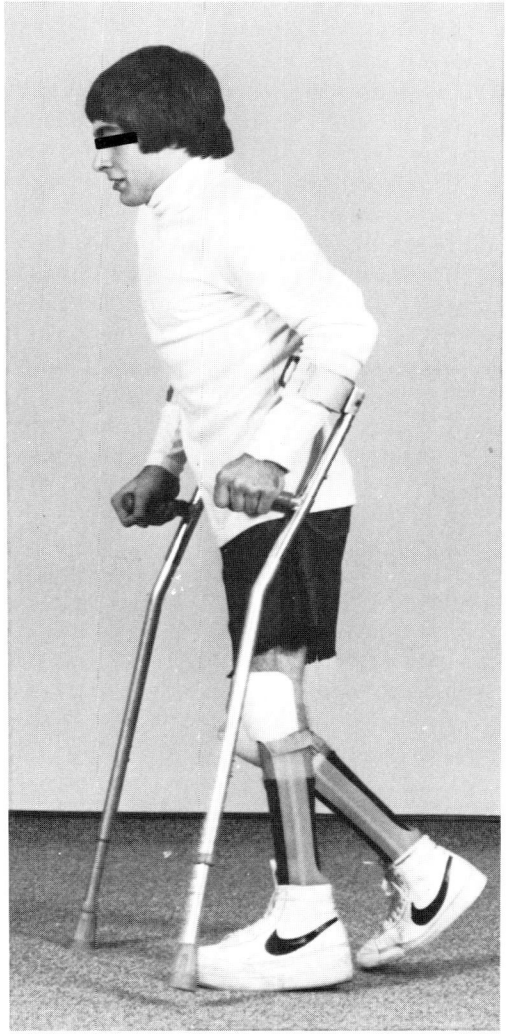

Fig. 10.2. The application of the ground reaction force to the anterior aspect of the knee provides a stabilizing knee-extension moment during the stance phase of gait. The Newington Children's Hospital's anterior floor reaction orthosis is used primarily with spastic diplegics who have no residual knee-flexion contracture.

are poor candidates for subtalar or triple arthrodeses, since these procedures may precipitate the development of neurotrophic changes in the remaining joints which must compensate for the motion sacrificed at the time of arthrodesis.

The level of the neurologic lesion provides the basis for the following outline of foot deformities. The discussion of upper motor neuron disorders will be followed by presentations of lesions at the different levels of the motor unit.

Cerebral palsy (upper motor neuron)

Cerebral palsy foot deformities result from dynamic muscle imbalance. No deformities are present at birth. Changes in muscle tone, the effect of gravity, and positioning during the first few months of life lead to postural and eventually fixed acquired deformity. Additional factors, including weightbearing, the position of the other lower extremity joints, and the presence or absence of equilibrium reactions, further alter the foot deformities which require orthopaedic management.

The incidence of cerebral palsy remains constant at 1–2 per 1,000 live births in the Western World (Jones 1975). The ability to control Rh factor incompatibility has led to a remarkable decrease in the number of athetoid patients. Conversely, the increased survival rate of premature infants has led to a dramatic increase in spastics, especially diplegics. Nearly all cerebral palsy patients have feet of normal length.

Types of cerebral palsy (Chapter 1)

Spasticity, the most common form, results from an insult to the pyramidal–extrapyramidal system which decreases cortical control over selective muscle function and limits lower extremity activities to gross motor patterns. Extensor tone dominates the lower limb and is expressed as plantarflexion at the ankle joint. The extensor position is enhanced in weightbearing because of stimulation of the hyperexcitable muscle spindles in the plantar intrinsic musculature.

Diplegia represents the most common group and becomes clinically evident during the second half of the first year when extensor tone spreads into the lower extremities. Motor milestones are delayed and most diplegics begin to ambulate between 2 and 3 years of age. The presence of extensor tone coupled with overactive plantarflexors may lead to a fixed equinus. Young patients combine an unsteady upright posture with typical ligamentous laxity. Their standing stability is increased by the resulting adaptive hindfoot equinovalgus and forefoot pronation. Postural forefoot pronation favours peroneal overactivity which leads to a secondary hindfoot eversion which then permits further contraction of both the heel cord and peronei and a fixed equinovalgus deformity results.

Infantile presentation of spastic *hemiplegia* includes a lack of reciprocal kicking or a tendency for unilateral fisting of one hand. The average age of ambulation is 21 months. Most commonly, an equinovarus deformity develops due to overactivity of the triceps surae and tibialis posterior coupled with a minor limb length difference. The rare patient with a significant limb length difference may develop both hindfoot and forefoot equinus. The shorter limb is effectively a balance limb which accepts less weight in stance than the longer limb.

A minority of patients with *total body involvement* will ambulate.

Movement disorders result from lesions in the basal ganglia. Athetosis describes gross, uncoordinated movements most visible in the proximal joints. The patient is unable to maintain stable extremity positioning in space and is further handicapped by abnormal involuntary movements present only when the patient is awake. Dystonia (tension athetosis) clinically mimics spasticity. Repeated examinations demonstrate a dramatic decrease in the apparent hypertonicity. Failure to recognize this small group of patients results in serious postoperative problems, particularly following ill advised heel cord lengthening.

Management

Most foot surgery is performed for patients who are either ambulatory or have the potential to walk with or without crutches. Ideally, surgery is performed between ages 5 and 7 years under one general anaesthetic (Bleck 1979). Nonambulatory patients with fixed soft tissue contractures which interfere with function are also candidates for surgery. The patient with a significant equinus that interferes with pivot transfer technique is an example.

Equinus

Surgery is indicated when the triceps surae contracture does not permit the foot to be brought to neutral dorsiflexion when measured with the hindfoot in an inverted position even when the knee is flexed. Lengthening of the gastrocnemius-soleus muscle also decreases the exaggerated heel cord stretch reflex. Overlengthening favours dorsiflexion overactivity and the development of a calcaneal deformity and is most likely to occur when an isolated heel cord lengthening is performed in the presence of concomitant untreated hip- and knee-flexion contractures.

Techniques for Z-lengthening of the heel cord   The tendon sheath of the Achilles tendon is identified and incised through a medial longitudinal incision. A coronal lengthening is recommended. The anterior half of the tendon is divided near its insertion. The proximal transverse incision divides the superficial half of the tendon, thus permitting the residual exposed surface to be covered by the thick distal calf subcutaneous fat. When a varus element is present, the tendon is lengthened in the sagittal plane and the distal incision is made medially near the insertion of the calcaneus to decrease the secondary invertor activity of the triceps surae. Conversely, the distal incision is placed laterally when the foot has an equinovalgus deformity. The foot is manually dorsiflexed to neutral and then permitted passively to assume an equinus position while the tendon repair is performed with nonabsorbable mattress sutures. Passive dorsiflexion to neutral documents that sufficient muscle tension remains in the triceps surae and that no dorsiflexion can occur. Postoperatively, a long leg cast is applied with the knee in slight flexion and the foot in neutral position. The cast may be shortened in 3 weeks to permit knee rehabilitation. An ankle–foot orthosis and regular shoes are then employed. The goal for spastic diplegic and hemiplegic patients is to have them free of braces for daytime activities 6 months after the introduction of full-time use of the orthosis. Continuous nighttime splinting is recommended during the growth years. Recurrent equinus occurs in less than 10% of patients with this programme (Sharrard & Bernstein 1972).

Gastrocnemius lengthening   Electromyographic evaluation permits distinction between gastrocnemius and soleus spasticity. Isolated gastrocnemius phase distortion or clonus can be improved by gastrocnemius recession, whereas combined soleus and gastrocnemius overactivity require heel cord lengthening. Baker (1956) describes a 'tongue in groove' method of lengthening the aponeurotic tendon of the gastrocnemius which includes dissection of the central aponeurotic tendon of the soleus. This rarely indicated procedure causes extensive scar formation because of the amount of muscle stripping required and has a higher rate of recurrence than Z-lengthening of the heel cord.

Soleus neurectomy   This rarely indicated procedure has its only application when there is a severe functional equinus or clonus and is not appropriate when the triceps surae has a fixed contracture. Precise identification of the motor nerves to the soleus by means of electrical stimulation with a coated needle and clinical assessment after the introduction of 2 mm of procaine through this needle, should be prerequisites before formal surgical resection of the motor nerves is carried out.

Equinovarus deformity

Equinovarus deformity develops in hemiplegics or nonambulatory patients with total body involvement. Serial corrective long leg casts followed by the use of straight last shoes with a Denis Browne bar offer an effective management programme in young, total body involved patients.

Mild fixed equinovarus deformity in the ambulatory young hemiplegic patient can be managed by combining an intramuscular lengthening of the tibialis posterior with a heel cord lengthening. Should fixed forefoot equinus deformity develop in the skeletally immature patient, a staged intrinsic release and posterior tibial lengthening followed by a split anterior tibial tendon transfer (SPLATT procedure) has proved effective (Hoffer *et al.* 1974). Posterior tibial transfer is not recommended because of the high incidence of iatrogenic equinovalgus deformities which result. The split anterior tibial transfer is performed in skeletally immature patients with spastic hindfoot varus who demonstrate inappropriate anterior tibial continuous activity on electromyographic testing.

Technique of the SPLATT procedure The insertion of the tibialis anterior tendon is identified through an incision placed over the dorsomedial aspect of the first metatarsus. The tendon frequently can be split bluntly through its natural divison and the lateral half isolated by a nonabsorbable suture. An anterior distal calf incision permits the passage of a hemostat beneath the dorsal retinaculum into the first incision. The suture is brought into the second wound while it bluntly splits the tendon. The lateral half of the anterior tibial tendon is then released at its insertion. A third incision is made over the cuboid and the freed lateral half of the tendon is passed subcutaneously into a drill hole made through the bone. A button placed on a nonweightbearing area of the medial longitudinal arch serves as the fixation point for the nonabsorbable Bunnel woven suture in the transferred tendon. Following 5 weeks of immobilization in a short leg cast, the patient employs an ankle–foot orthosis. Daytime orthotic control is necessary for 6 months and prolonged use of a night-time orthosis is recommended.

Split posterior tibial tendon transfer Green *et al.* (1983) and Kaufer (1977) have reported favourable results of combining a split posterior tibial transfer with heel cord lengthening in children with a flexible spastic equinovarus gait whose electromyograms demonstrate disphasic activity of the posterior tibial muscle. Normally, that muscle is not active during the swing phase of gait. The split posterior tibial tendon transfer maintains the plantarflexion strength of the posterior tibial muscle and, therefore, avoids the potential complication of a calcaneal deformity when the transfer is combined with a heel cord lengthening.

Technique of split posterior tibial tendon transfer The tendon is split longitudinally at its insertion at the navicular and the plantar half dissected from the bone. A second incision in the posteromedial distal calf exposes the posterior tibial tendon which is then split longitudinally to the musculotendinous junction. By blunt dissection, the freed half of the tendon is passed laterally deep to the neurovascular structures and the long toe flexor tendons. The peroneus brevis tendon is identified and its sheath split longitudinally through an incision made directly posterior to the lateral malleolus. A tendon passer is used to assist in transferring the freed half of the posterior tibial tendon into the open sheath of the peroneus brevis tendon. A fourth incision exposes the insertion of the peroneus brevis at the base of the fifth metatarsal bone. The distal stump of the posterior tibial tendon is brought into the wound and sutured to the peroneus brevis tendon by weaving it in and out of the tendon. Tension is adjusted to permit the hindfoot to rest in a neutral position at the conclusion of surgery. The heel cord lengthening precedes the procedure described. Postoperatively, a weightbearing, long leg cast is used for 4 weeks and then a short walking cast is applied for an additional 4-week period. No further immobilization is recommended.

Calcaneal osteotomy The Dwyer (1959) technique can be used to correct rigid hindfoot varus or valgus deformity in growing children. The procedure is most commonly used in managing heel varus and may be combined with a release of the intrinsic muscles and plantar fascia. A laterally based closing wedge resection is used when the heel is of adequate height and size. An incision placed a half inch below the palpable peroneal tendons is used for exposure. The wedge to be removed rarely exceeds a quarter inch. Two parallel osteotomies outline the lateral aspect of the wedge and are directed to meet at the medial aspect of the os calcis. An effort is made to retain the medial cortex as an intact hinge. Placing an awl in the tuber assists in the satisfactory closure of the osteotomy site. Stability is achieved by using a Kirschner wire or staple.

Equinovalgus deformity

Equinovalgus deformity is most common in ambulatory spastic diplegics or paraplegics. Heel cord lengthening and longterm use of a UCBL shoe insert are recommended when the valgus is flexible. Soft tissue surgery has proved ineffective with a fixed deformity and, therefore, a subtalar extra-articular arthrodesis combined with a heel cord lengthening is the procedure of choice in patients over 3 years of age (Grice 1952). The Dennyson modification (Dennyson & Fulford 1976) of the subtalar extra-articular arthrodesis is recommended.

Techniques of the subtalar extra-articular arthrodesis An Ollier incision extending from the midline of the dorsum of the ankle to the peroneal tendons beneath the lateral malleolus is used. The contents of the sinus tarsi are sharply freed up and reflected distally. A small curette is used to decorticate the cancellous bone on the medial aspect of the undersurface of the neck of the talus and nonarticular calcaneal surface. The lateral cortical bone in this area is preserved to permit four-cortex fixation with the Sherman screw which is used for rigid internal fixation. The anterior surface of the talar neck is exposed by blunt dissection between the tendon of the extensor digitorum longus and the anterior tibial neurovascular bundle.

A Kirschner wire is drilled across the neck of the talus into the calcaneus, exiting through the inferolateral cortex of the calcaneus. Radiographic verification of the reduction and measurement for the length of the Sherman screw are obtained. An awl is used to begin a second talar neck site and an appropriate length screw introduced until its head bites into the superior surface of the talus. The Kirschner wire is then

removed. The sinus tarsi is filled with autogenous iliac cancellous chips and its contents reattached. The author prefers to delay weight-bearing for 6 weeks and then continue plaster immobilization until an oblique radiograph demonstrates satisfactory incorporation of the graft into both bones of the hindfoot (Fig. 10.4). Longterm use of an ankle–foot orthosis is recommended in the skeletally immature patient.

Triple arthrodesis This procedure is reserved for patients who are nearing skeletal maturity. Radical capsulotomies are required to mobilize the bones of the hindfoot and to permit limited bony resection to avoid excessive shortening of the foot in length and height which may create footwear problems. Both the calcaneocuboid and talonavicular joints require staple fixation in these patients.

Bunions

Painful hallux valgus develops as a secondary deformity in ambulatory patients with severe equinovalgus feet. The overactive peroneus longus everts the hindfoot and forefoot, shifting the peroneal sheath origin of the adductor hallucis proximally and laterally, thus increasing its mechanical advantage. The great toe pronates and moves laterally because of increased weight-bearing on its medial and inferior surfaces. The McKeever metatarsophalangeal arthrodesis (McKeever 1952, Renshaw *et al.* 1979) is recommended.

Hereditary spinal and cerebellar degenerative disease (upper and lower motor neuron)

These patients frequently combine both peripheral and central nervous system involvement which is slowly progressive over decades. Friedreich's ataxia is the most common form of spinal cerebellar degenerative disease and usu-

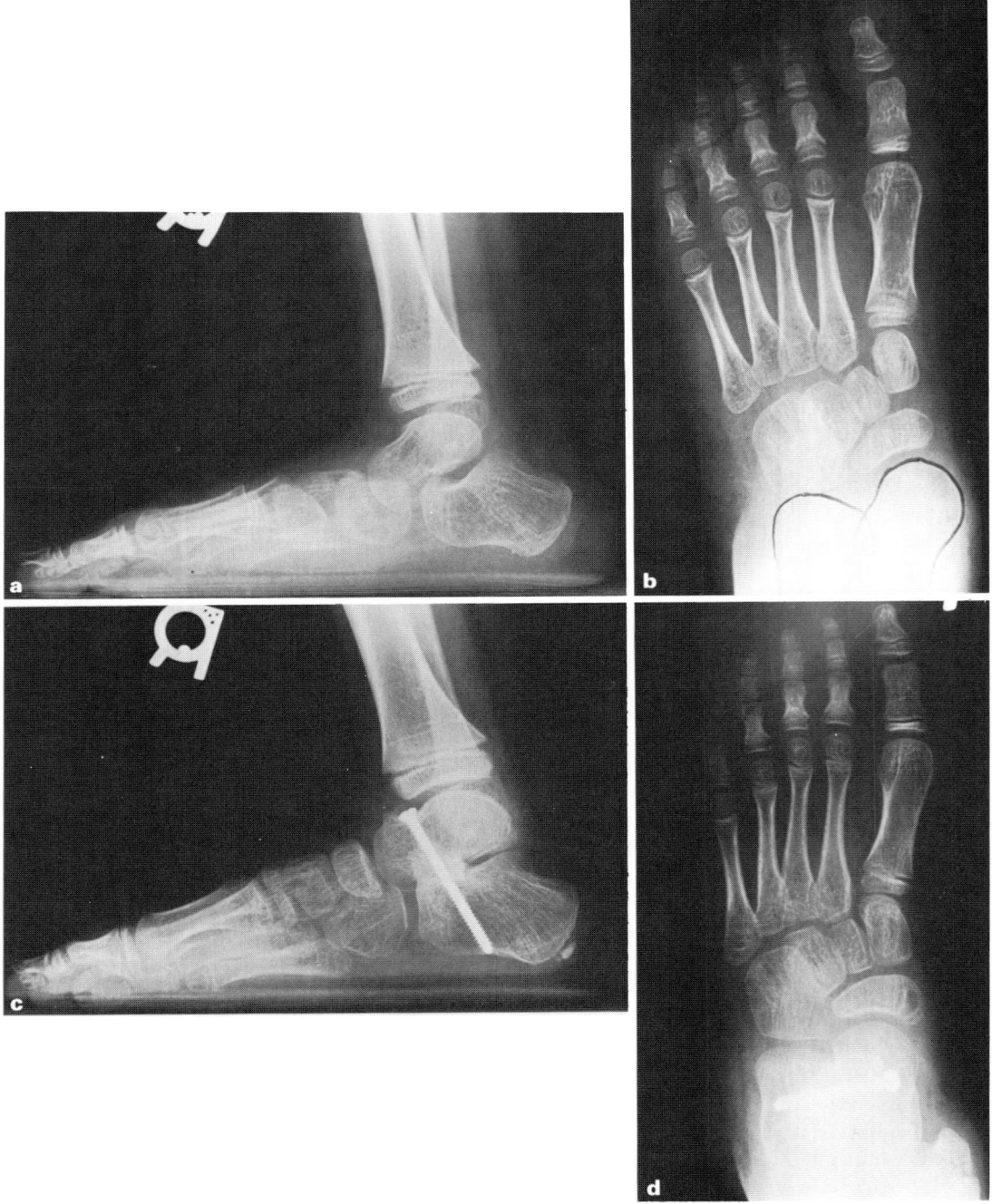

Fig. 10.4. (a) and (b) X-rays of an equinovalgus deformity in a 10-year-old spastic diplegic patient. (c) and (d) Correction following subtalar arthrodesis.

ally presents with an unsteady gait before the age of 10 years. A positive Romberg sign, unsteady widebased gait, and decreased vibration and position sense are present early. Distal weakness of the lower extremities and intrinsic muscles of the feet is out of proportion to the degree of severity of the disease. Late in the first decade, the foot develops a cavus deformity which is symmetric and progressive. Initially flexible, it soon becomes fixed and may develop a heel varus component. Intrinsic muscle wasting adds to the extrinsic muscle imbalance and contributes to the developing cavus. A Dwyer calcaneal closing wedge osteotomy with plantar intrinsic release (Dwyer 1959) and the longterm use of an ankle–foot orthosis has been effective. Eventually, a triple arthrodesis may be required for stabilization (Levitt *et al.* 1973). The gains from this procedure must be carefully weighed since there is considerable risk that the patient will suffer loss of ambulation following the period of immobilization. Jones and Hibbs procedures (Jones 1916, Hibbs 1919) coupled with arthrodeses of interphalangeal joints may eventually be needed for painful clawed toes in the adult patient.

Myelomeningocele (upper and lower motor neuron)

The neurologic involvement of the lower limb in myelomeningocele patients combines lower and upper motor neuron lesions. A minority of patients present with a complete loss of motor and sensory function below a specific segmental level. More commonly, the interruption of the long spinal tracts is accompanied by the presentation of reflex activity in isolated caudal segments. The lower lumbar and sacral nerve roots innervate the extrinsic and intrinsic muscles of the foot and ankle and are the neurologic levels most commonly involved in myelomeningocele.

Most myelomeningocele infants have foot deformities (Sharrard & Grosfield 1968). Muscle imbalance is the primary cause of the defor-

mity and results from imbalance between normal, flaccid, and spastic muscles. The feet are small, insensate, and frequently demonstrate vasomotor instability.

The rehabilitation goal is to obtain plantigrade, braceable feet when the child begins to stand at about 15 to 18 months of age. Muscle balance must be obtained to avoid recurrence or a secondary iatrogenic deformity. Inability to achieve a plantigrade position in an anaesthetic foot may lead to the development of pressure sores, cellulitis, or osteomyelitis. These complications generally respond to local management and rarely require ray resection or foot amputation.

Management

Treatment should be initiated in the newborn nursery with a series of manipulations and the application of serial plaster casts. The objective is to achieve and to maintain maximum possible correction until the foot is large enough to be shoed so orthotic control can be introduced.

Soft tissue procedures are recommended in the younger child. Surgery should be deferred until the infant is at least 9 months of age at which time a definitive assessment of muscle imbalance is possible. Accurate preoperative clinical and faradic evaluation is required for the selection of the appropriate transfer of a muscle under voluntary control. Deforming reflex muscles are tenotomized. Very deliberate surgery is required because of the small size of the hindfoot osseocartilaginous structures and the narrow joints surrounded by dense capsules. The surgeon must be aware that these cartilage cells have the dual responsibility for growth as well as articular function. Capsulotomies, tendon lengthenings, or tenotomies are performed through carefully planned surgical incisions. A loosely applied, bulky dressing and a posterior long leg plaster splint is used initially because of expected soft tissue swelling and can be followed several days later by the application of a well padded long leg cast which extends beyond the visualized anaesthetic toes to protect them from pressure sores.

Osseous surgery is limited to ambulatory patients in older age groups who require a stable plantigrade foot with good weight distribution between the hindfoot and forefoot during both stance and walking. Surgical procedures that do not include arthrodesis avoid excessive foot shortening and retain joint motion and proprioception. Bony deformities must be corrected before tendon transfers can be performed. Many of the specific tendon and bony surgical techniques are discussed in other sections of this chapter.

Equinovarus deformity

This common problem results from an imbalance of the paralyzed dorsiflexors and peroneus muscles and the retained activity of the tibialis anterior and posterior muscles (Smith & Duckworth 1976). Capsulotomies of the posterior ankle, subtalar, and talonavicular joints are required as well as lengthening of the Achilles tendon, tibialis posterior, and long toe flexors. The tibialis anterior may be transferred laterally into the third cuneiform. Talectomy offers an alternative in the severe equinovarus foot but remains successful only when muscle balance is achieved (Menelaus 1971).

Equinus deformity

Equinus can result either from a flail foot or from an extremity that retains unopposed reflex activity in the triceps surae and long toe flexors. Paralytic equinus can be prevented by proper physical therapy and the use of shoes with a plantar stop brace. Equinus exceeding 40 degrees may require a percutaneous tenotomy of the Achilles tendon. Reflex equinus deformity is more difficult to manage and recurrences are frequent. Radical excision of the Achilles tendon and the long toe reflexors may be carried out but repeated procedures may be required.

Equinovalgus deformity

Overactivity of the peroneus muscles and a shortened Achilles tendon lead to this deformity. Surgery is delayed until after the age of one year when the peroneus longus is transferred to augment the paretic tibialis posterior and its distal stump anastomosed to the mobilized peroneus brevis. The Achilles tendon is lengthened through a separate incision.

Valgus deformity of the hindfoot in an older child requires careful assessment. Limited experience at Newington Children's Hospital with both extra-articular subtalar arthrodesis and triple arthrodesis performed for low-level lumbar myelomeningocele patients suggests that satisfactory longterm plantigrade feet can be

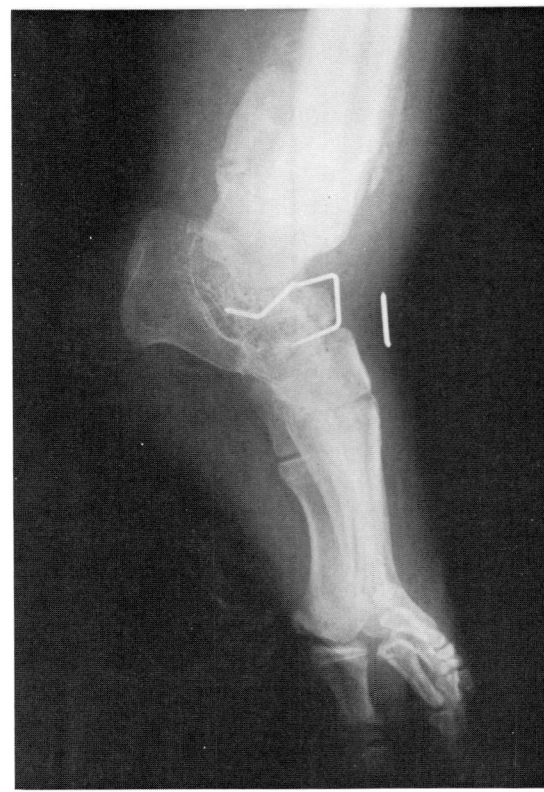

Fig. 10.5. A triple arthrodesis in a 13-year-old myelomeningocele patient resulted in talar avascular necrosis and a neurotrophic fracture through the distal tibial growth plate.

obtained. Patients who lack proprioception generally do not benefit from arthrodeses and demonstrate a higher rate of nonunion and neurotrophic ankle joint changes (Fig. 10.5) than in other foot deformities.

A weightbearing anteroposterior roentgenogram of the ankle joint distinguishes ankle valgus from true hindfoot valgus. Ankle valgus in the young child may be managed by tenodesis of the tendo calcaneus to the fibula (Dias 1978). Stapling of the medial part of the distal tibial epiphysis is recommended when the child is between ages 8 to 12 years (Burkus *et al.* 1983). Supramalleolar osteotomy is reserved for patients nearing skeletal maturity because of risk of affecting the distal tibial epiphysis (Sharrard & Webb 1974).

Calcaneus deformity

This rare deformity results from unopposed function of the ankle and toe dorsiflexors. After initial treatment with manipulations and casting, the patient at one year of age may undergo transfer of the combined tendons of the tibialis anterior and peroneus tertius through the interosseous membrane to the os calcis. The remaining long toe extensors are tenotomized. The heel cord may require shortening. Bracing is required, limiting ankle dorsiflexion to 10 degrees.

Congenital convex pes valgus

This rigid deformity is caused by strong evertors and dorsiflexors of the foot that overpower the paretic tibialis posterior (Drennan & Sharrard 1971). Surgical correction can be performed through a one stage procedure that combines soft tissue releases and tendon transfers. The technique described under arthrogryposis is complemented by the tendon transfer of the peroneus longus to the navicular to augment the paretic tibialis posterior. Longterm use of UCBL shoe inserts is recommended.

Arthrogryposis multiplex congenita (congenital anterior horn cell)

Arthrogryposis is a rare disorder characterized by nonprogressive multiple rigid joints present at birth. The pathophysiology of this clinical syndrome has not been established and the name remains descriptive. The presence of normal sensation and the histologic demonstration of an absent or decreased number of anterior horn cells in the lumbar and cervical enlargements localize the site of the lesion.

Diarthrodial joints are freely movable and are characterized by a prominent joint cavity between the mobile skeletal parts which are held with a peripheral fibrous capsule. The joint cavity arises in the third month from clefts in the dense mesenchyme located circumferentially between the prospective bones. These clefts progress in a central direction until they meet. The sleevelike capsule is derived from the denser peripheral tissue that borders the cavity and its fibres are continuous with the perichondrium. Joints develop in arthrogryposis but the periarticular soft tissue structures becomes fibrotic, leading to the development of an incomplete fibrous ankylosis.

Clinical features

Limb involvement is usually quadrimelic, although there is a large group of patients who have only lower extremity involvement (Gibson & Urs 1970, Lloyd-Roberts & Lettin 1970). Involved limbs tend to have symmetrical rigid joints with the distal parts of the extremity more involved. The classic arthrogrypotic pedal deformities present at birth include talipes equinovarus (Fig. 10.6) and congenital convex pes valgus.

The diagnosis must be accurately established in the newborn period. Thorough evaluation should rule out more common congenital abnormalities. The back and neck are examined for evidence of spinal dysraphism and sacral agenesis. Radiographs may be necessary to rule

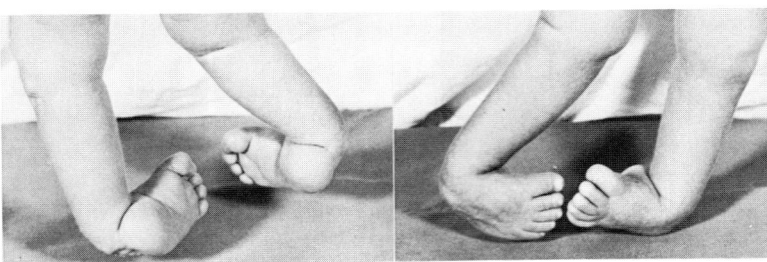

Fig. 10.6. Rigid talipes equinovarus deformity in an arthrogrypotic newborn. The deep skin clefts suggest that talectomy will be required for satisfactory plantigrade correction.

out spinal dysraphism, skeletal dysplasia, or Turner's syndrome.

Management

Neonatal foot deformities should be approached by serial manipulation and plaster casting. Arthrogrypotic foot deformities are usually severe and associated with very limited ankle and tarsal motion. Untreated, they result in difficulty in walking, shoe fitting, and may lead to the development of pain and ulceration with attempted weightbearing. The newborn plaster technique may partially correct the deformity but it will promptly recur when this nonsurgical treatment programme is interrupted.

Talipes equinovarus

Surgical correction should be performed before the young child begins to walk. The orthopaedic goal is to create a stiff plantigrade foot. Posteromedial release, tendon transfers, and tenotomies have proved ineffective. Talectomy, performed at 12–18 months of age, results in a satisfactory longterm plantigrade foot (Drummond & Cruess 1978). This procedure is one of the most difficult technical operations in paediatric orthopaedics.

Technique for talectomy   An Ollier incision is employed. A fine-tipped hemostat is used to define the individual joints, which are narrow and have a relative capsular thickening. The

ankle joint is first identified. The entire bone is enucleated. Meticulous attention to detail is required because small cartilaginous fragments left behind eventually ossify and may lead to a recurrent deformity. The posterior capsule is divided through the incision in order to be able to displace the foot posteriorly, thereby creating a heel. It is sometimes necessary to remove the navicular to gain sufficient posterior displacement. An Achilles tendon tenotomy is performed through a short separate posterior incision. The fibula or calcaneus may require careful shaving and remodelling to permit satisfactory calcaneal alignment in the ankle mortise. The calcaneus must be aligned with the ankle joint. A Kirschner wire is passed through the heel into the tibia and is removed after 3 weeks. Plaster immobilization is continued for 3 months and the foot is then held in a rigid ankle–foot orthosis, which extends the entire length of the foot to prevent paralytic forefoot equinus. Orthotic control is required until the child reaches skeletal maturity because recurrence of the deformity cannot be surgically corrected in the immature child. A supramalleolar osteotomy performed in childhood to correct a recurrent deformity would result in the migration of the compensatory tibial deformity into the diaphysis and create a bizarre new shape to that bone.

Congenital convex pes valgus

Two separate types of congenital vertical tali are recognizable. The more common form represents a dislocation of the medial longitudinal

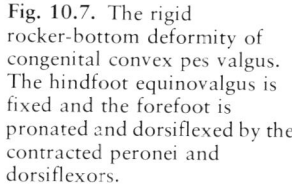
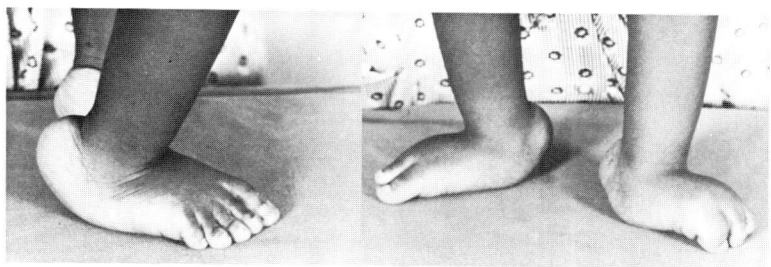

Fig. 10.7. The rigid rocker-bottom deformity of congenital convex pes valgus. The hindfoot equinovalgus is fixed and the forefoot is pronated and dorsiflexed by the contracted peronei and dorsiflexors.

arch at the talonavicular joint (Fig. 10.7) while the more severe form includes a dislocation of the lateral longitudinal arch through the calcaneocuboid joint (Drennan & Sharrard 1971). Both types of the deformity are rigid and require surgical correction. The surgery should be performed before the patient begins to ambulate. Correction must be complete or the deformity will recur.

Technique of surgical correction (Drennan 1976) A one-stage procedure employing the Cincinnati posterior incision is recommended (Crawford *et al.* 1982). The incision extends from the first cuneiform circumferentially to the cuboid on the lateral aspect of the foot. Radical capsular release of the posterior ankle, subtalar, and talonavicular joints are performed as well as complete release of the calcaneocuboid joint when indicated. All extrinsic muscles to the foot are tenotomized on both the anterior and posterior aspects of the ankle. No tendon transfers are performed in the arthrogrypotic vertical talus. The completely mobilized hindfoot bones require Kirschner wire fixation for stability. The first pin is passed through the heel into the os calcis and the talus to control hindfoot valgus and equinus. The foot alignment is then reassessed and a second Kirschner wire used to transfix the talonavicular joint (Fig. 10.8). The third wire stabilizes the calcaneocuboid joint and prevents pronation of the forefoot. A long leg plaster cast is required for 4 months and an ankle–foot orthosis employing the Gillette modification of the UCBL insert is then used (Colson 1979).

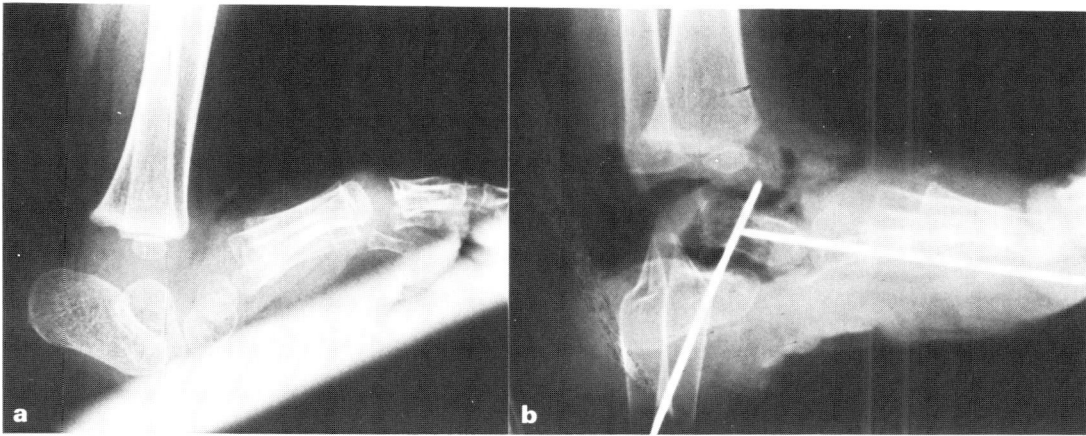

Fig. 10.8. (a) Congenital convex pes valgus.
(b) Intra-operative radiograph demonstrates correction of the plantarflexed talus and calcaneus. A third Kirschner wire through the calcaneocuboid joint was necessary to correct the persistent forefoot pronation.

Foot surgery in the older child

Triple arthrodesis with limited bone resection may be necessary in patients with residual deformities related to talipes equinovarus. A closing wedge or rotational supramalleolar osteotomy can be performed to correct a number of deformities in the area of the ankle joint in the adolescent. Most commonly, the wedge is based anteriorly and the varus may be corrected by including lateral resection.

Pantalar arthrodesis also has been carried out in skeletally mature patients as the recurrence of the deformity following triple arthrodesis usually is at the ankle. Occasionally, forefoot equinus develops causing a significant cavus which can be corrected either by a closing dorsal wedge osteotomy through the mid-foot or metatarsal osteotomies. On the rare occasions when calcaneovalgus occurs in the child with arthrogryposis, it presents no management problems and should be left untreated.

Table 10.1 Classification of spinal muscular atrophy based on maximum functional achievement

I	No sitting balance. Poor head control.
II	Sitting balance and head control.
III	Limited ability to walk, with or without orthoses.
IV	Walk, run, and climb stairs normally.

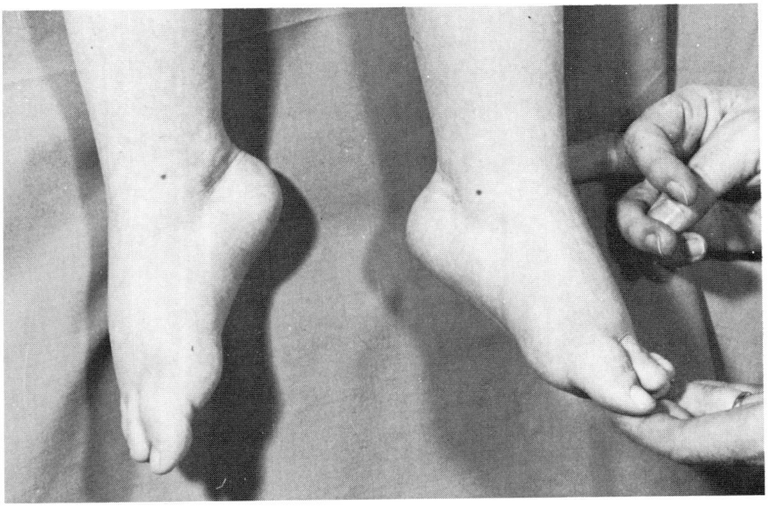

recessive pattern (Russman *et al.* 1983). The degree of clinical involvement can be used as a practical guide, both to prognosis and types of foot deformity (Table 10.1, Drennan 1983). Lower extemity contractures develop early and are most marked in the severely paralysed patient (Fig. 10.9, Evans *et al.* 1981). In infants with severe muscle weakness, foot deformities begin to develop during the first year of life. Significant foot contractures rarely develop in patients in Group III before they reach 10 years of age or before they have lost the ability to walk. Equinus deformity develops in approximately half of the patients in Group I and II.

Fig. 10.9. Gravity plays a major role in the development of fixed equinus contractures in patients with spinal muscle atrophy.

Spinal muscular atrophy (congenital anterior horn cell)

Spinal muscular atrophy is a progressive chronic degeneration of the anterior horn cells in the spinal cord and is transmitted by an autosomal

Forefoot equinus also may develop occasionally in Group IV patients.

Soft tissue surgery is recommended for correcting ankle and foot deformities and has been well tolerated by selected patients. Indications include relief of pressure that may lead to skin ulceration over the talar head or the fifth metatarsus, and to allow the application of normal footwear. The ability to wear shoes improves the appearance of the feet and allows them to be placed properly on a foot rest to distribute weight. Talectomies, as well as soft tissue releases, can be performed.

Poliomyelitis (acquired anterior horn cell)

Anterior poliomyelitis is an acute viral infection with localization in the anterior horn cells of the spinal cord, especially in the lumbar and cervical enlargements. Paralysis occurs twice as frequently in the lower extremity muscles when compared with those in the upper extremity. The tibialis anterior is commonly involved. The sacral nerve roots are spared, resulting in characteristic sparing of the intrinsic muscles of the foot. The major clinical recovery occurs during the first month following acute illness and is nearly complete by the sixth month.

Acute stage

The acute phase of poliomyelitis generally lasts 7–10 days. Muscles are tender, even to gentle palpation. Efforts to stretch irritated muscles may increase the reflex muscle spasm. Fixed contractures develop during the acute stage because of flexion and equinus positioning of the extremities. The combination of an irritated muscle and the force of gravity permit the foot to go into an equinus position and the antagonistic muscles are too weak to oppose the irritated muscle groups. The spastic triceps surae cause rapid development of a fixed equinus, preventing recovery of the overstretched dorsiflexors. This can be avoided by placing the feet in a supine patient against a padded foot board (Green & Grice 1951). Adequate space should be allowed at the lower end of the mattress to permit the foot to rest in a neutral position when the patient is placed in the alternate prone pos-

ition. Gentle passive range of motion, preceded by the application of moist heat, should be carried out on all joints several times a day. An active exercise programme should be discouraged until the muscles are no longer sensitive to touch.

Convalescent stage

The convalescent stage begins 2 days after the temperature returns to normal and progression of the paralysis stops. While this phase continues for 2 years, the spontaneous improvement in muscle strength is most rapid through the fourth month and much more gradual thereafter. An important exception is the triceps surae in which the end result is generally achieved by 18 months.

Orthopaedic objectives include obtaining maximum recovery of individual muscles, maintenance and restoration of normal range of motion, and prevention of deformities that do occur. Muscles must lose their sensitivity before a thorough assessment in grading of individual muscles can be accomplished. Serial assessments are the best guides to potential recovery and should be carried out monthly for 6 months and then every 3 months.

The physical therapy programme should be directed toward isolating and exercising individual muscles so that each can achieve maximum return of strength. The muscles must be made to work in a normal pattern of motor activity. Since the muscles fatigue quickly, after a few contractures, they must not be exercised beyond their capabilities or recovery will be inhibited. Bivalved casts or plastic orthoses are used to prevent overfatigue and maintain proper alignment of the extremity between physical therapy sessions. Vigorous passive stretching exercises and wedging casts may be necessary when mild to moderate degrees of contracture develop. Hydrotherapy may be an important adjunct in patients with extensive paralysis.

Bracing should be withheld as long as further recovery is anticipated and is designed to avoid the development of an abnormal gait. Dynamic-assist bracing is preferred. Early walking may benefit the patient who has mild paralysis, but may be contraindicated in those who have more involvement. Weakness in the foot dorsiflexors may require a posterior leaf spring type of ankle–foot orthosis. Accompanying weakness in the lateral flexors may be controlled by the use of a varus- or valgus-producing door with an ankle–foot orthosis.

Chronic stage

No improvement can be expected during this stage and the orthopaedic surgeon must manage the longterm residua which result from the muscle imbalance. Management is directed toward the achievement of maximum functional activity. Surgical means of obtaining muscle balance, prevention or correction of soft tissue deformity or secondary osseous complications, may be necessary (Green & Grice 1952). Growth in the immature patient also contributes to fixed deformity. The worse deformities occur with early age and severe muscle imbalance. Soft tissue surgery, especially tendon transfers, are emphasized in the young child. Bony procedures are postponed until skeletal growth is adequate. In this phase, use of orthoses is directed toward the patient's increasing functional activities, such as walking, and toward protecting paretic muscles from overstretching while augmenting the action of weakened muscles.

Management

Tendon transfers

A tendon transfer is performed when dynamic muscle imbalance is sufficient to produce deformity and orthotic management is required. Tendon transfers are performed to:

1   provide active motor power to replace the function of a paralyzed muscle;

2   eliminate the deforming effect of a muscle when its antagonist is paralyzed;
3   produce stability through better muscle balance.

The principles of muscle transfers must be followed (Herndon 1961). They include that the muscle being transferred should rate good or normal in strength and have sufficient motor strength to carry out the desired function. On the average, one grade of motor power is lost after muscle transfer. Strength and range of motion of the transferred muscle and the one being replaced must be similar. The potential loss of the original function resulting from tendon transfers must be balanced against the proposed gains. Free passive range of motion and absence of joint deformity are important. The transfer can improve the result of bony stabilization but cannot be expected to correct a fixed bony deformity. The tendon should be routed straight between its origin and new insertion and the transfer attached in sufficient tension to correspond to the normal physiologic condition.

Requirements for satisfactory longterm ambulation include a stable plantigrade foot which has the weight distributed evenly between the heel and forefoot during standing and ambulation. Muscle transfers are performed to achieve balance between dorsiflexors and plantarflexors as well as the lateral flexors, to prevent the development of contracture, and to reestablish a walking pattern (Broderick et al. 1952). No major fixed deformity is acceptable. Bony procedures are generally delayed until the patient nears skeletal maturation at approximately 12 years of age and are then carried out to correct or prevent deformity or to achieve bony stability.

Dorsiflexor paralysis

The majority of polio tendon transfers are performed for drop foot deformity. The ability to substitute muscle power sufficient to permit the toes to clear the ground avoids the need for ankle-foot orthoses.

Tibialis anterior paralysis

The resulting loss of dorsiflexor and invertor power results in the development of an equinovalgus deformity. Initially observed in swing phase, this insufficiency eventually is found in both phases of gait. Secondary toe deformities develop when the long toe extensors become overactive during the swing phase in an attempt to replace the paralyzed muscle. The functioning triceps surae contracts, causing an equinus contracture.

Initial orthopaedic management is directed toward correcting the equinus by passive stretching exercises and serial casts. Later, an anterior transfer of the peroneus longus to the base of the second metatarsal is recommended. The distal stump of the peroneus longus is sutured to the peroneus brevis to prevent the formation of a dorsal bunion. A second option would be recessing the extensor digitorum longus muscle to the dorsum and midfoot.

Occasionally the unopposed activity of the peroneus longus depresses the first metatarus and causes the formation of a cavovarus deformity. This may require a plantar fasciotomy and intrinsic release prior to tendon surgery. The peroneus longus should be transferred to the base of the second metatarsal and the extensor hallucis longus to the neck of the first metatarsal.

Paralysis of the tibialis anterior and posterior muscles

The combined paralysis of these muscles leads to more rapid development of hindfoot and forefoot equinovalgus. The tight heel cord must be stretched with serial casts to avoid surgical weakening of the triceps surae. The peroneus longus is transferred to the base of the second metatarsal to replace the tibialis anterior and one of the long toe flexors is substituted for the paretic tibialis posterior.

Paralysis of the tibialis posterior

This uncommon pattern results in hindfoot and forefoot eversion. The flexor hallucis longus and flexor digitorum longus have both been used successfully in tendon transfers. Axer (1960) recommended bringing the conjoined extensor digitorum longus and peroneus tertius tendon through a transverse tunnel in the talar neck and suturing the tendon back onto itself.

Paralysis of tibialis anterior, toe extensors, and peronei

Progressive severe equinovarus deformity results with the unopposed activity of the tibialis posterior and triceps surae. Passive stretching and corrective serial casts are recommended for the initial treatment. An intrinsic release may be necessary to control the forefoot equinus. A staged heel cord lengthening may be required with this type of deformity. Anterior transfer of the tibialis posterior through the interosseus membrane to the base of the third metatarsal is effective.

Paralysis of the peronei

This rare pattern results in severe hindfoot varus. Balance is restored by lateral transfer of the tibialis anterior to the base of the second metatarsal bone. If the tibialis posterior is strong the tendon should be anchored in line with the fourth ray.

Triceps surae muscle paralysis

Paralysis of the triceps surae leads to a rapidly progressive calcaneal deformity of the foot. The deformity increases as a result of unopposed dorsiflexor function combined with attenuation of the triceps surae. The patient cannot stabilize his calcaneus or transfer his body weight distal to the metatarsal heads and, thus, loses push-off power in walking. The foot shortens as the os calcis rotates into an increasingly more vertical position and a secondary forefoot equinus creates a cavus deformity (Green & Grice 1956).

The rapid development of this deformity necessitates the taking of serial standing roentgenograms. Surgical correction is required to prevent the development of the calcaneal deformity and to restore hindfoot plantarflexion. This deformity is the only absolute indication for tendon transfers in children under the age of 5 years (Goldner & Irwin 1948, Herndon et al. 1956). The type of transfer is determined by the degree of residual strength of the triceps surae and the pattern of remaining muscle function. When the remaining motor strength is rated fair, the posterior transfer of two or three muscles may lead to a normal gait. Complete triceps surae paralysis is managed by posterior transfer of as many muscles as are available. The presence of a fixed cavus deformity requires a plantar fasciotomy before a tendon transfer can be performed. A Mitchell posterior displacement osteotomy (Mitchell 1977) can be used in the correction of a calcaneocavus deformity (Fig. 10.10). This combines an extensive plantar release with an oblique transverse osteotomy which permits upward and backward displacement of the weight bearing part of os calcis.

can be used for dorsiflexion (Herndon et al. 1956). The transfer is performed through the interosseous membrane, the foot placed in a position of maximum plantarflexion to ensure attachment under appropriate tension, and the attenuated Achilles tendon may require shortening, which is accomplished by a Z-plasty.

Pure calcaneocavus develops when the invertors and evertors have balanced muscle strength. Posterior transfer of only one set of these muscles would lead to instability and iatrogenic secondary deformity. Transfer of the peroneus brevis and tibialis posterior to the heel controls the calcaneus and provides sufficient power to permit the patient to regain a normal gait pattern. Cavus with lateral imbalance requires transpositioning the active invertor or evertor to the heel. Calcaneocavovalgus is managed by transferring both peronei to the heel, whereas the tibialis posterior and flexor hallucis longus are the preferred muscle transfers for calcaneocavovarus deformity.

Flail foot

Equinus deformity may develop because of passive plantarflexion and retained function in the

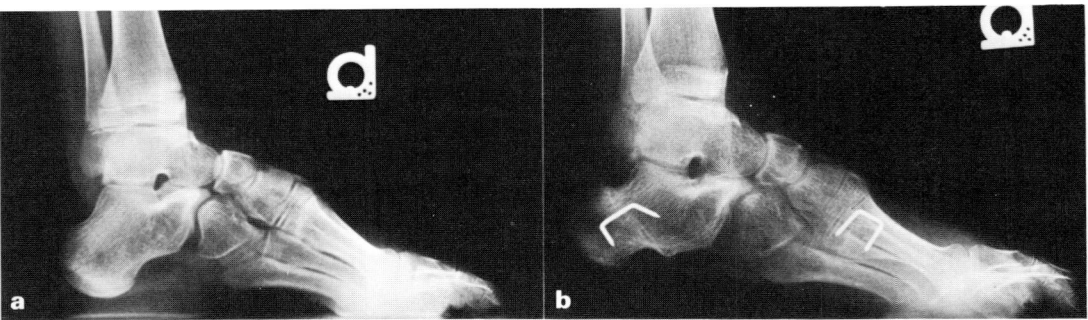

Fig. 10.10. (a) and (b) A Mitchell/Dwyer calcaneal osteotomy combined with a first metatarsal osteotomy effectively decreased the cavus deformity. Note the posterior migration of the fibula.

The tibialis anterior may be transferred posteriorly as early as 18 months after the acute stage of poliomyelitis (Peabody 1949). This can be carried out as an isolated procedure if the lateral stabilizers are balanced and strong toe extensors

intrinsic muscles, since sacral sparing is common in poliomyelitis. A formal release of the intrinsic muscles and plantar fascia may be performed through a lateral heel incision. Older patients may require a second stage midfoot wedge resection for forefoot equinus in order to be able to use a polypropylene ankle–foot orthosis.

Operations on bone

Bony procedures are performed to correct or prevent deformity or to achieve stability. Tendon transfers cannot be performed until structural bony deformity has been corrected. The rate of progression of the deformity as well as the age of the patient determine the type of correction. An excessively short foot would result from arthrodesis in the skeletally immature patient and, therefore, bony deformity in younger children is corrected by procedures not involving cartilage. Foot and ankle stabilization procedures include:

1   extra-articular subtalar arthrodesis;
2   triple arthrodesis;
3   anteroposterior bone blocks to limit ankle motion;
4   ankle arthrodesis.

These may be performed singly or in combination.

Extra-articular subtalar arthrodesis   Paralytic equinovalgus deformity secondary to paralysis of the tibialis anterior and posterior may initially be managed by a short leg brace with a varus-producing T-strap. Hindfoot and forefoot equinovalgus may develop and require surgical correction (Pollock & Carrell 1964). Grice (1952) originally described an extra-articular subtalar fusion for patients between the ages of 3 and 8 years. This procedure restored the height of the medial longitudinal arch. Currently, the Dennyson modification of the extra-articular subtalar arthrodesis (Dennyson & Fulford 1976) is recommended. The technique is described on page 177.

Triple arthrodesis   This procedure is indicated when most of the weakness and deformity occurs at the subtalar and midtarsal joints. Motion of the foot and ankle are reduced to

plantar- and dorsiflexion. Pre-operative assessment includes radiographic evaluation for stability of the talus in the ankle mortise.

Surgical goals include stable and static realignment of the foot, arrest of progressive deformity, elimination of pain and decrease of limp, removal of deforming forces, a normal appearing foot, and improvement in orthotic wear. At the time of surgical correction, the foot must be aligned with the ankle mortise and not with the knee. Associated rotational or angular deformity in the extremity should be corrected by a separate procedure (Pauker 1959).

Several different types of triple arthrodeses have been described (Dunn 1922, Ryerson 1923). The Hoke method (Hoke 1921) can be adapted for the correction of any of the variety of foot deformities and this technique is recommended. Hindfoot malalignment alters the specific operative technique (Fig. 10.11). In talipes equinovalgus, the medial longitudinal arch is depressed and the talar head plantarflexed and the forefoot abducted. The medial arch is restored by means of a subtalar joint wedge based medially which permits raising the talar head and shifting the sustentaculum tali beneath the talar neck and head. The forefoot pronation can be corrected by a midtarsal joint resection with the wedge again based medially. In talipes equinovarus, the enlarged talar head blocks dorsiflexion and lies lateral to the midline axis of the foot. Correction is obtained by a subtalar wedge based laterally combined with a midtarsal joint resection with the wedge based laterally.

Operative technique for Hoke triple arthrodesis   Exposure is gained by an incision at the midtarsal joint level extending laterally from the extensor digitorum longus tendon towards the calcaneocuboid joint and then curving laterally posteriorly to terminate one centimetre below and posterior to the lateral malleolus. No skin flaps are developed and the dissection is carried directly to bone. The contents of the sinus tarsi are sharply elevated in a single soft tissue pedicle based distally. Radical resection of

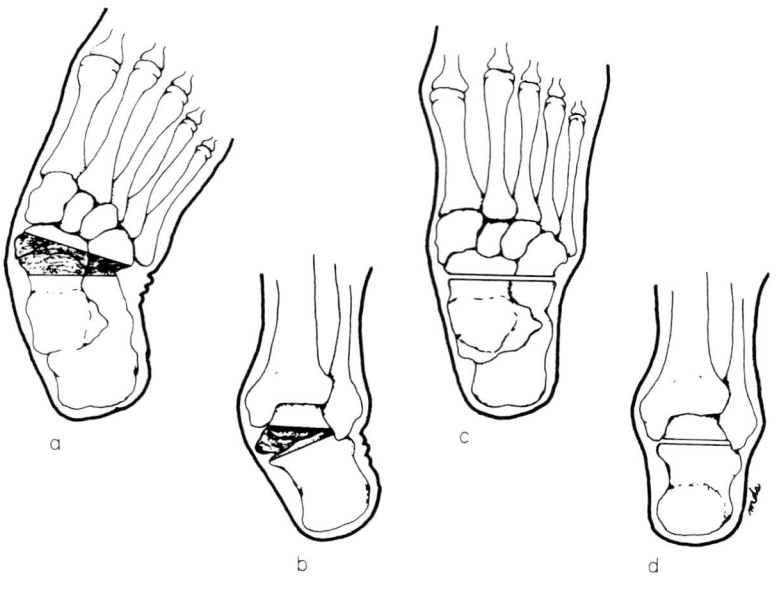

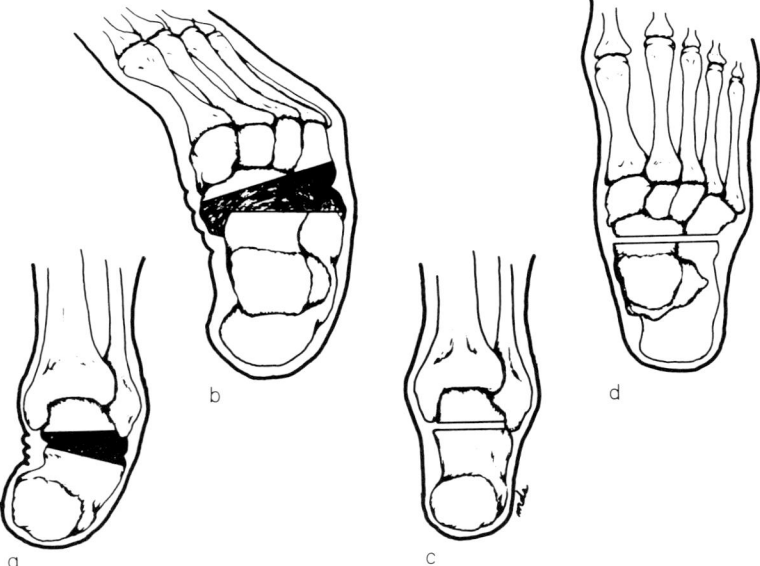

Fig. 10.11. (Top) Triple arthrodesis for valgus deformity. Forefoot abduction and heel valgus are corrected by wedge resection (a and b). The position of the bones after surgery is shown (c and d). (Bottom) Triple arthrodesis for varus deformity. Shaded areas (a and b) indicate wedge resections to correct forefoot inversion and heel varus. The position of the bones after surgery (c and d).

the capsules of all three joints permits mobilization of the bones of the hindfoot and decreases the amount of bone resection necessary for adequate correction. It is necessary to strip a short segment of the cuboid to allow adequate soft tissue retraction to expose the plantar surface of the calcaneocuboid joint. The cartilaginous surfaces of this joint are osteotomized and this is followed by excision of the talonavicular joint. Maximum bony contact of the talonavicular joint is insured by minimal decortication of the talar head and navicular in feet not requiring correction of valgus or varus. A severe valgus deformity may require an accessory incision for exposure of the talonavicular joint. The hook of the navicular must be resected flush with the navicular body in cases with severe varus or it will prevent lateral displacement of the forefoot.

The osteotome is next used to excise the articular surfaces of the anterior subtalar joint including the sustentaculum tali. The posterior subtalar joint capsule is excised along the calcaneal dome. Care is taken to separate the capsule from the anterior fibulocalcaneal ligament. Improved exposure of this joint is gained by removing the anterior lip of the posterior talar facet and by using a small laminar spreader in the sinus tarsi. The calcaneal wedge is removed *en bloc* with a wide osteotome. A limited wedge is removed from the posterior talar facet to avoid the possibility of talar avascular necrosis. Apposition of the bony surfaces is evaluated and any defects packed with chips of the removed bone to insure maximum bony contact. Staple fixation of an individual joint may be indicated. The sinus tarsi soft tissue pedicle is reattached and a single-layer closure of the subcutaneous tissue and skin is carried out.

The patient is then placed in a well-moulded long leg cast with the knee flexed to 45 degrees and both the plaster and sterile cast padding are divided down to the level of the skin to accommodate postoperative swelling. This opening must be packed with cast padding to avoid the development of window oedema. Postoperative use of slings on an overhead frame is recom-

mended until all swelling has subsided. Ten to fourteen days following surgery, the cast is changed under general anaesthesia and the patient then begins to walk with crutches. A short leg walking cast is applied after 6 weeks and is worn until there is radiographic evidence of solid union, which generally occurs at 10–12 weeks.

Talonavicular joint pseudarthrosis is the most frequent complication (Patterson *et al.* 1950). Degenerative arthritis caused by the increased stress on the ankle joint and anterior ankle subluxation may be indications for delayed ankle fusion (Flint & MacKenzie 1962, Pyka *et al.* 1964). Talar avascular necrosis is most common in adolescence and should be treated with nonweightbearing until the amount of vascular healing is evident.

The Lambrinudi drop foot arthrodesis is recommended for the rare patient with a fixed equinus deformity (Lambrinudi 1927, Fitzgerald & Seddon 1937, Hart 1940). This results from retained activity in the triceps surae coupled with inactive dorsiflexors and peronei. A physiologic bone block is created and the posterior talus abuts the undersurface of the tibia. The fixed plantarflexed position of the talus is retained and the rest of the foot is brought up to the desired degree of dorsiflexion. The procedure is not recommended for a flail foot (MacKenzie 1959) or if paralysis in the remainder of the limb will require bracing because of hip or knee instability. Anterior talar subluxation seen on a weightbearing lateral roentgenogram indicates the need for a two-stage pantalar arthrodesis.

Talipes calcaneus

Talectomy Astragalectomy performed for a calcaneus or a calcaneovalgus deformity provides stability and posterior displacement of the foot and is recommended for children between the ages of 5 and 12. The technique is described on page 182 (Whitman 1922, Thompson 1939, Leikkonen 1950, Holmdahl 1956). Longterm use of an ankle–foot orthosis is recommended since a tibiocalcaneal arthrodesis performed at skeletal maturity is the only alternative following the recurrence of this deformity (Carmack & Hallock 1947). Mitchell's posterior displacement osteotomy (Mitchell 1977) also has a definite role to play in the management of talipes calcaneus.

The skeletally mature patient can be effectively managed by the Elmslie double tarsal wedge osteotomy (Elmslie 1934, Cholmeley 1953). The first stage combines a release of the plantar soft tissues through a lateral calcaneal incision with a dorsal wedge excision arthrodesis of the talonavicular and calcaneocuboid joints to completely correct the cavus. Following 6 weeks of casting in marked dorsiflexion, a posterior excision wedge arthrodesis of the subtalar joint is carried out to correct the hindfoot calcaneus. The wedge extends to the point of the previous osteotomy. The bony surfaces are opposed by plantarflexing the foot and the redundant Achilles tendon surgically shortened. The tenotomized long toe flexors are also inserted into the Achilles tendon.

Ankle fusion and pantalar arthrodesis

Ankle fusion has been carried out most commonly for a dangle or flail foot. The Charnley compression arthrodesis (Charnley 1951) is recommended. The ankle joint is exposed by an anterior incision and all dorsal soft tissue structures are divided. Both malleoli and the distal tibia are osteotomized in a horizontal plane. The foot is placed in the desired position, and appropriate correction obtained through a talar wedge resection. The talar Steinmann pin is placed anterior to the talar axis to increase compression and counterbalance the activity of the Achilles tendon. The tibial Steinmann pin is located at a point determined after the compression clamps have been applied, confirming that the pins will be parallel. The pins are maintained for 8 weeks and an additional 4 weeks of plaster immobilization is indicated for a flail foot with paralysed quadriceps to eliminate the need

for a long leg brace (Hamsa 1936). A strong gluteus maximus is required to begin toe-off at the end of stance phase in a knee that has full extension. The ankle should be fused in 10 degrees of equinus to produce the backward thrust on the knee joint necessary for stable weightbearing (Waugh *et al.* 1965). Complications of both ankle and pantalar arthrodeses include pseudarthroses, painful plantar callosities secondary to unequal weight distribution, and excessive heel equinus leading to increases pressure on the forefoot.

Claw-toe deformity may develop when long toe extensors are used to substitute for severely weakened dorsiflexors during swing phase (Dickson & Diveley 1926). Marked deformity occurs when an Achilles tendon contracture is present. Correction of fixed ankle equinus and appropriate tendon transfers are required to restore active ankle dorsiflexion. The Jones transfer (Jones 1916) of the extensor hallucis longus tendon to the neck of the first metatarsus coupled with a Hibbs transfer (Hibbs 1919) of the extensor digitorum longus is recommended when the residual clawing is the result of ankle dorsiflexion insufficiency. The claw-toe deformity may also develop when the long toe flexors are used to substitute for a paretic triceps surae in the toe-off phase of stance. This can be corrected by a Girdlestone–Taylor transfer of the long toe flexors into the dorsal hood of the extensor tendon (Taylor 1951).

Cavus deformity

The pathogenesis of pes cavus in poliomyelitis is obscure. Fixed soft tissue cavus deformity should be corrected before adaptive bony changes have occurred (Steindler 1920, Dekel & Weissman 1973, Samilson & Dillin 1983). The author prefers an Elmslie lateral heel incision (Elmslie 1934) extending from the tuber of the os calcis to the calcaneocuboid joint. A release of the plantar fascia and intrinsic muscles as well as the plantar ligaments is carried out. The procedure is designed to lengthen the medial longitudinal arch and this lateral incision is performed without creating excessive tension on the skin closure. A series of short leg casts, which include an absence of moulding on the plantar surface, and utilization of double thickness felt under the forefoot are required. A walking boot with a rubber platform placed beneath the forefoot is applied 2 weeks following surgery and is worn for an additional 3 weeks.

Bony procedures that may be performed include the Dwyer calcaneal osteotomy (Dwyer 1959) coupled with a plantar release. A Cole midfoot dorsal tarsal wedge osteotomy (Cole 1940) is effective for severe cavus deformity.

Posterior bone block This rarely performed procedure is limited to patients who require a drop foot brace for excessive ankle plantarflexion. It is useful in patients with a completely flail foot and weak quadriceps muscle who may be made brace-free by a combination of a triple arthrodesis and a posterior bone block. The procedure is contraindicated in fulltime brace users. Both Campbell (1923) and Inclan (1949) have described operative techniques. Longterm review of the bone block suggests that degenerative arthritis of the ankle joint and avascular necrosis of the talus develop in many patients (Ingram & Hundley 1951). Therefore, the procedure has fallen into disfavour.

Hereditary motor and sensory neuropathies (peripheral nerve)

Peripheral neuropathies that demonstrate peroneal muscular atrophy and weakness as prominent features early in the course of the disease have recently been classified by Dyck & Lambert (1968). Included are patients previously termed having peroneal muscular atrophy (Charcot–Marie–Tooth disease: Charcot & Marie 1886, Tooth 1886) or familiar interstitial hypertrophic neuritis (Déjérine–Sottas disease:

Déjérine & Sottas 1893). Life expectancy is normal. Patients demonstrate slow progression of weakness and cavus formation (Sabir & Lyttle 1983) with minor sensory abnormalities and generally have a positive family history. There may be a wide variation, both in the degree of severity and length of feet, within a given family. The length of the foot reflects the severity of the neurologic deficit. Females tend to have a more severe form.

These patients achieve independent bipedal gait before requiring orthopaedic intervention. Diminished proprioception decreases their standing balance. The progressive nature of the neuromuscular disease underlines the need for constant reassessment of their peripheral neurologic status and pedal deformity. Postoperative management must be carefully planned before surgery.

Weakness in the peronei permits the lateral malleolus to migrate posteriorly, thereby giving the ankle joint itself a lateral disposition (Fig. 10.12). The ankle malalignment may be accepted when there is the planned postoperative use of a rigid ankle–foot orthosis. Patients who are considered potentially brace-free at the conclusion of foot surgery, may require a supramalleolar osteotomy before corrective bony and tendon surgery is performed in the foot (McNicol *et al.* 1983). This is also true for patients who will use a posterior leaf spring design orthosis or have orthotic problems because of the prominence of the lateral malleolus in an abnormally posterior position (Fig. 10.13). There is a high incidence of early degenerative arthritis in the unprotected, malaligned ankle joint following triple arthrodesis (Fig. 10.14). Recurrent deformity is prevented by using an ankle–foot orthosis extending to the toes.

Dyck's classification (p. 72)

Type I includes the hypertrophic neuropathy of Charcot–Marie–Tooth disease as well as hereditary areflexic dystaxia (Roussy–Lévy syn-

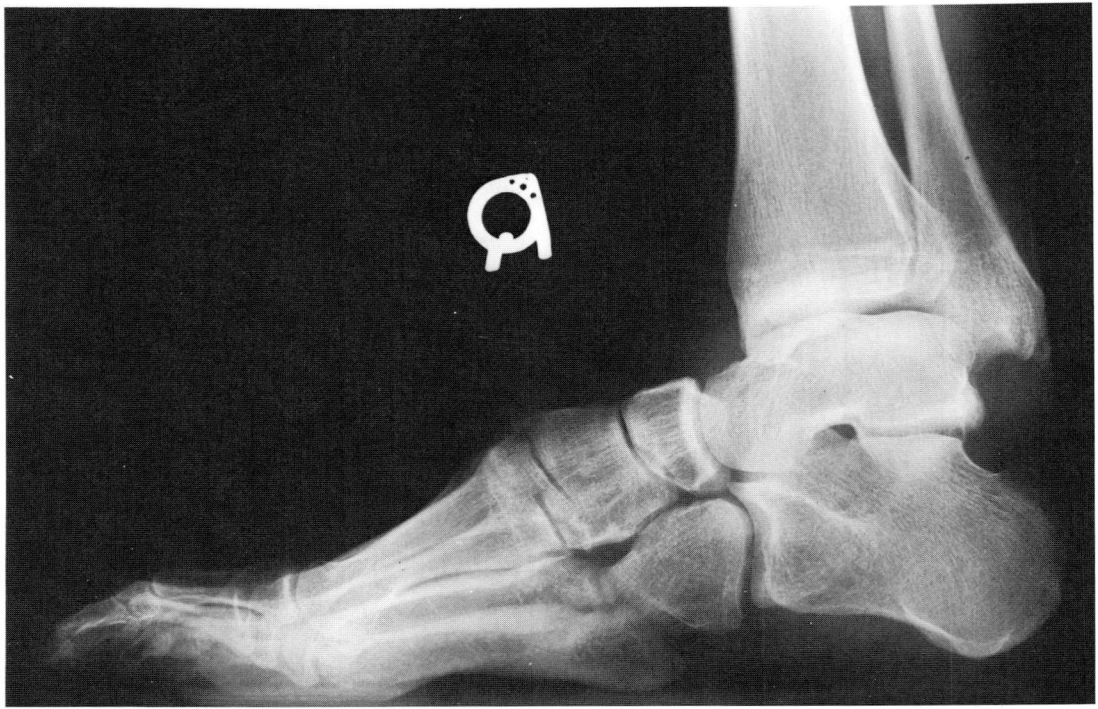

Fig. 10.12. Ankle malalignment results from peroneal weakness and contributes to the development of degenerative disease of the ankle.

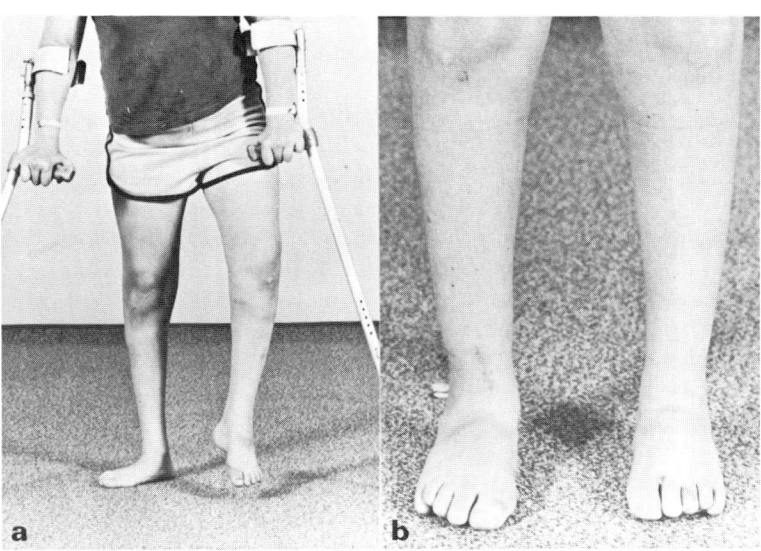

Fig. 10.13 A derotational supramalleolar osteotomy corrects excessive ankle external rotation. (a) Prior to surgery. (b) After derotational supramalleolar osteotomy.

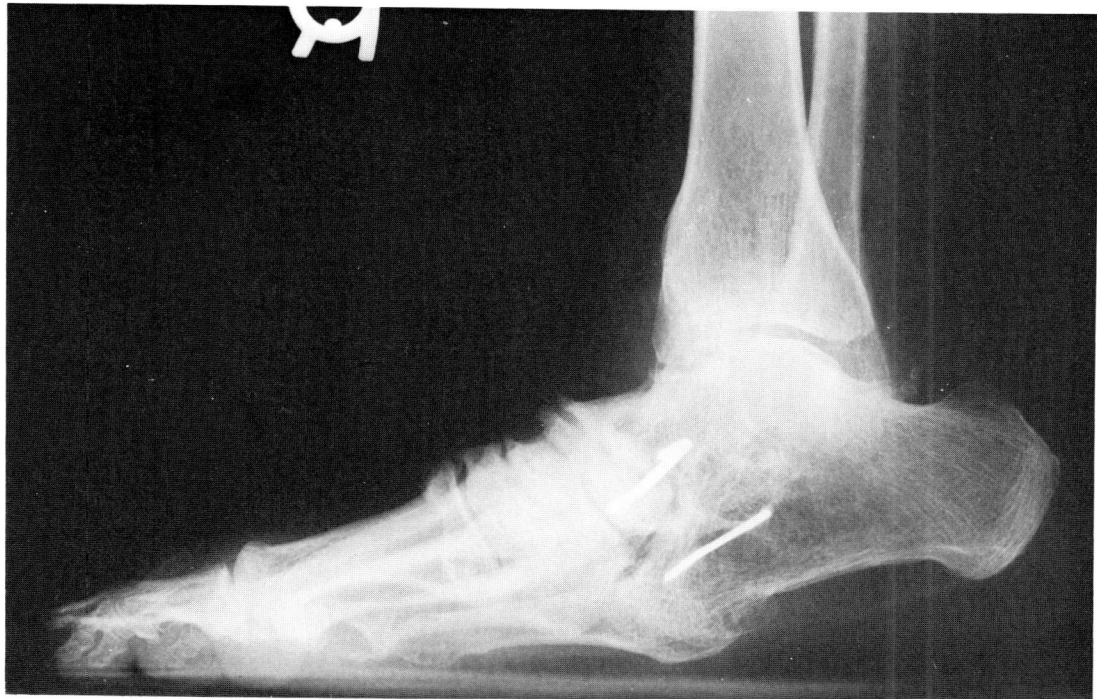

Fig. 10.14. A long-term follow-up radiograph shows residual hindfoot equinus following a triple arthrodesis and the resulting degenerative joint disease.

drome: Roussy & Lévy 1926). Symptoms develop in the second decade of life as peroneal muscle involvement becomes more pronounced and an equinocavovarus deformity gradually develops. Discomfort beneath the lateral metatarsal heads with weightbearing and difficulty in running may be noted. Physical assessment demonstrates wasting and weakness of the peronei and dorsiflexors and, in particular, the extensor digitorum brevis. Sensory deficit is minor. Motor nerve conduction velocities of half the normal value are the most significant laboratory finding. Eventually, all muscles distal to the knee joint become involved and the patient may develop a dramatic slap-foot gait.

The young child who presents with tight heel cords may be managed by serial walking casts followed by the use of short leg night splints. Forefoot equinus may require an intrinsic release

when the plantar fascia can be palpated as being a restrictive band. Mild osseous equinovarus deformity with early cavus is corrected by a Dwyer calcaneal osteotomy combined with a plantar fascial release (Washington *et al.* 1979). In the adolescent, when the tibialis anterior muscle becomes weak, the tibialis posterior muscle may be transferred to the dorsum in combination with the Dwyer osteotomy. Foot stabilization by triple arthrodesis (Fig. 10.15) remains the definitive method for longterm surgical management and may be performed after skeletal growth is complete (Levitt *et al.* 1973). Triple arthrodesis may also be combined with a first and second metatarsal osteotomy for equinus of the medial longitudinal arch. A posterior tibial transfer is generally necessary 6 weeks after the arthrodesis (Fig. 10.16).

Type II is equivalent to the neuronal form of Charcot–Marie–Tooth disease. Nerve con-

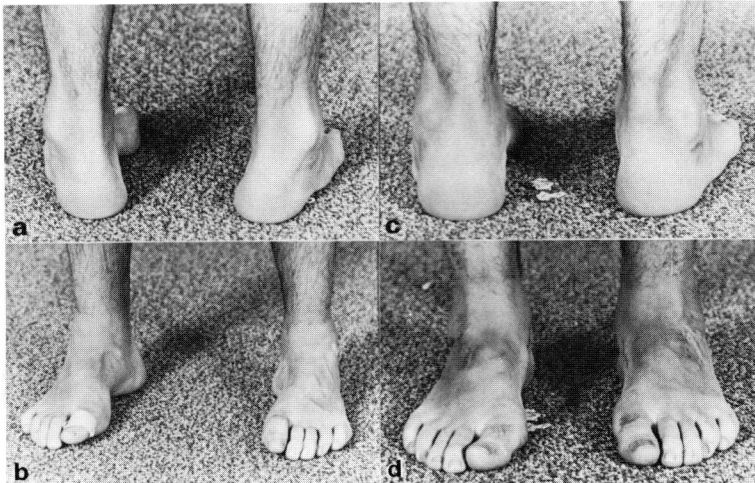

Fig. 10.15. (a) and (b) Equinovarus in a patient with Type I peripheral neuropathy. (c) and (d) Correction of deformity by triple arthrodeses.

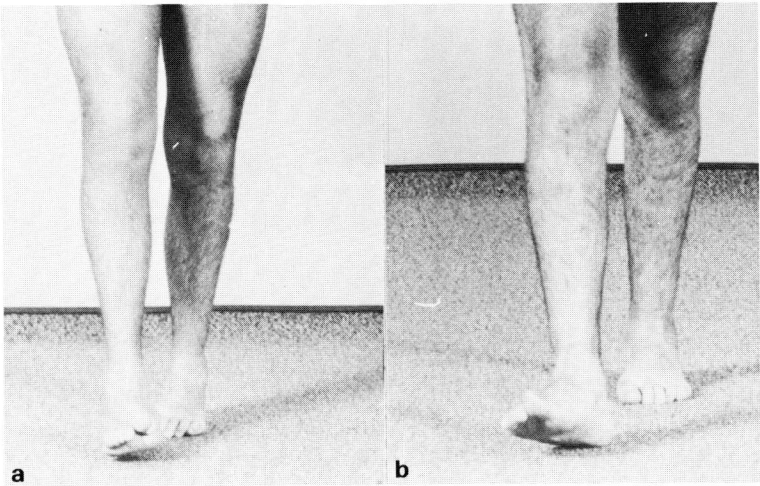

Fig. 10.16. (a) Inversion of the foot at the time of heel strike. (b) The correct position of the foot following posterior tibial transfer.

duction velocities are either slightly reduced or may be normal. Muscle weakness in the lower extremity generally begins during the third decade of life and spreads in a centripetal fashion to include the distal third of the quadriceps and hamstrings.

Weakness of the plantar flexors is common and results in a hindfoot calcaneus. The combination of a dangle foot and lack of knee stabilizers may lead to genu recurvatum requiring the use of a unilateral KAFO (Fig. 10.17). A

Mitchell posterior calcaneal displacement osteotomy coupled with metatarsal osteotomies has proved effective in managing these patients who frequently have very short feet.

Type III patients have a markedly slow conduction time and were previously termed Déjérine–Sottas disease.

Type IV (Refsum's disease) is due to an elevation of serum phytanic acid. These patients have deformities similar to Type I and the treatment is similar to that described above.

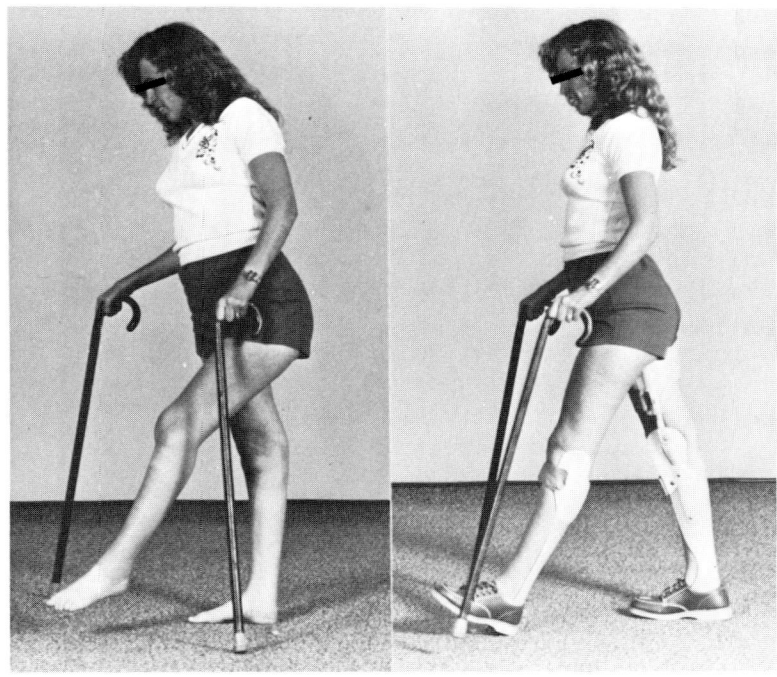

Fig. 10.17. A right knee–ankle–foot orthosis with hyperextension stop effectively controls genu recurvatum. Adults find bilateral long leg braces excessively cumbersome and, therefore, a short leg brace was used on the less involved limb.

Hereditary sensory and autonomic neuropathy

Hereditary sensory and autonomic neuropathy and the term congenital indifference to pain are both used in current neurologic literature (Dyck *et al.* 1983). This rare condition is characterized by a normal threshold for perception of ordinary painful stimuli but the patient fails to demonstrate the usual objective and subjective responses. Both soft tissue and osseous mutilation occur. Minor injury causes local damage which the patient cannot fully appreciate and, therefore, the healing process is unduly shortened. Many of these patients will develop neurotrophic changes in the weightbearing joints because of repeated abnormal stresses and trauma (Rose 1953). Haemarthrosis and secondary ligamentous laxity are accompanied by hyperemia and resulting bone resorption and atrophy. Complete joint destruction is common

(Fig. 10.18). Protective lower extremity orthoses and occasionally arthrodeses are necessary. Longterm follow-up of an initially successful major joint fusion of the lower extremity may reveal the delayed development of a pseudarthrosis. Other orthopaedic complications include unsuspected dislocations, fractures, septic arthritis, and chronic osteomyelitis of the long bones. Appropriate roentgenograms of the involved limb are required whenever the clinical examination reveals the presence of erythema, warmth or swelling.

Progressive muscular dystrophy (skeletal muscle)

Foot deformities are very common in the sex-linked muscular dystrophy group. The Duchenne patient frequently achieves delayed independent ambulation and may also present as a toe walker. The boy is able to walk initially, but never runs and may have difficulty climbing stairs (Drennan 1983). Symmetrical pelvic girdle weakness becomes evident in the first decade of life. Generally before the age of 8 years, increasing quadriceps weakness leads to the development of functional toe walking gait which allows the weightline to pass in front of the knee joint and thereby stabilizing that joint in extension. Retained strength in the triceps surae and tibialis posterior eventually cause the equinus deformity to become fixed and a varus element develops, making standing and walking precarious (Fig. 10.19).

become candidates for lower extremity surgery accompanied by orthotic control (Spencer & Vignos 1962). Loss of ambulation generally occurs after the quadriceps can no longer fully extend the knee against gravity. Measurements for knee–ankle–foot orthoses are obtained before surgery, or if the cast is changed at 2–3 weeks (Chapter 6).

Equinovarus deformity

Equinovarus deformity is corrected by transfer of the tibialis posterior to the second cuneiform

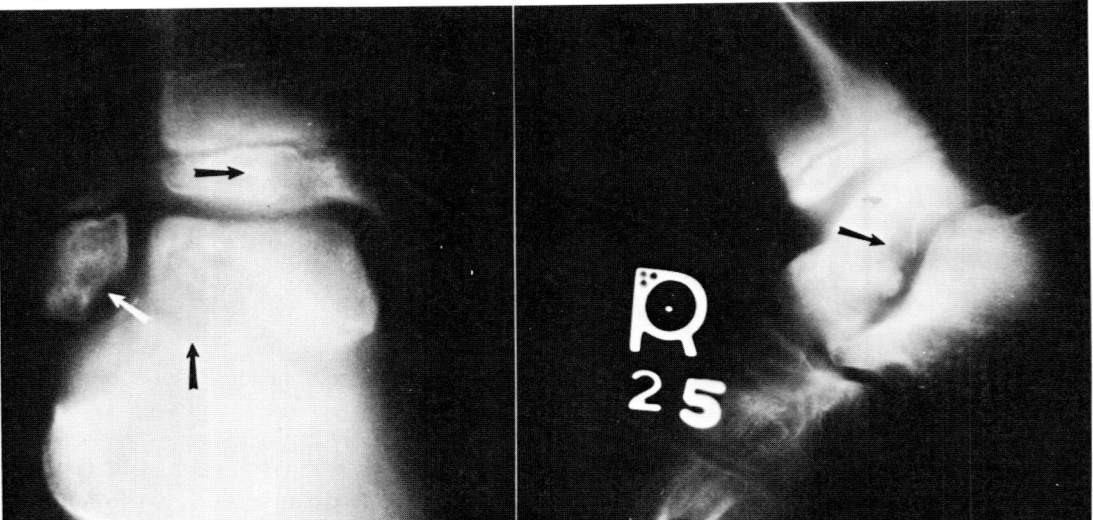

Fig. 10.18. Patient with sensory neuropathy. The arrows show the avascular necrosis in the distal tibia and fibula, and talus. The patient eventually underwent talectomy and has developed a stable tibiocalcaneal ankylosis.

Prophylactic night-time bracing has not been effective. The equinovarus deformity may develop asymmetrically as muscle imbalance is added to the static plantarflexed position. Full knee extension and ankle flexion to neutral continue in the dominant weightbearing limb while the extremity used for balance during stance more rapidly develops a heel cord contracture that is accompanied by mild knee and hip flexion contractures.

Patients threatened with loss of ambulation

combined with a heel cord lengthening. It is usually carried out in boys between 8 and 12 years and results in an additional 3–5 years of assisted independent ambulation.

Operative procedure for equinovarus deformity The procedure is performed bilaterally. The initial incision over the insertion of the tibialis posterior permits the freeing of the tendon from its navicular insertion while maintaining its length. Longitudinal traction is

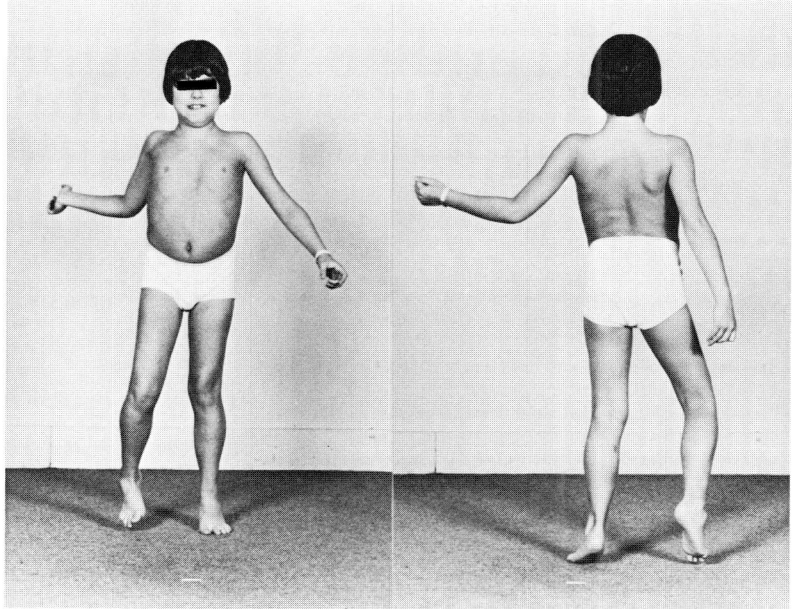

Fig. 10.19. The precarious left foot stance and the poor prepositioning of the right foot during swing phase are demonstrated in an 11-year-old patient with Duchenne muscular dystrophy.

applied to the tip of the freed tendon. The muscle belly of the tibialis posterior is located in the posterior calf by palpation. The second incision is made over the muscular tibialis posterior in an area proximal to the superior crural retinaculum. The freed tendon is advanced and the heel cord is lengthened. A third incision over the distal anterior leg permits dissection between the tendons of the tibialis anterior and extensor hallucis longus. Having bluntly swept aside the neurovascular structures, the interosseous membrane is exposed and a generous window is made just proximal to the tibiofibular syndesmosis. The periosteum is not violated to avoid heterotopic bone formation. The tibialis posterior is brought through the window and the first two incisions are closed. The fourth incision over the second cuneiform is in direct line with the third toe. Osteoperiosteal flaps are created and a tunnel through the bone is directed toward the apex of the medial longitudinal arch. The tendon is passed superficial to the crural ligaments into the final field. A sturdy woven Bunnell suture is passed through the tunnel and the plantar skin with two Keith straight needles. The suture is tied over a felt pad and button, which

are placed on the nonweightbearing plantar surface of the medial longitudinal arch. Long leg casts are applied with the feet at right angles.

Management postoperatively is enhanced by the use of a Circ-o-lectric bed. After 24 hours, the patient is begun tilting for short periods to avoid pedal swelling. The angle of the bed is increased until the patient is able to assume a vertical position. His rehabilitation is then transferred to physical therapy for the use of the parallel bars for gait training. Alternatively, standing with the help of the physiotherapist is started within 12–18 hours of surgery (Chapter 6). Patients usually achieve a satisfactory ambulatory pattern with a rollator 7–10 days following surgery and discharge from the hospital is possible. Five weeks following surgery, the patient is re-admitted for the application of the previously measured orthoses. The physical therapy programme is resumed at this time.

Equinus contracture

Equinus deformity of the forefoot may rarely develop as an isolated deformity in the more severely affected young Duchenne patient. A plantar release made through a lateral incision is recommended and rarely is serial casting required postoperatively as an adjunct. This deformity is more common in patients with Becker's type of muscular dystrophy (Bradley *et al.* 1978).

Equinus of both the hindfoot and forefoot may develop in ambulant patients and may be improved by the combination of an intrinisic release followed by a Cole midfoot wedge tarsectomy and staged heel cord lengthening. Patients with more precarious gait are best managed by intrinsic release and staged heel cord lengthening. Those who are barely able to walk with bracing may benefit from a simple heel cord tenotomy. Equinovarus deformity is rare in these patients and should be managed by a simple tenotomy of the heel cord and posterior tibial tendons.

Infantile myotonic dystrophy

Approximately half of the infants with myotonic dystrophy have a particularly rigid form of talipes equinovarus which has been associated with hydramnios and decreased fetal movement (Bell & Smith 1972, Carroll *et al.* 1975, Harper 1979). Serial plaster casts may be tried but the infant patient generally requires a complete posteromedial release. In the older child with myotonic dystrophy, a variety of other foot deformities may be encountered unilaterally or bilaterally. Forefoot equinus may require intrinsic release and the longterm use of an ankle–foot orthosis. Peroneal muscle weakness and a secondary talipes equinovarus can be managed by a Dwyer calcaneal osteotomy combined with a split anterior tibial transfer. Persistent forefoot adduction may require metatarsal osteotomies. These patients are sensitive to anaesthetics, particularly respiratory depressants which may cause sudden death.

References

AXER A. (1960) Into-talus transposition of tendons for correction of paralytic valgus foot after poliomyelitis in children. *Journal of Bone and Joint Surgery*, **42A**, 1119–42.

BAKER L.D. (1956) A rational approach to the surgical needs of the cerebral palsy patient. *Journal of Bone and Joint Surgery*, **38A**, 313–23.

BELL D.B. & SMITH D.W. (1972) Myotonic dystrophy in the neonate. *Journal of Pediatrics*, **81**, 83–6.

BLECK E.E. (1979) *Orthopaedic Management of Cerebral Palsy*, p. 187. W.B. Saunders Co., Philadelphia.

BRADLEY M.A., JONES M.Z., MUSSINI J.M. & FAWCETT P.R. (1978) Becker-type muscular dystrophy. *Muscle and Nerve*, **1**, 111–32.

BRODERICK T.F., REIDY J.A. & BARR J.S. (1952) Tendon transplantation in the lower extremity. A review of end results in poliomyelitis, II. Tendon Transplantations at the knee. *Journal of Bone and Joint Surgery*, **34A**, 909–14.

BURKUS J.K., MOORE D.W. & RAYCROFT J.F. (1983) Valgus deformity of the ankle in myelodysplastic patients. Correction by stapling of the medial part of the distal tibial physis. *Journal of Bone and Joint Surgery*, **65A**, 1157–62.

CAMPBELL W.C. (1923) An operation for the correction of 'drop-foot'. *Journal of Bone and Joint Surgery*, **5**, 815.

CARMACK J.C. & HALLOCK H. (1947) Tibiotarsal arthrodesis after astragalectomy, a report of eight cases. *Journal of Bone and Joint Surgery*, **29**, 476–82.

CARROLL J.E., BROOKE M.H. & KAISER K. (1975) Diagnosis of infantile myotonic dystrophy. *Lancet*, **2**, 608.

CHARCOT J.M. & MARIE P. (1886) Sur une forme particuliére d'atrophic musculaire progressive, souvent familiale, débutant par les pieds et les jambes et atteignant plus tard les mains. *Revue de Médecine* (Paris), **6**, 97.

CHARNLEY J. (1951) Compression arthrodesis of the ankle and shoulder. *Journal of Bone and Joint Surgery*, **33B**, 180–91.

CHOLMELEY J.A. (1953) Elmslie's operation for the calcaneus foot. *Journal of Bone and Joint Surgery*, **35B**, 46–9.

COLE W.H. (1940) The treatment of claw-foot. *Journal of Bone and Joint Surgery*, **22**, 895.

COLSON J.M. (1979) An effective orthotic design for controlling the unstable subtalar joint. *Orthotics and Prosthetics*, **33**, 39–49.

CRAWFORD A.H., MARXEN J.L. & OSTERFELD D.L. (1982) The Cincinnati incision: A comprehensive approach for surgical procedures of the foot and ankle in childhood. *Journal of Bone and Joint Surgery*, **64A**, 1355–8.

CREGO C.H. JR. & McCARROLL H.R. (1938) Recurrent deformities in stabilized paralytic feet. A report of 1100 consecutive stabilizations in poliomyelitis. *Journal of Bone and Joint Surgery*, **20**, 609.

DÉJÉRINE J. & SOTTAS J. (1893) Sur la néurite interstitielle hypertrophique et progressive de l'enfance. *Comptes redus des Séances de la Société de Biologie et des ses filales.* (Paris), **45**, 63.

DEKEL S. & WEISSMAN S.L. (1973) Osteotomy of the calcaneus and concomitant plantar stripping in children with talipes cavo-varus. *Journal of Bone and Joint Surgery*, **55B**, 802–08.

DENNYSON W.G. & FULFORD G.E. (1976) Subtalar arthrodesis by cancellous grafts and metallic internal fixation. *Journal of Bone and Joint Surgery*, **58B**, 507–10.

DIAS L.S. (1978) Ankle valgus in children with myelomeningocele. *Developmental Medicine and Child Neurology*, **20**, 627–33.

DICKSON F.D. & DIVELEY R.L. (1926) Operation for correction of mild claw foot, the result of infantile paralysis. *Journal of the American Medical Association*, **87**, 1275.

DRENNAN J.C. (1976) Management of myelomeningocele foot deformities in infancy and early childhood. *American Academy of Orthopaedic Surgeons Instructional Course Lectures*, **25**, 82.

DRENNAN J.C. (1983) *Orthopaedic Management of Neuromuscular Disorders*. J.B. Lippincott, Philadelphia.

DRENNAN J.C. & SHARRARD W.J.W. (1971) The pathological anatomy of convex pes valgus. *Journal of Bone and Joint Surgery*, **53B**, 455–61.

DRUMMOND D.S. & CRUESS R.L. (1978) The management of the foot and ankle in arthrogryposis multiplex congenita. *Journal of Bone and Joint Surgery*, **60B**, 96–9.

DUCKWORTH T. (1983) The hindfoot and its relation to rotational deformities of the forefoot. *Clinical Orthopaedics and Related Research*, **177**, 39–48.

DUNN J. (1922) Stabilizing operations in the treatment of paralytic deformities of the foot. *Proceedings of the Royal Society of Medicine*, **15**, 15.

DWYER F.C. (1959) Osteotomy of the calcaneum for pes cavus. *Journal of Bone and Joint Surgery*, **41B**, 80–6.

DYCK P.J. & LAMBERT E.H. (1968) Lower motor and primary sensory neuron diseases with peroneal muscular atrophy. Part I. Neurologic, genetic and electrophysiologic findings in hereditary polyneuropathies. Part II. Neurological, genetic, and electrophysiologic findings in various neuronal degenerations. *Archives of Neurology*, **18**, 603–18; 619–25.

DYCK P.J., MELLINGER J.F., REAGAN T.J., HORWITZ S.J., MCDONALD J.W., LITCHY W.J., DAUBE J.R., FEALEY R.D., GO V.L., KAO P.C., BRIMIJOIN W.S. & LAMBERT E.H. (1983) Not 'indifference to pain' but varieties of hereditary sensory and autonomic neuropathy. *Brain*, **106**, 373–90.

ELMSLIE R.I. (1934) *In* TURNER G.G. (ed.) *Modern Operative Surgery*, 2nd ed. Cassell, London.

EVANS G.A., DRENNAN J.C. & RUSSMAN B.S. (1981) Functional classification and orthopaedic management of spinal muscular atrophy. *Journal of Bone and Joint Surgery*, **63B**, 516–22.

FITZGERALD F.P. & SEDDON H.J. (1937) Lambrinudi's operation for drop-foot. *British Journal of Surgery*, **25**, 283.

FLINT M.H. & MACKENZIE I.G. (1962) Anterior laxity of the ankle. A cause of recurrent paralytic drop foot deformity. *Journal of Bone and Joint Surgery*, **44B**, 377–83.

GAGE J.R. & DRENNAN J.C. (1983) Orthotics in cerebral palsy. *In* THOMPSON G.L. (ed.) *Comprehensive Management of Cerebral Palsy*, pp. 205–13. Grune & Stratton, New York.

GIBSON, D.A., URS N.D.K. (1970) Arthrogryposis multiplex congenita. *Journal of Bone and Joint Surgery*, **52B**, 483–93.

GOLDNER J.I. & IRWIN C.E. (1948) Paralytic deformities of the foot. *American Academy of Orthopaedic Surgeons Instructional Course Lectures*, **5**, 190.

GREEN W.T. & GRICE D.S. (1951) The treatment of poliomyelitis: Acute and convalescent stages. *American Academy of Orthopaedic Surgeons Instructional Course Lectures*, **8**, 261.

GREEN W.T. & GRICE D.S. (1952) The management of chronic poliomyelitis. *American Academy of Orthopaedic Surgeons Instructional Course Lectures*, **9**, 85.

GREEN W.T. & GRICE D.S. (1956) The management of calcaneus deformity. *American Academy of Orthopaedic Surgeons Instructional Course Lectures*, **13**, 135.

GREEN N.E., GRIFFIN P.P. & SHIAVI R. (1983) Split posterior tibial-tendon transfer in spastic cerebral palsy. *Journal of Bone and Joint Surgery*, **65A**, 748–54.

GRICE D.S. (1952) An extra-articular arthrodesis of the subastragalar joint for correction of paralytic flat feet in children. *Journal of Bone and Joint Surgery*, **34A**, 927–40.

HAMSA W.R. (1936) Panastragaloid arthrodesis. A study of end-results in eighty-five cases. *Journal of Bone and Joint Surgery*, **18**, 732.

HART V.L. (1940) Lambrinudi operation for drop-foot. *Journal of Bone and Joint Surgery*, **22**, 937.

HARPER P.S. (1979) *Myotonic Dystrophy*, 12th ed., W.B. Saunders, Philadelphia.

HERNDON C.H. (1961) Tendon transplantation at the knee and foot. *American Academy of Orthopaedic Surgery Instructional Course Lectures*, **18**, 145.

HERNDON C.H., STRONG J.M. & HEYMAN C.H. (1956) Transposition of the tibialis anterior in the treatment of paralytic talipes calcaneus. *Journal of Bone and Joint Surgery*, **38A**, 751–60.

HIBBS R.A. (1919) An operation for 'claw-foot'. *Journal of the American Medical Association*, **73**, 1583.

HOFFER M.M. (1976) Basic considerations and classification of cerebral palsy. *American Academy of Orthopaedic Surgeons Instructional Course Lectures*, **15**, 96.

HOFFER M.M., REISWIG J.A., GARRETT A.M. & PERRY J. (1974) The split anterior tibial tendon transfer in treatment of spastic varus of the hindfoot in childhood. *Orthopaedic Clinics of North America*, **5**, 31–8.

HOKE M. (1921) An operation for stabilizing paralytic feet. *American Journal of Orthopaedic Surgery*, **3**, 494.

HOLMDAHL H.C. (1956) Astragalectomy as a stabilizing operation for foot paralysis following poliomyelitis; results of a follow-up investigation of 153 cases. *Acta Orthopaedica Scandinavica*, **25**, 207–27.

INCLAN A. (1949) End results in physiological blocking of flail joints. *Journal of Bone and Joint Surgery*, **31A**, 748–54.

INGRAM A.J. & HUNDLEY J.M. (1951) Posterior bone block of the ankle for paralytic equinus. An end-result study. *Journal of Bone and Joint Surgery*, **33A**, 679–91.

INMAN V.T. (1969) UCBL axis control system and UCBL shoe insert. *Bulletin of Prosthetic Research*, **10**, 11.

JONES M.H. (1975) Differential diagnosis and natural history of the cerebral palsied child. *In* SAMILSON R.L. (ed.) *The Orthopaedic Aspects of Cerebral Palsy*, pp. 5–25. J.B. Lippincott, Philadelphia.

JONES R. (1916) The soldier's foot and the treatment of common deformities of the foot. *British Medical Journal*, **1**, 749.

KAUFER H. (1977) Split tendon transfers. *Orthopaedic Transactions*, **1**, 191.

LAMBRINUDI C. (1927) New operation on drop-foot. *British Journal of Surgery*, **15**, 193.

LEIKKONEN O. (1950) Astragalectomy as ankle stabilizing operation in infantile paralysis sequelae. *Acta Chirugica Scandinavica*, **100**, 668–70.

LEVITT R.L., CANALE S.T., COOKE A.J. JR. & GARTLAND J.J. (1973) The role of foot surgery in progressive neuromuscular disorders in children. *Journal of Bone and Joint Surgery*, **55A**, 1396–410.

LIN R.S. (1982) Application of the varus T-strap principle to the polypropylene ankle foot orthosis. *Orthotics and Prosthetics*, **36**, 67–70.

LLOYD-ROBERTS G.C., LETTIN A.W.F. (1970) Arthrogryposis multiplex congenita. *Journal of Bone and Joint Surgery*, **52B**, 494–508.

MACKENZIE I.G. (1959) Lambrinudi's arthrodesis. *Journal of Bone and Joint Surgery*, **41B**, 738–48.

MCKEEVER D.C. (1952) Arthrodesis of the first metatarsophalangeal joint for hallux valgus, hallux rigidus and metatarsus primus varus. *Journal of Bone and Joint Surgery*, **34A**, 129–34.

MCNICOL D., LEONG J.C.Y. & HSU L.C.S. (1983) Supramalleolar derotation osteotomy for lateral tibial torsion and associated equinovarus deformity of the foot. *Journal of Bone and Joint Surgery*, **65B**, 166–70.

MENELAUS M.B. (1971) Talectomy for equinovarus deformity in arthrogryposis and spina bifida. *Journal of Bone and Joint Surgery*, **53B**, 468–73.

MITCHELL G.P. (1977) Posterior displacement osteotomy of the calcaneus. *Journal of Bone and Joint Surgery*, **59B**, 233–5.

PATTERSON R.L., PARRISH F.F. & HATHAWAY E.N. (1950) Stabilizing operations on the foot. A study of the indications, techniques used, and end results. *Journal of Bone and Joint Surgery*, **32A**, 1–26.

PAUKER E. (1959) Correction of the outwardly rotated leg from poliomyelitis. *Journal of Bone and Joint Surgery*, **41B**, 70–2.

PEABODY C.W. (1949) Tendon transposition in the paralytic foot. *American Academy of Orthopaedic Surgeons Instructional Course Lectures*, **6**, 179.

POLLOCK J.H. & CARRELL B. (1964) Subtalar extra-articular arthrodesis in the treatment of paralytic valgus deformities. A review of 112 procedures in 100 patients. *Journal of Bone and Joint Surgery*, **46A**, 533–41.

PYKA R.A., COVENTRY M.B. & MOE J.H. (1964) Anterior subluxation of the talus following triple arthrodesis. *Journal of Bone and Joint Surgery*, **46A**, 16–24.

RENSHAW T.R., SIRKIN R.B. & DRENNAN J.C. (1979) The management of hallux valgus in cerebral palsy. *Developmental Medicine and Child Neurology*, **21**, 202.

ROSE G.K. (1953) Arthropathy of the ankle in congenital indifference to pain. *Journal of Bone and Joint Surgery*, **35B**, 408–10.

ROUSSY G. & LÉVY G. (1926) Sept cas d'une maladie familiale particulaire: Troubles de la marche, pieds, bots et aréfléxie tendineuse généralisée, avec accessoirement, légère maladresse des mains. *Revue Neurologique* (Paris), **54**, 427.

RUSSMAN B.S., MELCHREIT R. & DRENNAN J.C. (1983) Spinal muscular atrophy: The natural course of disease. *Muscle and Nerve*, **6**, 179–81.

RYERSON E.W. (1923) Arthrodesing operations on the feet. *Journal of Bone and Joint Surgery*, **5**, 453.

SABIR M. & LYTTLE D. (1983) Pathogenesis of pes cavus in Charcot–Marie–Tooth disease. *Clincial Orthopaedics and Related Research*, **175**, 173–8.

SALTIEL J. (1969) A one-piece laminated knee locking short leg brace. *Orthotics and Prosthetics*, **23**, 69.

SAMILSON R.L. & DILLIN W. (1983) Cavus, cavovarus, and calcaneocavus. An update. *Clinical Orthopaedics and Related Research*, **177**, 125–32.

SHARRARD W.J.W. & GROSFIELD I. (1968) The managment of deformity and paralysis of the foot in myelomeningocele. *Journal of Bone and Joint Surgery*, **50B**, 456–65.

SHARRARD W.J.W. & BERNSTEIN S. (1972) Equinus deformity in cerebral palsy. A comparison between elongation of the tendo calcaneus and gastrocnemius recession. *Journal of Bone and Joint Surgery*, **54B**, 272–6.

SHARRARD W.J.W. & WEBB J. (1974) Supra-malleolar wedge osteotomy of the tibia in children with myelomeningocele. *Journal of Bone and Joint Surgery*, **56B**, 458–61.

SMITH T.W.D. & DUCKWORTH T. (1976) The management of deformites of the foot in children with spina bifida. *Developmental Medicine and Child Neurology (Supplement)*, **37**, 104–10.

SPENCER G.E., JR. & VIGNOS P.J. JR. (1962) Bracing for ambulation in childhood progressive muscular dystrophy. *Journal of Bone and Joint Surgery*, **44A**, 234–42.

STEINDLER A. (1920) Stripping of the os calcis. *Journal of Orthopaedic Surgery*, **2**, 8.

TAYLOR R.G. (1951) The treatment of claw toes by multiple transfers of flexors in to extensor tendons. *Journal of Bone and Joint Surgery*, **33B**, 539–42.

THOMPSON T.C. (1939) Astragalectomy and the treatment of calcaneovalgus. *Journal of Bone and Joint Surgery*, **21**, 627.

TOOTH H.H. (1886) *The Peroneal Type of Progressive Muscular Atrophy*. H.K. Lewis & Co., London.

WASHINGTON J.S., SCRANTON P.E. JR. & MARTINEX A.J. (1979) Charcot–Marie–Tooth disease: Clincial presentation, histopathology, and treatment. *Orthopaedic Surgery*, **2**, 314.

WAUGH T.R., WAGNER J. & STINCHFIELD F.E. (1965) An evaluation of pantalar arthrodesis. A follow-up study of one hundred and sixteen operations. *Journal of Bone and Joint Surgery*, **47A**, 1315–22.

WHITMAN A. (1922) Astragalectomy and backward displacement of the foot. An investigation of its practical results. *Journal of Bone and Joint Surgery*, **4**, 266.

Chapter 11
The Management of
Upper Limb Problems

N. J. BARTON

Introduction

It has been said that the hand is the cutting edge of the brain. Certainly the strong connection between the two is shown by the enormous cerebral representation for the hand, both as a motor and sensory organ. Indeed, we have more grey matter in the brain manipulating the thumb alone than in the total control of the chest and abdomen.

In consequence, disorders at any point from the cerebral cortex to the sensory nerves in the fingertips interfere with the function of the hand, both as an informant of the brain and as the executive of its desires.

It is useful to start by considering which manifestations of neurological disorders cannot be helped by local surgical treatment within the upper limb, and which may. There is, for example, nothing that peripheral surgery can do to improve involuntary movements such as *tremor, ataxia,* or *chorea. Writer's cramp* may present to the orthopaedic or hand surgeon, but is similarly unsuited to operative treatment: this condition is now regarded as a segmental dystonia, like torticollis, (not a psychological disorder) and may be helped by appropriate drugs. *Epilepsy* obviously affects the upper limbs during the fits, but may indirectly be associated with lasting abnormalities: posterior dislocation of the shoulders caused by a fit, or the proved association with Dupuytren's contracture (James 1969).

Psychiatric problems may also manifest themselves in the hand, though the patient, having deflected his problems into his hand, usually appears normal in his behaviour. There are four main types of presentation (Osborne 1983):

1 *Hysterical contracture of the fingers.*   This is typically a flexion contracture of the ulnar fingers (so that the patient has visible deformity and disability) but with sparing of the index finger and thumb (so that the patient is not too disabled). The degree of flexion is not altered by movements of the wrist (Simmons & Vasile 1980).
2 *'Functional' pain or paraesthesiae.*   The most common manifestation of this is pain in the wrist in girls or young women, akin to the non-organic anterior knee pain often experienced by such patients. The symptoms may be induced by problems with boy-friends or parents, or by the stress of impending examinations in which case the pain prevents the patient from writing.
3 *Bizarre forms of paralysis.*
4 *Persistent oedema.*   This can, of course, be produced by letting the hand hang down continuously and never using it, but it has been shown that in some cases the patient creates oedema by tying something around the arm to act as a venous and lymphatic tourniquet (Smith 1975). It is likely that many cases of Secretan's disease (oedema on the back of the hand following a minor injury and progressing to dense fibrous tissue binding down the extensor tendons and preventing flexion) are of this type.

Whatever the form, a hysterical hand is very hard to treat. Physical treatment, or even excessive investigation, merely focuses the patient's mind even more strongly upon the hand, and unfortunately this type of patient, lacking overt psychiatric problems, seldom responds well to psychiatric treatment (Louis *et al.* 1985), though prolonged courses of hypnosis may lead to some improvement. Some of these patients are on the borderland of malingering (Asher 1972, Spiegel & Chase 1980) and it is desirable that they should all be subtly offered some gain to set against the loss of their symptoms, although if compensation is involved the medical profession may not be able to offer as much as the legal profession.

Dystonia and athetosis are conditions in which the affected part makes uncontrollable writhing movements, which are rapid in athetosis and slow in dystonia. These movements may be the result of head injury, cerebral palsy, or Wilson's disease, and are not amenable to relief by extremity surgery: indeed athetosis is a contraindication to arm surgery in cerebral palsy. There are a few very uncommon situations where surgery may help. Pollock (1962) has reported good relief of painful dystonic shoulder movements in spastic hemiplegics by division of the anterior nerve roots of the third cervical to the first thoracic nerve. This is an extreme measure as it leaves an arm which is flail, but a useless arm may be preferable to one which is a menace. The rare idiopathic condition called dystonia musculorum deformans, which usually affects children, may stop progressing and become static, at which stage the orthopaedic surgeon may be able to help by correcting contractures. The author has seen a patient whose unceasing athetoid movements caused osteoarthritis of the shoulder which needed arthrodesis to relieve the pain.

Loss of sensitivity in the hand is just as disabling as paralysis but much harder to treat. It is well known that, even if a hand has normal motor function, any part which is anaesthetic will be little used or not at all: the anaesthetic finger is left sticking out while the other fingers grip something, and the patient with median nerve anaesthesia uses the ring and little fingers for manipulation. This is because cutaneous sensation is an important part of proprioception in the hand, and the manipulation of small objects (such as buttons, or the winding knob of a watch) require these afferent impulses to control

the movement and ensure that the correct amount of pressure is applied. This explains why patients with severe carpal syndrome sometimes drop things. The anaesthetic hand is a blind hand.

If the sensory deficit is due to some removeable cause, such as nerve compression, that should be treated and, provided there has not been too much delay, a full recovery can be expected. If the peripheral nerve has been cut, it should be sutured as accurately as possible, using magnification; if it has been damaged over a distance of up to 10 cm, the damaged section should be excised and grafts used to bridge the gap. In special circumstances, sensitive skin can be moved from a less important to a more important area (Omer 1980). The best known example is the neurovascular island flap from the ring finger to a reconstructed thumb, but the brain continues to regard this skin as belonging to the ring finger. However, it is now possible, with microsurgical techniques, to move free flaps of skin and suture their sensory nerve to a nerve at the recipient site, thus avoiding the misplaced perception.

In children, excellent results can be obtained from nerve suture, but adults never completely regain normal sensation. They should obtain protective sensation, but what is wanted is fine discriminatory sensation. One of the difficulties is that there is no satisfactory way of measuring sensation, and even if we can't do anything to improve sensation, we must always think about it, as the presence or absence of useful sensation may determine the functional result of an operation to improve motor power.

Moberg (1976) pointed out that the way in which a surgeon needs to assess sensation is quite different to the way in which this is done by a neurologist, and is worth quoting at length:

'The prominent British neurologist, Sir Russell Brain, said that the neurologist is concerned with sensibility primarily for the purpose of localizing lesions in the nervous system and determining their nature. His methods of investigation are therefore more rough and ready and have been adopted for their practical value for *his* immediate purpose. The purpose, however, of the hand surgeon is totally different. He must establish the value of the remaining afferents for gripping, proprioception, and other hand functions; thus his methods must be totally different. Of all the feeling, only a very limited part is of interest to him as useful. The hand surgeon's methods and tools must be entirely different from those of the neurologist. This applies also to other aspects of orthopaedic surgery.

'The most important part of hand exteroception and the only part worthwhile to register for useful function is the tactile gnosis, the high quality function which will let fingers and other parts of the hand *see* what they are doing.

'For the examination of useful sensibility, of all the tests evaluated by the author [Moberg], the only one which was found to be significant is the two point discrimination test now performed with a paper clip. All other tests for sensory function in reconstructive work, in my opinion, should be abandoned, including cottonwool and paper strip, pin prick, ordinary tuning fork, the difference between sharp and blunt, finger writing, the wrinkling skin test, and the two point discrimination test performed with sharp pointed compass. They are not only useless, they are even misleading.

'Though all the technical details necessary for accurate testing of two point discrimination need not be repeated here, one very important point, the amount of pressure applied, should be stressed. Deformation of the skin surface is admittedly a most important part of the stimulation upon which this test is built and deformation and motion of this surface is certainly a basis for the proprioceptive information the cutaneous afferents are able to transmit efficiently. A proper use of the two point discrimination test requires, therefore, that the pressure be minimal and the same every time. The rule is that where the limbs of the clip are put on the skin, blanching spots should be barely visible if at all. If too much pressure is applied, even receptors from an adjacent area of normal sensibility can be made to respond and their afferent impulses will be interpreted as coming from denervated receptors, and the test result will be totally unreliable.' (Moberg 1976)

The attraction of two-point discrimination is that it can be measured and a figure put on it. However, there is a danger, as in academic examinations, in measuring what is easy to measure rather than what is important. It has been shown by Wynn Parry (1981) that even two-point discrimination often has no correlation with the actual use of the part. This may be because two-point discrimination is usually measured in a static way whereas in normal life, when using the hand to feel something, one always *moves* the finger over the surface of the object. Dellon (1981), who has studied this subject in great detail, advocated the use of the moving two-point discrimination test, but this too has problems. Probably functional tests, as described by Wynn Parry (1981), are the most reliable, though they are very time consuming.

The truth is that sensory recovery is not a quantitative phenomenon. The patient does not regain 40% or 80% of normal sensation; he develops an *abnormal kind of sensation,* which is often not under-sensitive but over-sensitive and may be very unpleasant. Sensory re-education may help (Wynn Parry 1981), but if peripheral nerve surgery has failed or is inapplicable, or if the sensory loss is due to pathology in the central nervous system, then there is little that can be done except to educate the patient about the risk of unrealized injury, especially burns, so that the anaesthetic parts are not repeatedly damaged (Brand 1980).

Loss of sensitivity may also cause neuropathic joints; syringomyelia, for example, is often quoted as producing a neuropathic shoulder. In practice, this is seldom a problem in the upper limb, except in leprosy (Cochrane 1964).

Spastic paralysis is also a difficult problem.

Here again quantitative assessment is difficult as the familiar MRC scale of muscle power is not applicable, and the functional problem is complicated by lack of central control and often sensory defect. It is therefore not surprising that the types of tendon transfer which work so well in flaccid paralysis have proved disappointing in spastic conditions. Nevertheless there is sometimes a place for upper extremity surgery in these patients, provided that a very full assessment of the patient has been made, not just on one occasion but over a period.

Flaccid paralysis is the situation *par excellence* where surgery can help a great deal, but the problem to be solved and the manner of solving it vary with the cause and level of the lesion and these will be considered in turn.

From an anatomical point of view, one may classify neurological disorders affecting the upper limb into those where the primary pathology is in the brain, the spinal cord, the nerve roots, the region of the brachial plexus, or the peripheral nerves. The sympathetic nervous system will not be considered here, as post-traumatic sympathetic dystrophy (Sudeck's atrophy) is not really a neurological condition.

Disorders of the brain

As far as the upper limb is concerned, these usually produce a mainly spastic paralysis, but it may be flaccid or mixed spastic and flaccid. The situation is often further complicated by a sensory deficit and sometimes by mental defect.

There are three main types of brain damage having many points in common, but also differing in some important respects.

Cerebrovascular accidents

These usually affect older patients, who often make a good or even complete recovery. The place of surgery is thus palliative: either to tide the patient over a particular problem until he has recovered enough to control it, or to overcome some undesirable contracture. The patient's life-expectancy is often limited, and there is always a risk of another stroke, so reconstructive surgery to improve function is seldom applicable. The subject is more fully discussed in Chapter 12.

Head injury

Head injury from external trauma may cause permanent and sometimes tragic disability, often in a young or middle-aged person with many years of life ahead of them. The same may be said of the necessary injury caused by excision of a cerebral tumour. Treatment will consist, after the acute phase, of physiotherapy, retraining, and what social help is necessary. By about two years, the final state is likely to have been reached, both physically and mentally, and it is then worth considering whether surgical treatment may help, though it will do so only in a few cases.

Cerebral palsy

Cerebral palsy presents particularly complex problems, as there is no baseline of previously normal performance and, though the disorder itself is not progressive, the child will change with growth and intellectual development. It is therefore necessary to study the child over a period, with the help of a physiotherapist skilled in this specialized problem, to learn what the child can and cannot do, and have some idea of the prognosis. It must be remembered that the deformity varies according to circumstances and the excitement and activity of the child: this is why an assessment by an experienced physiotherapist is so important.

These aspects are considered in Chapter 2, but as most operations in cerebral palsy are carried out on the lower limbs, it is worth considering here the differences which apply in dealing with the upper limbs. These have been well described by Pollock (1962):

'A greater degree of neuromuscular co-ordination is required to thread a needle or to fasten small buttons than is demanded for such mass movements as standing or walking. It follows, therefore, when function forms the yardstick of the success or failure of an operation, that a greater degree of satisfaction will be gained by those who have had lower limb operations than is likely to be enjoyed by those who have had upper limb operations.'

However, Inglis and Cooper (1966) pointed out 'that many of these patients possess a relatively good opposite extremity and may require merely an assistive member or a posture or the right hand suitable for shaking hands'. It is essential to set realistic goals: if the aim is too high, both the surgeon and the patient will be disappointed. Swanson (1960), having seen about 300 spastic children, operated on the upper limbs in only 12, and this is probably a correct proportion.

Many patients can be ruled out as candidates for surgery because of:

1 Severe mental handicap.
2 Severe sensory defect. Sensation to pin-prick is usually normal, but is not what matters. The important thing to learn is the patient's ability to recognize (without seeing) various familiar objects placed in the hand, as this determines the capacity of the hand for practical functional use.
3 Athetosis.
4 Lack of voluntary motor control in the arm and hand.
5 Lack of desire to use the hand. If the affected limb has been 'forgotton' by the patient, and he never makes any attempt to use it, then it is unlikely that he will do so after an operation.

Although most experienced surgeons consider that each of the above factors makes the patient unlikely to benefit from an operation, it must be remembered that each one has been stated by some expert *not* to be a contraindication. This just shows how difficult is the subject. The surgeon would have to be very sure that the patient was ideal in every other way before operating in the presence of one of these deficits. The assessment of these children requires both time and knowledge; Goldner (1974) gave an excellent account of the special methods of examination required, and the concepts to be borne in mind when planning surgery. An inadequately thought-out operation will not merely fail to produce better function, but may make it worse. It is therefore wise to defer surgery until the child is old enough to cooperate. Zancolli (1979) classified the deformities as mild, moderate and severe. The severe ones are usually beyond surgical correction, and the mild ones often do not need it. It is the moderately severe

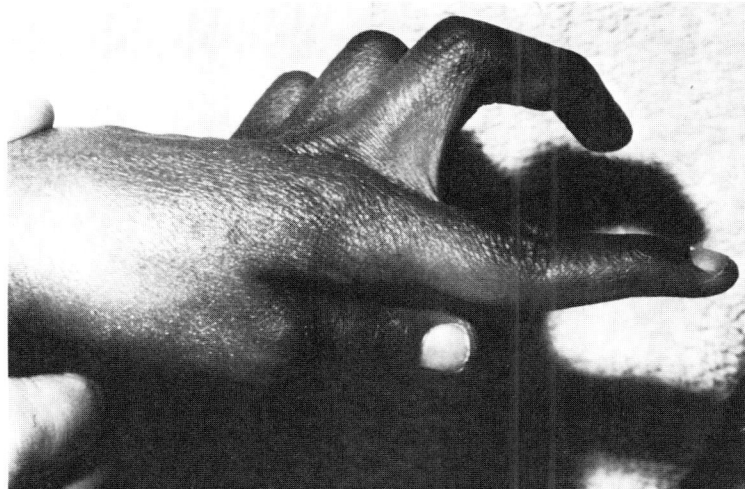

Fig. 11.1. Swan-neck deformity in cerebral palsy.

cases which are most likely to benefit from surgery.

What types of deformity occur? The following description applies mainly to cerebral palsy, but to some extent also to stroke and head injury patients.

Deformities of the arm

Three deformities may be seen: internal rotation of the shoulder, flexion of the elbow, and pronation of the forearm. These seldom require surgical correction. Pollock (1962) pointed out that 'in the hemiplegic patient the involved or assisting hand functions best in pronation'.

Deformity of the wrist

The flexion deformity of the wrist is the key to the whole problem as it determines not only the position of the hand but the function of the fingers and thumb. Generally it is due to spasticity of the wrist flexors, but the wrist extensors may be either relatively normal (and just overcome by the spastic flexors) or actually weak due to the admixture of flaccid paralysis which may be present in cerebral palsy. A median nerve block may make the picture clearer. This balance between flexors and extensors is the key to the problem, and the wrist is the key joint. One might compare the situation to a see-saw, which must have roughly equal forces on each side to work properly, but is more complicated because the long flexors and extensors of the fingers cross several joints which, if not properly balanced, will collapse into a Z deformity: thus it is more like a see-saw with one or more hinges in the middle.

If the deformity can be passively corrected, then transfer of flexor carpi ulnaris (which is used in radial nerve palsy) around the ulnar border of the wrist to extensor carpi radialis longus or brevis (opinions differ) produces good correction (Green & Banks 1962). It should be added that Samilson and Morris (1964), while

recommending this operation, noted that simple tenotomy of flexor carpi ulnaris seemed to be just as effective. This transfer has the added advantage of helping to overcome the pronation of the forearm and is logical, as it has been shown that, in the spastic arm, the flexor carpi ulnaris is electrically active in extension as well as flexion (Samilson & Morris 1964). Sharrard (1971) considered that this operation, unlike most in the spastic upper limb, should sometimes be carried out in early childhood if, in spite of good conservative management, a flexion deformity of the wrist was developing. An alternative tendon to use as the transfer is brachioradialis, but it may be wise to save that for the thumb (see below).

If there is a flexion contracture of the wrist, so that it cannot be passively extended, some sort of release will be necessary to straighten it. However, this must be approached with the utmost caution. In this position, neither the finger flexors nor the wrist extensors can act to full advantage, and assessment of their power is very difficult. Still more important, if there is spasticity of the long flexors of the fingers and thumb, increasing the extension of the wrist will make these tighter and increase the flexion of the fingers and thumb. Arthrodesis of the wrist, once popular, may be even worse, because many patients can only obtain active flexion and extension of their fingers by a tenodesis effect produced by flexion and extension of the wrist. No such operation should be performed without a preliminary trial period in a plaster-cast with the wrist as fully extended as possible, as this may worsen function of the hand. On those rare occasions when the spastic wrist is arthrodesed, the bone should be shortened considerably to avoid tightening the long flexors of the digits.

Deformities of the hand

Many patterns are possible, but the most common are flexion of the fingers and flexion–adduction of the thumb or, alternatively, swan–neck deformity of the fingers (Fig. 11.1) and the

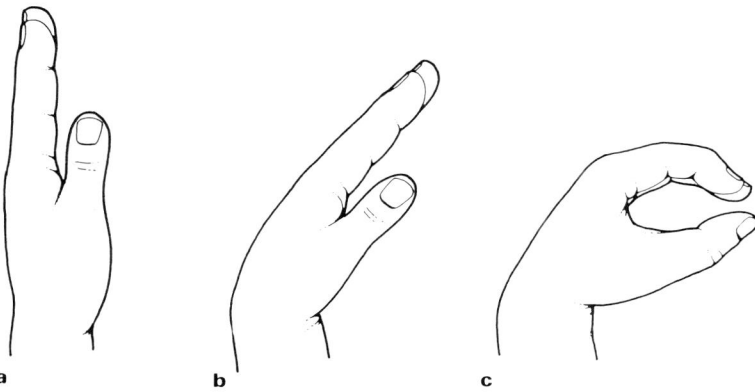

Fig. 11.2. Zancolli's classification of cerebral palsy:
(a) Fingers can be extended when wrist is straight.
(b) Fingers can be extended when wrist is flexed. (This may be divided into two subgroups: see text.)
(c) Even with the wrist flexed the fingers cannot be extended.

corresponding hyperextension of the metacarpophalangeal joint of the thumb.

No definitive correction of these should be carried out until the final position of the wrist has been decided and achieved, as this will alter the balance of the extrinsic muscles acting on the digits.

Flexion of the fingers

This may be so severe that the fingernails dig into the palmar skin and damage it, but the usual problem is that the patient can't open his hand to grasp. It is not much use being able to flex the fingers to hold something, unless they can first be extended sufficiently to get them around the object to be grasped.

The flexor tendons to the fingers cross the wrist joint, and the deformities of the wrist and fingers are closely interlinked. Zancolli (1979) distinguished different grades of severity (Fig. 11.2). If the patient *can actively extend the fingers fully with the wrist in a neutral position,* surgical treatment is not needed. The patients who are most amenable to improvement by operation are those in whom *the fingers can only be extended when the wrist if flexed.* These may be divided into two subgroups: in the first, the patient can *actively* extend the wrist when the fingers are flexed. This means that the extensors

of the wrist are active, that the spasticity of the wrist flexor muscles is not very important, and that the principal spasticity is located in the flexor muscles of the fingers. Treatment may therefore be confined to lengthening the finger flexors. The technique for this will be considered later. In the second subgroup, the patient, even with the fingers flexed, actively extend the wrist. This means that the extensors are themselves weak and need to be reinforced by one of the methods described above. In more severe cases, *the fingers cannot be extended even when the wrist is flexed,* and operation to reduce strength in the flexors may produce a less awkward and better looking hand, but little improvement in function.

It is easy enough to lengthen the flexors by tendon lengthening, but in so doing the power of grasp is weakened. Zancolli (1979) described a method of lengthening the flexors within their muscle substance which, he stated, preserved the force of grasp. Inglis and Cooper (1966) recommended a more proximal procedure, releasing the origin of the flexor muscles and allowing them to slide distally (Fig. 11.3). The flexor muscle mass includes pronator teres, the wrist flexors, and flexor pollicis longus which are simultaneously released. Eighteen patients were reviewed after this operation, and all gained better control of the hand and improved appearance, with grasp which was excellent in nine and good so far in eight.

Thumb-in-palm deformity

This deformity seriously interferes with function, since the thumb is not only useless itself but gets in the way of the fingers and may even provoke a gripping reflex in them.

Again it is difficult to know whether the deformity is due mainly to weakness of the extensors, or to overactivity of either the flexors or the adductor of the thumb. Ulnar nerve block will eliminate adductor spasm.

longus, or to the 'de Quervain's tendons' abductor pollicis longus and extensor pollicis brevis.

If there is a fixed contracture, this must first be released. Matev (1963) stressed that it is not only the adductor pollicis which must be released, but also the first dorsal interosseous, and the flexor pollicis brevis. He found that proximal release of these muscles from their origins (similar to the flexor–pronator slide mentioned above) was superior to divison of the tendons at their insertion on the sesamoids, as some muscle power was retained. Once this has been done, it will become clear whether a cautious lengthening of the flexor pollicis longus tendon is also needed.

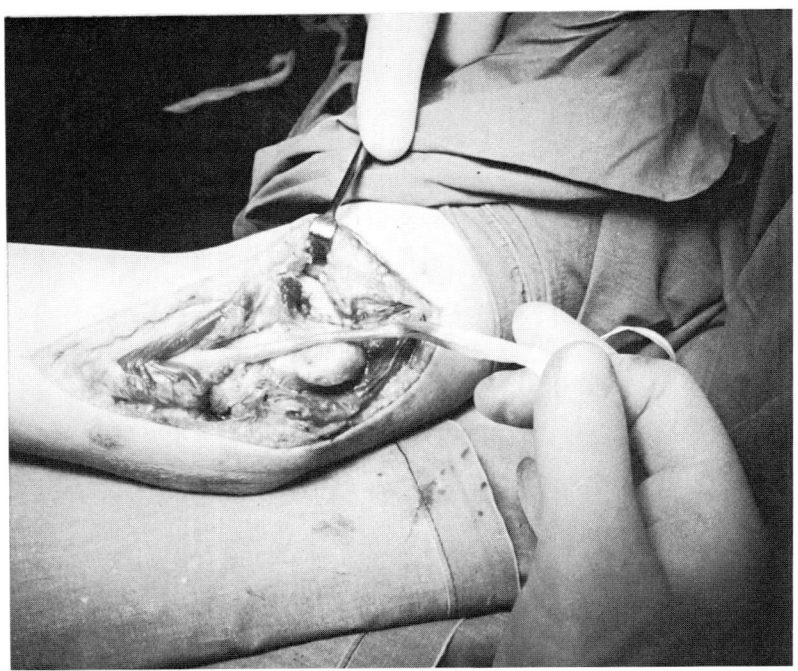

Fig. 11.3. Flexor slide operation for cerebral palsy; the common flexor origin has been detached and allowed to slide distally.

If passive extension can be achieved, by serial splintage if necessary, a tendon transfer is indicated to maintain it. Swanson (1960) recommended flexor carpi radialis as the donor; brachioradialis is probably better, as it is usually under voluntary control and has an adequate excursion provided that it is freed throughout its length, as described by McCue *et al.* (1970). The transfer may be to the re-routed extensor pollicis

Swan-neck deformity of the fingers

This deformity (Fig. 11.1) is seen in patients with less severe muscle imbalance who are therefore more likely to be helped by surgical procedures. It may also develop after operations to weaken the flexors or strengthen the long extensors. Swanson (1960) has described in detail the cause and management of this deformity in cerebral palsy. It is not, as stated by some authors, due to spasticity of the intrinsic muscles: contraction or contracture of these muscles produces flexion of the metacarpophalangeal joints and extension of the interphalangeal joints, but not swan-neck deformity (Heywood 1979). In patients with cerebral palsy, the intrinsic element can be largely eliminated by blocking the ulnar nerve (Caldwell *et al.* 1969); usually this does little to reduce the swan-neck deformity, which is mainly due to spasticity of the extrinsic long extensors, but it simplifies assessment of the problem. The most effective treatment seems to be tenodesis of the flexor digitorum superficialis tendon to hold the proximal interphalangeal joint in 20° or 30° of flexion (Swanson 1960).

Hyperextension of the metacarpophalangeal thumb joint

This similar deformity can be dealt with simply and satisfactorily by fusion of the metacarpophalangeal joint.

Finally, any operation in a spastic limb is likely to require a longer period of postoperative immobilization than would the same procedure in a flaccid limb; for example, it is wise to keep tendon transfers in plaster for six weeks, to avoid the spastic muscles pulling the suture-line apart.

Disorders of the spinal cord

Poliomyelitis

There are still millions of people throughout the world suffering from the effects of poliomyelitis. It is true that an orthopaedic surgeon working in an industrialized country in the northern half of the Western hemisphere will encounter few of them, but it behoves him to have a good understanding of this condition and its management for two reasons:

1 Air travel makes it easy for patients from the Third World to travel to the West, either as immigrants or to seek treatment. Moreover, there is no certainty that our programmes of immunization will continue to be as effective as they are now: new strains of virus may develop and, because the disease is now rare, parents may stop bothering to have their children immunized.

2 Many of the basic operations of orthopaedic surgery, for example tendon transfers, were worked out and developed for poliomyelitis patients, and the general principles underlying these operations are seen most clearly in this condition.

The muscular paralysis usually affects isolated groups of muscles in a predictable pattern for which standard methods of treatment have been evolved. The frequency of permanent paralysis in the muscles of the upper limb is shown in Table 11.1 (Sharrard 1957). Note that this is not the same as the pattern of original paralysis,

Table 11.1 Frequency of permanent paralysis in muscles of the upper limb in 149 patients with poliomyelitis. These figures are derived from Sharrard (1957) but presented differently; shown here is the proportion of patients with permanent paralysis in whom the particular muscle group was affected. The figures therefore do not add up to 100.

Muscle	% of patients
Thenar muscles	19
Deltoid	17
Interosseous and hypothenar muscles	10
Triceps	10
Wrist flexors	9
Infraspinatus	9
Wrist extensors	7
Pronators	7
Latissimus dorsi	7
Elbow flexors	7
Extensors of thumb	6
Pectoralis major	6
Flexor pollicis longus	5
Extensor digitorum longus	5
Flexors of finger	3
Trapezius	1

which is much more extensive; in Sharrard's 149 patients, 841 muscle groups in the upper limb were initially paralysed, but only 195 permanently, and it is those which are analysed in Table 11.1. There was also a difference in the pattern: for example, pectoralis major was often paralysed initially but usually recovered. Sharrard showed that the muscles most prone to lasting paralysis in poliomyelitis were those innervated by motor axons whose anterior horn cells were confined to a short length of the spinal cord. In contrast, if there is a longer column of anterior horn cells, it is likely that some will be spared and the muscle supplied will retain some function: as little as 20% of surviving anterior horn cells can produce muscle power of grade 4. Pectoralis major, supplied through C5, 6, 7, 8 and T1, is a good example.

Because the areas of paralysis are isolated, nearby muscles which are working normally are available for transfer. Further advantages are that poliomyelitis is not complicated by any sensory loss, and stiffness is seldom a problem unless long-standing muscle imbalance has led to contractures. The problem in the upper limbs is usually a clear-cut and relatively simple matter of weakness or complete paralysis.

For a full account of the orthopaedic management, the reader is referred to the chapter by Sharrard (1971) in his textbook on paediatric orthopaedics.

In the upper limb, the operations most often applicable in poliomyelitis are tendon transfers. There are five prerequisites to be established before such an operation is undertaken (Bunnell 1964):

1   Any contracture must be corrected first; no tendon transfer can overcome a contracture or can work unless there is good movement of the joints concerned.
2   The muscle whose tendon is to be transferred must be strong enough to do the job. It is likely to lose one grade on the MRC scale as a result of being transferred, so it must start as grade 5 if it is to end as grade 4 which is, in most situations, the minimum power to be useful. It must also, obviously, be a muscle which is surplus to requirements, or can be made surplus to requirements, so that no significant disability will result from moving it. However, there are some operations, such as transfer of pronator teres to the radial wrist extensors, after which the original function will be retained and the new one added.

3   The transferred tendon must have a large enough amplitude of excursion to provide the function needed. This is a complex subject; the author has seen a patient with no functioning finger flexors who had been treated by transfer of a radial wrist extensor to the flexor digitorum profundus tendons and obtained full active flexion of the fingers, despite the fact that the wrist had virtually no movement so there could be no tenodesis effect. It appears that some muscles have a greater *potential* amplitude of contraction than they use in their normal situation, and that it is the length of the individual muscle fibres which is the determining factor. Brand *et al.* (1981) published detailed figures of the fibre lengths and potential strengths of all the muscles below the elbow, and this thoughtful paper is well worth studying.
4   A straight line of pull is desirable, and where possible the transferred tendon should run in subcutaneous fat and not through fascial windows to which it may adhere.
5   'A muscle-tendon unit cannot provide two different degrees of power and amplitude by acting on two recipients of different excursions' (Bunnell 1964).

It is not possible to consider here every conceivable operation to improve function in the upper limb stricken by polio, but three of the most common problems in the upper limb requiring surgical treatment will be discussed. These are paralysis of opposition, paralysis of the elbow flexors, and paralysis of the deltoid.

Paralysis of opposition

It is possible to hold the thumb in an opposed position by inserting a bone graft between the first and second metacarpals, but this is unsatisfactory, especially in patients whose legs are also paralysed and who have to use crutches, which press on the bone graft.

A much better solution is by a tendon transfer to provide active opposition. It happens that, in polio, the thenar muscles are often paralysed but the flexor digitorum superficialis is nearly always still active, so the operation that became standard was transfer of the flexor digitorum superficialis to the thumb, passing it around some form of pulley on the ulnar side of the wrist to ensure that the tendon approached the thumb from the correct direction for the purpose.* Many variations of the operation have been worked out (Brand 1977). A more proximal pulley gives better palmar abduction and a more distal one better adduction, so the patient's main need must be identified. In a poliomyelitis patient, the need is usually for palmar abduction and pronation to contribute to the compound movement which moves the thumb into opposition with the fingers.

The results of transfers to provide opposition are usually good in poliomyelitis. When there is median nerve paralysis secondary to nerve division at the wrist, the superficialis transfer is unsuitable as the flexor digitorum superficialis tendons have often been damaged too, but it has been found that the spare extensor tendons to the index (Burkhalter et al. 1973) or little finger (Schneider 1969) can be used very satisfactorily to provide opposition, with the advantage that the grip is not weakened. In fact, they work so well that their use should be considered in poliomyelitis, especially in the supple oriental hand in which excision of superficialis often leads to a swan-neck deformity unless special measures are taken to prevent this (Ranney 1976).

The other intrinsic muscles of the hand are also frequently paralysed, but the effect is not so disabling and surgical treatment is less often necessary. The type of operations which may be done are considered later in relation to leprosy.

Paralysis of the elbow flexors

If the hand is normal, but the patient cannot flex his elbow, there is great restriction of what he can do with his hand. Although he can grasp something, he cannot lift it or move it from place

to place. For this reason, although the biceps and brachialis (which are the principal elbow flexors) are seldom permanently paralysed by polio (Table 11.1), severe disability results when these muscles are affected. The triceps is more often paralysed, but for most individuals loss of active flexion is the greater handicap, as the elbow can be extended by gravity.

A variety of different muscles and tendon transfers have been used to provide flexion. The simplest, and usually the best, is Steindler's operation in which the common flexor origin at the elbow is moved a short distance up the humerus so that contraction of these muscles flexes the elbow as well as the wrist and fingers. This often results in some loss of extension at the elbow but, perhaps for that reason, gives powerful flexion. This power is even greater if the extensor muscle origin on the lateral side of the elbow is similarly transposed upwards. The disadvantage of the procedure is that the hand clenches when the elbow if flexed, but usually both actions are required at the same time so no difficulty results.

Alternatively, the pectoralis major may be used to flex the elbow. In Clark's operation, the *origin* of the lateral part of the pectoralis major is detached from the lower ribs and external oblique muscle. This part of the muscle is then separated from the rest (while preserving its neurovascular pedicle) and the strip of freed muscle passed down the front of the upper arm to be attached to the biceps tendon; unlike most tendon transfers, the insertion is not disturbed. Brooks and Seddon devised a different method of using pectoralis major, in which its tendon of *insertion* was detached from the humerus and sutured to the biceps tendon, using the tendon of the long head of biceps to span the gap. They compared their results with those of the Steindler and Clark procedures and found that, on the whole, the latter were better (Segal et al. 1959). However, the two forms of pectoral transfer are not really alternatives; the Brooks–Seddon operation is designed for patients in whom the lower part of the pectoralis major is paralysed and therefore cannot be transferred. Both often

---

* It will be noted that this is an unavoidable exception to the general rule that transferred tendons should run in a straight line.

produce unwanted movements of the shoulder, especially internal rotation so that, when the elbow is flexed, the hand comes across the chest instead of up to the mouth. This may need to be corrected by an external rotation osteotomy of the humerus, or by arthrodesis of the shoulder.

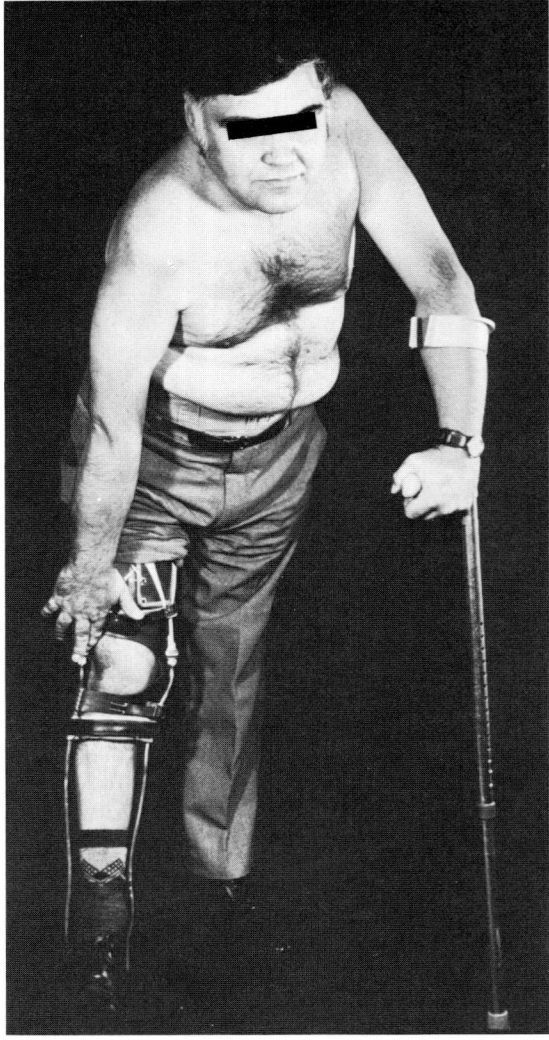

Fig. 11.4. This man with old poliomyelitis has paralysis of the elbow flexors. However, he has learned to live with this and any operation to improve active elbow flexion would be likely to cause some loss of extension. As can be seen in the picture, he needs full extension of the elbow to lock his caliper; such an operation might handicap him rather than help him.

For this reason, the Steindler operation, if possible, is the first choice.

Other transfers to restore elbow flexion are more notable for their ingenuity than their value to the patient: for example the sternomastoid transfer which flexes the elbow when the head is turned to the opposite side, a most unhelpful combination of actions. With the advent of free tissue transfers using microvascular anastomosis, it became possible to move muscles almost anywhere, but as far as is known these methods have not yet been applied in poliomyelitis and the necessity to divide and suture the motor nerve must diminish the likely final strength.

It must be stressed that surgery should not be undertaken if it may result in some loss of function (Fig. 11.4).

Paralysis of the deltoid

In most cases the muscles connecting the shoulder-girdle to the trunk are still working, and arthrodesis of the shoulder therefore allows the patient to control movements of the humerus. This procedure gained a bad reputation because the shoulder was often fused in excession internal rotation and abduction, but Barr *et al.* (1942) reviewed 101 patients and found that arthrodesis gave satisfactory results, even in girls, if done in the proper position of about 45° abduction, 20° flexion and 20° internal rotation.

They also reviewed 62 assorted muscle transfers around the shoulder in polio, and found that the results were only satisfactory in patients who had fair power in the deltoid before operation.

Tetraplegia

In injury of the spinal cord, the damage may be partial or complete. If partial, there is usually enough recovery to eliminate the need for surgery. If complete, there is severe disability which will be permanent. The degree of severity depends on the level of the lesion; the more proximal the damage, the more extensive the paralysis and anaesthesia, and in cervical cord injuries, which now constitute about half the admissions to spinal injury units, the result is tetraplegia.* In fact these patients have two-and-two-halves-plegia; their lower limbs are completely paralysed and their upper limbs partly paralysed. The question is whether the remaining muscular activity in the upper limbs can be redeployed to better advantage.

Before about 1945, the patients usually died. Once they began to have a future, largely due to the work of Guttman (1973), the question arose as to whether anything could be done to reduce their disability. The prospect of facing life as a tetraplegic is so appalling that one cannot imagine which aspects would be more tolerable, or less intolerable, than others:

1 loss of use of the lower limbs;
2 loss of normal bladder and bowel function;
3 loss of use and feeling of the sexual organs;
4 loss of use of the arms and hands.

Hanson and Franklin (psychologists, not surgeons) asked this question in 1976 to 74 male tetraplegics: 75% said that the function they would most like to regain was normal use of their upper limbs; 19% chose control of their bowel and bladder; and 4% use of their lower limbs. Sex came last, at 1.3%.

Obviously it is impossible to restore *normal* use of the arms and hands, but one might be able to provide a little function and, as Bunnell (who was among the first to try) used to say, 'to the patient who has nothing, a little is a lot'. The tendon transfers which had proved so effective in poliomyelitis were therefore applied in tetraplegic patients. However, tetraplegia is very different to poliomyelitis, partly because the cord damage is less patchy and there are usually fewer working muscles available for transfer, but mainly because in spinal cord injury there is also loss of sensation. This has two effects. First,

there are all the problems of pressure sores and other inadvertent damage to anaesthetic parts. Second, even if normal muscular action could be restored, normal prehension would not, because sensory feedback is an essential component; the fingers would remain like those in a complete median nerve lesion, only used to a limited extent. For this reason, these operations were not very helpful to the patients, and were condemned by the doctors responsible for their total care: Guttman, for example, declared (on his experience of two patients) that surgery had no part to play in restoring function in the upper limb, and such was his authority that this view was widely accepted.

Another approach was by the provision of active splints or orthoses, pioneered by Nickel *et al.* (1963) at the Rancho Los Amigos Hospital for Rehabilitation at Downey, near Los Angeles. A simple example of this is the finger hinge hand. The critical level in tetraplegia is C6; if this is intact, then at least extensor carpi radialis longus will be working, and if the patient can actively extend the wrist this movement can be harnessed, through a series of mechanical linkages, to flex the fingers against the thumb. In practice, the splints proved rather cumbersome, but sometimes enough contracture developed in the long flexors of the fingers to allow wrist extension to give some flexion by the tenodesis effect without any splint.

In about 1972 Erik Moberg, on his retirement from his post as Professor of Orthopaedic Surgery in Gothenburg, Sweden, applied himself to this problem. His experience and conclusions have been described in a book published in 1978 which is essential and fascinating reading for any surgeon considering operating on the upper limbs of a tetraplegic patient, or indeed for anybody involved in the care of such patients. In this short chapter it is only possible to pick out a few key points.

To describe a patient as having 'a C7 lesion' is useful as a rough shorthand expression to give some idea of the situation, but is imprecise and even misleading, because in about half the patients the degree of involvement differs in the

---

* The term 'tetraplegia' is preferable to 'quadriplegia', because in the former both elements are derived from Greek, whereas the latter is a mixture as 'quadri-' is Latin.

right and left upper limbs, and the levels of motor and sensory involvement may not be the same. The orthopaedic surgeon needs to be much more thorough and exact. He must *spend a long time assessing* the patient and deciding which muscles are active, what sensation is present, and what functions it may be possible to achieve. Moberg stated that 'the examination of the patient's upper limbs for the first time by a trained examiner usually takes about 1½ hours'. He also stressed that this examination should always take place with the patient in a wheelchair (Fig. 11.5).

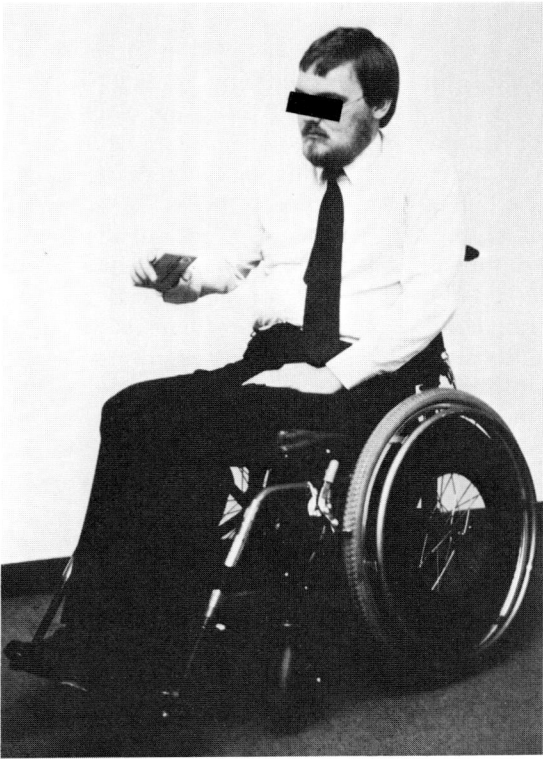

Fig. 11.5. Tetraplegia. The patient's function must be assessed very carefully, with the patient in a wheelchair.

The patients are classified into 'two main groups based on the afferent stimuli to control grip; ocular only, or ocular and cutaneous sensibility in the hand'. Each of these main groups is subdivided into subgroups based on the avail-able muscles working at grade 4 (because nothing less is of practical use)

0   nothing below elbow
1   brachioradialis
2   also radial wrist extensors
3   also pronator*

In planning treatment, Moberg's greatest contribution was to *define attainable and useful goals*. These were:

(i)   *Some grip with one hand*

He abandoned attempts to restore normal pulp-to-pulp pinch between the thumb and the index and middle fingers, and aimed instead at *key pinch*, between the pulp of the thumb and the radial border of the index finger. This is less precise but stronger and easier to achieve. Moberg considered that we use key pinch in about half our gripping actions; tetraplegics will not be picking up pins because of the sensory loss; they want to hold a piece of bread or a book. His method of achieving key pinch was by:

1   Arthrodesis of the interphalangeal joint of the thumb, so that the action of flexor pollicis longus is transferred to the metacarpophalangeal joint. (In practice, formal arthrodesis may be unnecessary, and the joint can simply be stabilized by a longitudinal threaded Kirschner wire which has the advantage that the procedure is reversible.)
2   Release of the fibrous flexor sheath of flexor pollicis longus, by a sort of extended trigger thumb operation, to further enhance flexion at the metacarpophalangeal joint.
3   Tenodesis of flexor pollicis longus to the front of the radius, so that extension of the wrist pulls it tight and moves the thumb as desired.

---

* Moberg's classification continued with another five subgroups, not applicable to post-traumatic tetraplegia, but worth considering in the whole context of this chapter:
4   also flexor carpi radialis
5   also extensor digitorum longus
6   also extensor pollicis longus
7   also some of the long finger flexors
8   also intrinsic muscles.

4 If necessary, the provision of a wrist extensor by transfer of brachioradialis.

(ii) *Active power of extension of the elbow*

It is no use being able to grip if the hand cannot be brought to the object to be gripped and then moved to place the object. When standing, elbow flexion is generally used for this purpose, but if confined to a wheelchair the perspective is different and the individual usually reaches *up* to things. For this purpose the elbow needs to be extended against gravity and against the weight of the object to be picked up. Furthermore, strong elbow extension assists in transfer from a wheelchair to a bed or car, and even if the patient can only partly lift his/her bottom off the chair, this will diminish the danger of pressure sores. The operation to achieve elbow extension uses as motor the posterior part of the deltoid muscle, which is supplied by C5 and therefore working (as patients with injuries above that level seldom survive for long). The deltoid is too short to reach to the triceps tendon and the gap is bridged by tendon grafts, a large supply of tendons being available in the useless lower limbs.

Lamb and Chan (1983) have reviewed 41 tetraplegic patients who have had reconstructive surgery in the upper limb. They use a different, and more practical classification, but again based on the available working muscles. Most of their patients had, in addition to shoulder abduction and elbow flexion, active wrist dorsiflexion, pronation and supination. Another large group also had flexor carpi radialis and elbow extension; these only needed hand surgery. Unlike Moberg, Lamb preferred active tendon transfers, usually extensor carpi radialis longus to flexor digitorum profundus, and brachioradialis to flexor pollicis longus. The aim, however, was the same; a key grip to give the patient greater independence. Twelve of the patients were followed up for over ten years, and the average follow-up was 7½ years. The results were good, not only in theory but also in practical functions such as holding cups, washing themselves, combing their hair, turning taps, propelling a wheel-chair and using a telephone.

Although the paralysis is usually mainly flaccid, in some patients there is a considerable element of spasticity, and the problem must be approached differently, along the lines described above for cerebral palsy.

It is quite clear that the lives of these unfortunate patients can often be improved considerably by carefully considered and carefully performed surgery. The value of deltoid transfers is perhaps still open to question, but surgical restoration of a key pinch, where appropriate, should now be regarded as a routine part of rehabilitation.

Other disorders of the spinal cord

Cervical disc lesions may produce a myelopathy, and of course rheumatoid arthritis may produce instability of the cervical spine causing neurological impairment. Here the orthopaedic surgeon is able to deal with the problem at its source.

Syringomyelia is a dilatation of the central canal of the spinal cord, producing flaccid paralysis and anaesthesia. The latter may manifest itself as a neuropathic joint, typically the shoulder, which paradoxically may be painful enough to require operation. Apart from this, the surgeon's role is likely to be limited to amputating fingers which have been irretrievably damaged by burns resulting from the loss of sensation. Patients with traumatic paraplegia due to thoracolumbar fractures may also develop a cystic dilation in the cervical cord, causing neurological impairment in the upper limbs on which they are so dependent. This requires urgent decompression, and doctors treating such patients must be on the lookout for this little-understood condition.

Transverse myelitis produces an effect similar to injury of the spinal cord, but the prognosis is uncertain. About 50% will later develop multiple sclerosis, but in others the disease process seems to be short-lived and the patient may be a candidate for reconstructive surgery if there is partial function in the upper limbs.

Friedreich's ataxia causes major orthopaedic problems in the form of scoliosis and foot deformities (Chapter 6), but the hands are seldom affected enough to need surgery.

Similarly peroneal muscular atrophy (Charcot–Marie–Tooth disease) results in wasting of the small muscles of the hand but function usually remains adequate.

Motor neuron disease progresses rapidly to death in a few years, and the surgeon can offer no more help than the physician. In spinal muscle atrophy (Chapters 5 and 6), there is proximal muscle weakness resembling that seen in muscular dystrophies, but the hands are little affected.

Nerve root lesions

The nerve roots may be compressed by a tumour as they leave the spinal canal, but far the commonest cause of trouble is a cervical disc lesion. The diagnosis and management of these is beyond the scope of this book, and for a full account the reader is referred to the monograph by Jeffreys (1980).

It is, however, appropriate to stress that cervical disc lesions are even more common than the carpal tunnel syndrome, and that the diagnosis of a peripheral nerve compression cannot be made until a cervical cause has been eliminated. C6 and 7 lesions must be distinguished from median nerve lesions, and C8 root pathology from affections of the ulnar nerve. In most cases, this can be done on the history and examination; for example, carpal tunnel syndrome usually causes painful pins-and-needles, whereas a cervical disc causes a feeling of 'deadness'. If the patient indicates the *back* of the hand as the site of symptoms, the origin is more likely to be cervical.

X-rays of the cervical spine will not help in locating the source of the symptoms, as degenerative changes are so common in the general population. Heller *et al.* (1983) found radiological cervical spondylosis was just as frequent in control patients having barium meals as

in patients with pain in their neck or arm: in fact over 60% of the control patients aged over 60 had radiologically marked disc changes. The *severity* of the disc changes did tend to be worse in patients with painful necks, but it was the only difference between the two groups; the severity of apophyseal joint changes was the same.

However, if the clinical evidence points to the neck, it seems wise to obtain radiographs as occasionally there may be a more serious pathology such as infection or tumour, for which neither physiotherapy nor a collar would be the best treatment. This is so rare that Heller *et al.* (1983) who found no such unexpected pathology in any of the 1263 cervical spines X-rayed, doubted whether routine radiology for this purpose was justified. The present author considers that even one missed but treatable infection is too high a price to pay. Trauma is, of course, a different problem, in that X-rays are mandatory.

Unfortunately, since cervical spondylosis and carpal tunnel syndrome are both common, there are undoubtedly some patients who have both; indeed it is thought that a mild degree of compression (not in itself enough to be symptomatic) may, if occurring at two levels, summate to cause symptoms distally. Such cases are difficult to work out, and nerve conduction studies may be required to establish whether or not there is significant slowing of conduction through the carpal tunnel. If so, then one should decompress the median nerve at that level, so that at least half the trouble is relieved (Upton & McComas 1973).

This double pathology may be the explanation for those occasional patients who, after carpal tunnel compression, declare their symptoms to be relieved but return two or three months later saying that they are not better after all.

Brachial plexus lesions

Injuries

Open

Lacerations of the nerves forming the brachial plexus are, happily, rare in Britain, but in countries where stabbing and slashing are more common, these injuries are sometimes encountered.

Immediate motor and sensory loss indicates that the nerves have been cut and they should be repaired like any other peripheral nerves, though of course the anatomy is more complicated and the procedure lengthy. In many cases the area will have to be explored anyway to repair the damaged blood vessels, and the time to repair the nerves is then, as later re-exploration in the scarred area around the vessels is distinctly hazardous. In view of the long distance from the injury to the sensory and motor endings in the forearm and hand, recovery is slow and usually imperfect, but much better than nothing.

Sometimes the paralysis does not develop until later, though it may progress to complete sensory and then motor loss. This is usually due to compression of the plexus by a false aneurysm of the subclavian or axillary artery resulting from the original wound. Arterial repair should be combined with neurolysis and will lead to complete recovery in most cases (Boome 1982).

Closed

Closed injuries of the brachial plexus are not very common either, but each one is a tragedy because the prognosis is poor and the patient is usually an energetic young man. The diagnosis is often overlooked because of other injuries, especially a head injury to which may be attributed the lack of movement in the arm. All patients unconscious after a car or motor-cycle accident should have the areas above and below the clavicle examined for swelling or bruising.

Nobody has more experience of brachial plexus lesions than Narakas, of Lausanne, Switzerland, who has treated 1068 patients and operated on 329. Only surgical exploration can define the pathology exactly, and Narakas suggested, as a useful approximation, the 'Law of the Seven Seventies':

1 70% of traumatic brachial plexus lesions are due to road traffic accidents;

2 70% of these road traffic accident victims are cyclists or motor cyclists;
3 70% of these patients have multiple injuries (which often lead to delay in diagnosis and, therefore, delay in treatment of the brachial plexus injury);
4 In 70% of them, the brachial plexus lesion is above the clavicle;
5 70% of patients with supraclavicular lesions have one or more roots avulsed from the spinal cord*;
6 70% of the root avulsions affect the lower roots, i.e. C7, C8, and T1, or C8 and T1.
7 70% of the patients with lower root avulsion will experience persisting pain.

The typical patient, then, is a young man knocked off his motorcycle and who has torn the upper trunks and avulsed the lower roots of the brachial plexus (Fig. 11.6). If the dominant arm is affected, the injury is even more devastating. Can anything be done to help?

Reconstruction of the brachial plexus itself

In the past, attempts at surgical repair proved unsatisfactory. However, the prognosis without operation is so bad that recent years have seen a new wave of attempts at surgical reconstruction of the plexus, using the operating microscope and modern techniques of nerve suture and grafting.

The upper trunks are usually so badly torn and stretched that direct repair is impossible and it is necessary to excise the damaged segments and recreate that part of the brachial plexus with nerve grafts. The lower roots have, in most cases, been avulsed from the spinal cord, so that no kind of proximal suture is possible, but what can be done is a nerve transfer; the distal segment is re-innervated from a nerve which normally goes elsewhere but whose function can be sacrificed, for example intercostal, the long thoracic, or the spinal accessory.

The timing of the operation is important; in

* This is indicated by Horner's sign.

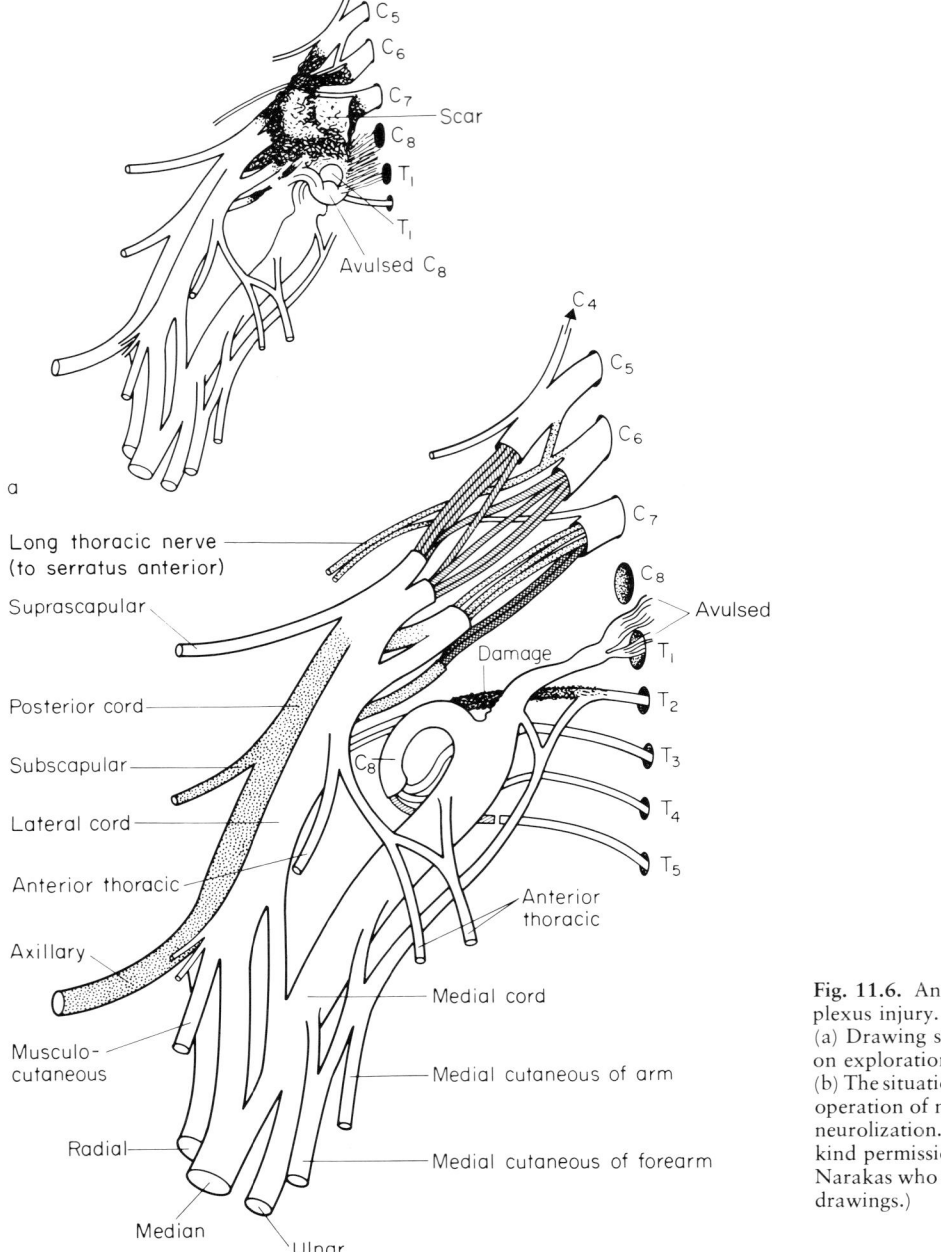

a

b

Fig. 11.6. An old brachial plexus injury.
(a) Drawing showing findings on exploration.
(b) The situation at the end of an operation of nerve grafting and neurolization. (Reproduced by kind permission of Dr A. Narakas who made the original drawings.)

broad terms, the sooner the better. If there is vascular damage requiring immediate repair, the nerves should be reconstructed at the same procedure; this will be an extremely lengthy operation, but is better than later re-exploration in a scarred area with a considerable risk of damaging the major blood vessels. If the vessels do not need immediate exploration, the operation can be delayed for a few days or even weeks, to allow for treatment of other injuries and to plan the operation for a convenient day.

ing normal power and function and allowing the patient to resume manual work, were only obtained in injuries of the suprascapular, axillary and musculocutaneous nerves near their origin. For the majority of injuries, affecting the more proximal part of the brachial plexus, surgery is often effective in restoring shoulder movement, sometimes effective in improving arm movement, and never effective in restoring function to the small muscles of the hand or fine discriminatory sensation in the hand.

Table 11.2 The results of surgical repair of brachial plexus injuries. (Modified from Sedel 1982.)

Grade	Usefulness of limb Function	Operated (43 patients) %	Conservative (49 patients) %
1	Manual work with normal strength	14	0
2	Able to do or help in everyday activities such as cutting meat or tying shoes	14	18
3	Only functions as hook or paperweight	28	35
4	Useless though it may have some movement	25	4
5	No movement and no use	19	43

In those patients in whom operation is performed after some delay and a stretched nerve is surrounded by scar tissue, neurolysis alone may produce considerable benefit, but should probably be limited to external neurolysis (i.e. incision or excision of the scarred and constricting epineurium, as opposed to separating and freeing each individual fascicle of the nerve).

Narakas (1985) has documented his findings and reported the results of this type of surgery in detail. About 60% of patients with supraclavicular lesions obtained what he classed as a fair result; active abduction of the shoulder between 50° and 85°, with some external rotation; elbow flexion, against gravity but not resistance, to between 90° and 115°; a hand with a weak grip, with a few fingers capable of holding a light object given to it, and protective sensation at least in the median nerve territory.

Whether this is enough to provide some useful function will depend upon the patient's personality and requirements. In about one case in seven, the results are better than this and definitely worthwhile. Excellent results, approach-

Sedel (1982) has reported similar results from similar operative procedures. His most important conclusion was that no patient was made worse by the operation, and there was a greater number of useful limbs in the patients treated surgically than in a group of similar patients managed conservatively (Table 11.2).

Another approach is to accept that the ulnar nerve will never be any use, and employ a length of ulnar nerve on a vascular pedicle to bridge the gap in the upper trunks to re-innervate the median nerve. This, of course, requires microvascular suture. As yet, it is too soon to assess the clinical results of this technique.

A direct surgical approach has also been applied to obstetrical injuries of the brachial plexus (Fig. 11.7). The essential thing here is to distinguish between those which will recover spontaneously and those which will not. Assin (1983) surveyed 300 babies and divided them into three groups as regards prognosis:

1 Those who start recovery within 3 weeks will recover completely and need no surgery.

2   Those who start recovering after the third week and continue recovering, will have a fair result which can be improved by tendon transfers.

3   Those who have not started to recover within 2 months are not likely to do so later. In these the brachial plexus should be explored immediately.

It is likely, however, that not only the frequency but the severity of these injuries varies considerably from one area to another, as obstetric techniques certainly vary. Hardy (1981) followed up 36 babies and found that nearly 80% had made a complete recovery by 13

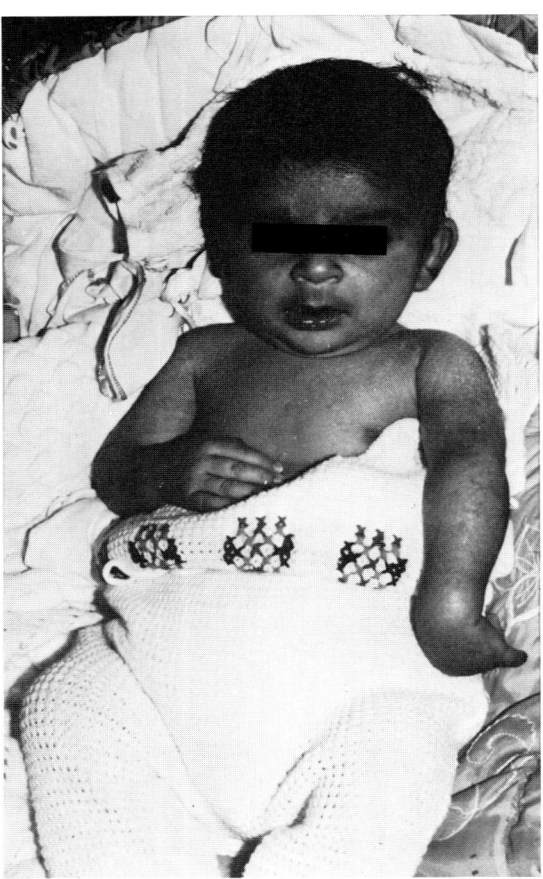

Fig. 11.7. Typical position of limb in Erb's palsy. Damage to C5, C6 and C7 nerve roots has caused paralysis of the abductors and external rotators of the shoulder, the flexors of the elbow, the supinators of the forearm and the extensors of the wrist. If this fails to recover, surgery may be indicated.

months, and none of those with significant residual defect had severe sensory or motor deficits in the hand. The residual defects affecting the shoulder and upper arm are more amenable to later correction by local surgery.

Late reconstructive surgery in the arm

Various prognostic tests have been devised, but none is completely reliable (Rorabeck & Harris 1981). Only the passage of time will give a certain answer.

If all that is possible has been done to promote recovery and a reasonable time has passed to allow that recovery to occur, but (as is usually the case) there remains considerable disability, consideration should be given to methods of minimizing the residual disability.

The key factor, as in any neurological loss in the hand, is the quality of sensation: if this is good, restoration of movement can lead to improvement of function, but if sensation is poor (and the other arm is normal) little use will be made of the injured arm.

At one time it was advised that in complete lesions, the arm should be amputated and the shoulder arthrodesed to allow a prosthetic arm to be controlled by intact proximal muscles inserted on the scapula, and this should be done early before the patient had developed a one-handed mentality. However, follow-up of these patients revealed that many were not making much use of the prosthesis and, since at least one patient with poor prognostic signs made a nearly complete recovery, early amputation is no longer recommended (Ransford & Hughes 1977). In fact, amputation should probably seldom be done at all even at a later stage.

What, then, can we do to improve motor function? If there is useful function in the hand, but paralysis of the biceps prevents the patient from putting his hand where he wants it, an orthosis can be fitted over the arm and elbow flexion produced by a cable, operated by movement of the other shoulder, as for an artificial arm. Alternatively, tendon transfers can be carried out (Fig. 11.8). Those which may be used to restore elbow flexion have been described above in connection with poliomyelitis, or one may transfer both ends of latissmus dorsi on an intact neurovascular pedicle (Takami *et al.* 1984). If the final lesion is only partial, tendon transfers in the hand and arm, of the type which will be considered for peripheral nerve lesions, may be appropriate, though the results are not as good as when similar operations are carried out for more distal nerve injuries; this may be partly because of greater sensory deficiency, and partly because of cross-innervation in the recovered nerves.

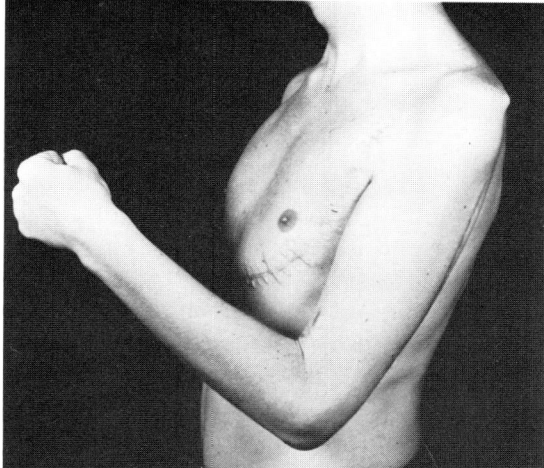

Fig. 11.8. This patient had an upper brachial plexus injury causing paralysis of elbow flexion but leaving a good hand. He has been successfully treated by Clarke's transfer of the outer part of the pectoralis major into the arm. The posterior scar which is just visible is from a subsequent external rotation osteotomy of the humerus to enable him to flex his hand towards his mouth rather than across his chest.

The problem of pain

This may be the most intractable problem of all. It usually starts a few weeks after the injury, and is most common in those patients with root avulsion. Narakas (1981) has found that some 50% of these patients have substantial relief of pain following reconstructive surgery to the brachial plexus, and this may occur within a few days or weeks of the operation, which is hard to understand (except where neurolysis has been done).

The surgeon must understand that amputation is not the answer; the pain is experienced centrally and continues even after the arm has been amputated (Ransford & Hughes 1977). If reconstructive surgery to the brachial plexus is not available or has not been successful, a non-surgical solution must be sought.

Superior thoracic aperture syndromes

This rather clumsy term is used since the aperture in question is sometives called the thoracic outlet and sometimes the thoracic inlet. Arterial blood and motor nerve conduction go one way, while venous blood and sensory impulses proceed in the opposite direction.

The aperture at issue is the circle formed by the first ribs on each side and completed by the first thoracic vertebra behind and the manubrium sterni in front. The lower roots of the brachial plexus, together with their accompanying vessels, emerge from this opening and pass outwards across the top of the first rib between the scalene muscles.

Between about 1920 and 1950, many patients with pain or tingling in their arm were diagnosed as having nerves compressed in this area by various structures, especially a cervical rib or fibrous analogue, and had operations carried out to relieve this.

In 1947, Brain published a paper showing that the familiar syndrome of noctural acroparaesthesiae in middle-aged women was due to compression of the median nerve in the carpal tunnel and could be relieved by dividing the flexor retinaculum. It soon became obvious that many of the patients previously diagnosed as having superior thoracic aperture syndromes really had peripheral compression of the median or other nerves.

The older diagnoses, superior in the anatomical if not the scientific sense, thus fell into abeyance, and nowadays many surgeons never consider them.

Where does the truth lie? The answer depends upon who is asked, though the difference may be more a matter of emphasis. Few would be so bold as to say that superior thoracic aperture syndromes never occur, and even their strongest proponents would not claim that they are common. Nevertheless, there is a real divergence of opinions as to their incidence. King and Bonney (1983) reviewed 82 patients who underwent such operations in a 16-year period. This is far more than have been done in most centres, but whether these authors overdiagnosed such disorders, or the patients were referred from a wide area, or others underdiagnosed them is hard to say. Gilliatt (1979) quoted Kremer as saying that he had seen 600 patients with carpal tunnel syndromes and, in the same period, only 12 patients with neurological deficits due to cervical ribs.

Various different compressing structures have been described. Those above the neurovascular bundle, such as scalenus anterior, will affect the upper trunks of the plexus, and the symptoms may be made worse by elevating the arm. Alternatively the plexus may be affected by something below it, such as a cervical rib or, more often, a sharp-eged fibrous band extending from a long down-curving transverse process of C7, or from a rudimentary cervical rib, downwards to the first rib. This will affect the lower roots of the brachial plexus, and the symptoms may be made worse by downward traction of the arm.

The diagnosis of these conditions is further confused by variability not only in the distribution of the symptoms but in their character. It is often stated that they produce vascular symptoms with changes of colour or temperature in the hand, especially when there is a large cervical rib. Vascular surgeons, however, are loth to operate on such patients unless there is definite evidence of ischaemia, embolism or aneurysm. King (1984) stated that the vascular symptoms in such patients were intermittent and more like Raynaud's disease than the effects produced by blockage of a major artery; he suggested that they may be due to disturbance of the sympathetic nerves to the arm. Dawson *et al.* (1983) claimed that the symptoms were essentially neurological in type; paraesthesiae, pain and muscle weakness. Muscle weakness and wasting involve the small muscles of the hand because these are supplied by the T1 nerve root, which is closest to the cervical rib or fibrous band. For some reason, the thenar muscles are affected first and worst, and this may lead to a wrong diagnosis of carpal tunnel syndrome (Gilliatt 1979), though patients with a superior thoracic aperture syndrome are not woken at night by painful paraesthesiae. As in carpal tunnel syndrome, the sensory symptoms may not be accompanied by a demonstrable sensory deficit; when present, this is found on the inner side of the forearm (i.e. the T1 dematome), not usually extending into the hand. Nerve conduction studies are necessary to sort out these cases.

In King and Bonney's series the best results were obtained after excision of the cervical rib, but this does not mean that every patient with neurological symptoms in the arm and who has a cervical rib should have it removed, as they are not necessarily the cause of the trouble, and although the radiological abnormality is often bilateral, the symptoms seldom are. A smaller proportion of their patients was improved by removal of fibrous bands or the first rib, though in other series removal of fibrous bands has been the most rewarding (Gilliatt 1979).

It seems reasonable to suggest that one should keep these diagnoses in the back of one's mind, particularly in dealing with patients whose symptoms or signs are not typical of the more common conditions. One should consider them if the patient does not respond to treatment (whether conservative or operative) for a peripheral nerve lesion, though of course it should be a general principle that when any patient fails to improve as expected, one must ask oneself if the diagnosis was correct.

Peripheral nerve lesions

This is, of course, an enormous field. This chapter, however, is concerned with the surgical management of these conditions and for this purpose they may be divided into three groups.

(i) Peripheral neuropathy as a manifestation of systemic disease

The orthopaedic surgeon must never forget that what seems to be an isolated peripheral nerve lesion may be the first or only manifestation of a generalized disorder. In Britain the commonest instances are diabetes, alcoholism and neuralgic amyotrophy. Surgery has little to offer in the management of these conditions, except that carpal tunnel syndrome is probably more common in diabetes than in the general population (but must, of course, be distinguished from diabetic neuropathy).

World-wide, however, the commonest cause of peripheral neuropathy is probably *leprosy*. There are about ten million people in the world suffering from this disease, and many of them can be helped by the surgeon. The nerves usually affected are those which lie subcutaneously, possibly because they are at a lower temperature; thus the ulnar nerve at the elbow is often involved, causing paralysis of the intrinsic muscles in the hand, and there is a major field of surgery in restoring this function. This will be considered below under ulnar nerve lesions. Other forms of neuritis in leprosy were described by Cochrane (1964).

The surgeon may also be asked to do a nerve biopsy, the usual choice being the superficial radial nerve at the wrist, where it may be palpably thickened. This nerve can be sacrificed without causing serious problems but, using the operating microscope, it is possible to remove only one or two of its constituent fasciculi, thus diminishing the area of anaesthesia produced. It must be remembered that if there is median and ulnar nerve anaesthesia, the radial nerve sensation may extend on to the palmar surface of the thumb and this priceless survival must not be jeopardized.

One of the most important aspects of treatment in leprosy is education of the patient in how to avoid damage to his anaesthetic extremities. The toes do not drop off because the disease rots them; they drop off because they are repeatedly injured and then become infected. This is avoid-able. To a lesser extent, the same applies to the hand. Though this is not a surgical treatment, it is treatment in which the surgeon should play a part.

(ii) Peripheral nerve compression

This may be an external force (such as a crutch or the arm of a chair), internal compression by a displaced fracture or by a tumour, or one of the nerve compression syndromes (Spinner 1972, Dawson *et al.* 1983). Whatever the cause of compression, if it is removed without undue delay, recovery can be anticipated and subsequent reconstructive surgery is rarely required.

(iii) Interruption of the nerve pathway

This is usually by injury (i.e. the nerve is cut or torn) but occasionally by other types of pathology such as neurofibroma. Following division of a nerve the main changes occur distal to the cut, but the proximal axon is also affected. Demyelination occurs back to the node of Ranvier proximal to the lesion, and changes also take place in the nucleus of the cell, the commonest being chromatolysis, but the cell may die and connecting neurones may show changes.

The surgeon's concern is with the process of regeneration. Work using the scanning electron microscope (Van Beek *et al.* 1982) has shown that regeneration can begin very early, while degeneration is still taking place. It also showed that the myelin tubes remained intact, patent, but 'empty' for a surprisingly long time and that regeneration nerve sprouts did not grow down the empty tubule but infiltrated themselves between the neurolemmal membrane and the old myelin tube. Lundborg *et al.* (1982a) suggested that a cut nerve secreted some chemical substance which, if it remained concentrated around the cut end of the nerve, promoted repair. Its effect is similar to that of nerve growth factor, a protein known to promote growth of sympathetic and sensory neurones, but it is not the same as nerve growth factor.

The primary treatment is by direct repair or grafting of the nerve. With the operating microscope, we can repair individual fascicles within the nerve, but since a nerve contains thousands of axons we shall never be able in any practicable manner to repair the individual axons. It seems that further improvements in the results of nerve repair are more likely to be achieved by biological factors than by striving still further for perfect mechanical alignment.

The techniques of nerve repair are beyond the scope of this book. However, if a direct nerve suture is impossible for any reason, or if it has been done with limited success, the surgeon must consider whether what would otherwise be permanent disability can be decreased by some form of reconstructive surgery, not to the nerve itself, but to the parts whose movement it controls.

It is helpful to consider the different types of paralysis on an anatomical basis.

The spinal accessory nerve

This is the only one of the cranial nerves whose disorders come within the ambit of the orthopaedic surgeon. In its passage down the side of the neck, it emerges from under cover of the sternomastoid (which it supplies) and lies superficial for a short distance before disappearing under the trapezius muscle (which it also supplies). This exposed section of the nerve is sometimes damaged in operations on the posterior triangle of the neck, usually biopsies of lymph nodes (King & Motta 1983).

The spinal accessory nerve is joined, beneath the anterior border of trapezius, by branches from the third and fourth cervical nerves which may contribute to the innervation of trapezius. In consequence, division of the accessory nerve above this level does not necessarily mean complete paralysis and subsequent wasting of trapezius, though it is weakened. In clumsy operations on this area, however, these fine cervical branches may also be damaged.

The presenting symptoms of trapezius paralysis is usually aching around the shoulder, due to loss of the normal elevating action of the trapezius and fatigue of the muscles attempting to compensate for this. This may also lead to traction on the brachial plexus causing paraesthesia. The patient will still be able to shrug his shoulders with levator scapulae, but there is limitation of abduction, due to lack of stabilization of the scapula (Fig. 11.9).

If the injury is diagnosed early, the nerve can be repaired or grafted. In later cases, satisfactory relief of symptoms may be achieved by Henry's operation in which two slings of fascia are used to hold the scapula up and in, towards the spinal column.

The long thoracic nerve of Bell

This is the most proximal branch of the brachial plexus, arising from the roots of C5 and 6 soon after their emergence from the intervertebral foramina. It runs down the outer side of the chest wall, lying on the surface of and supplying the serratus anterior, whose function is to hold the scapula against the chest wall during movements of the shoulder joint.

Paralysis of the muscle causes winging of the scapula, but also limits shoulder movement because of lack of stabilization of the scapula. Winging of the scapula must be distinguished from displacement of the scapula due to scoliosis or in Sprengel's shoulder.

The nerve is rarely involved in brachial plexus lesions but, if it is affected, indicates a hopeless prognosis because the upper roots have been avulsed. During its long course thereafter, the nerve is vulnerable to injury during operations on the axilla, for example radical mastectomy. It is also liable to paralysis in poliomyelitis.

Isolated paralysis of the serratus anterior, for no apparent reason, is seen from time to time, and usually recovers spontaneously, though this may take up to two years (Foo & Swann 1983).*

---

* These authors observe that 'it is a remarkable coincidence that the long thoracic nerve of Bell should suffer from a similar affliction to the facial nerve where the paralysis is known as Bell's palsy'.

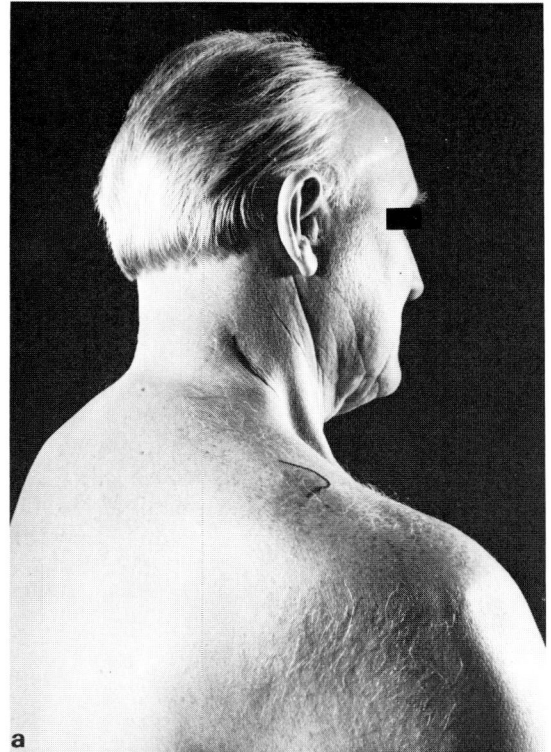

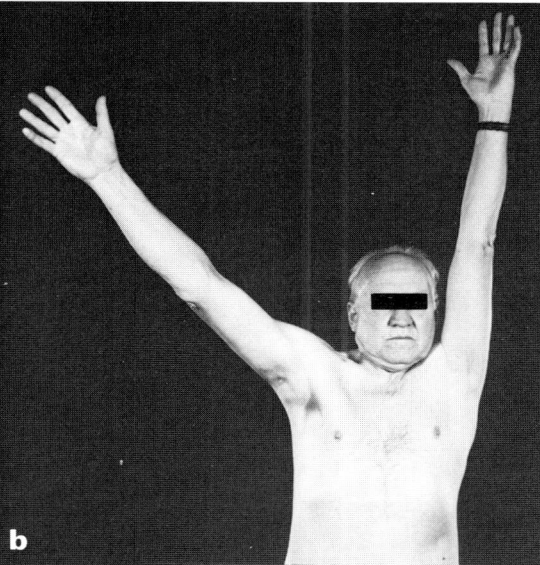

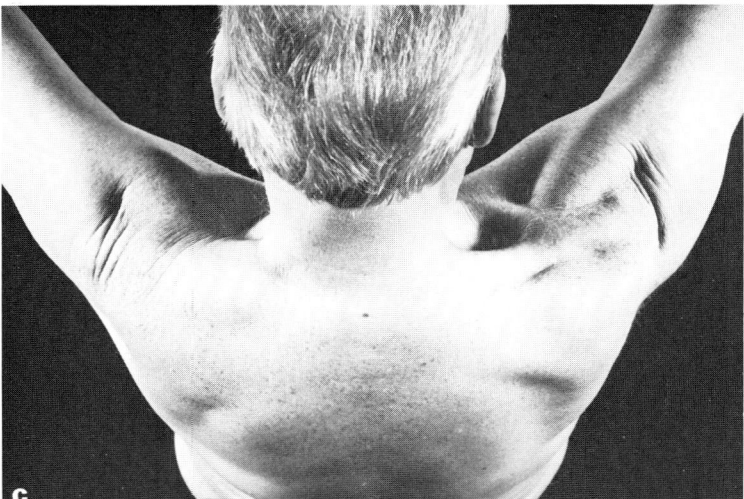

Fig. 11.9. (a) The upper mark indicates the scar from an operation which damaged the spinal accessory nerve; the lower mark outlines the superior pole of the scapula, unusually prominent because of the wasting of the trapezius.
(b) The patient can, with effort, abduct the right arm fairly well, but he cannot keep it up for long.
(c) In active abduction the wasting of trapezius is evident; the levator scapulae can be seen stabilizing the scapula. On the opposite side it is concealed by the normal trapezius muscle.

It appears that this is usually a manifestation of neuralgic amyotrophy, a condition with which an orthopaedic surgeon needs to be familiar, because the patient may present in an orthopaedic clinic with a painful shoulder. In contrast to the commoner types of pathology around the shoulder, which are merely painful, this condition may be agonizing; in the absence of injury, only acute calcification in the tendons of the rotator cuff causes shoulder pain as severe as this. During the subsequent few weeks, the smaller muscles around the shoulder (especially the spinati) become wasted, but it is worth making the diagnosis before this, as systemic steroids bring relief within a day or two. The nature of neuralgic amyotrophy remains obscure, but current neurological opinion is that most cases are due to some form of allergic reaction to a preceding viral infection, though some cases follow injections, for example of antitetanus serum. The upper branches of the brachial plexus are particularly affected and there is a curious tendency to affect the right shoulder, even in left handed people. The condition is often provoked by unusual or excessive muscular activity, which in the past was interpreted as causing a temporary compression neuropathy.

For the rare cases in which paralysis persists, various muscle transfers have been devised using the sternal part of pectoralis major, teres major, or the rhomboids. In facioscapulohumeral muscular dystrophy, which affects the serratus anterior muscle itself, fusion of the scapula to the ribs has been found to be effective, and is justifiable because the condition progresses very slowly and sufferers live for many years.

Suprascapular nerve

This nerve, which is quite large, comes off the upper trunk of the brachial plexus and runs laterally beneath the trapezius before passing through the suprascapular notch, deep to the suprascapular ligament. Having thus reached the supraspinous fossa, it supplies the supraspinatus muscle and then passes downward, lateral to the root of the spine of the scapula, into the infraspinous fossa where it supplies infraspinatus.

Supraspinatus assists in abduction of the glenohumeral joint, both directly and indirectly by holding the head of the humerus in towards the glenoid so that the deltoid can function more effectively. The myth that it *initiates* abduction should have been laid to rest many years ago. Inman *et al.* (1944) showed that it acts simultaneously with deltoid throughout the entire range of abduction of the shoulder, and Linge & Mulder (1963) confirmed this by temporarily paralysing the suprascapular nerve with local anaesthetic. Their subjects (including those in whom infraspinatus as well as supraspinatus were paralysed) could still abduct their arm through a full range, using deltoid, but this deltoid-only abduction was weak in power and tired quickly, after which the patient resorted to excessive scapulothoracic rotation in a vain attempt to hold the arm up, and the shoulder assumed the hunched position seen also in large tears of the supraspinatus tendon.

Paralysis of the supraspinatus is rare, but can occur in open wounds, following a fracture of the scapula which enters the suprascapular notch, or from external compression. The latter is illustrated in Fig. 11.10. In theory, this patient should have been able to abduct the arm with deltoid alone; why he could not do so is obscure, but it may be that other nerves and muscles were compressed at the same time. A compression syndrome of the suprascapular nerve has also been described. It may be precipitated by cross-body adduction of the arm and is said to cause burning or aching pain behind the shoulder, with weakness and wasting of supraspinatus and infraspinatus (Swafford & Lichtman 1982).

Loss of supraspinatus action is usually due to degenerative tears in the supraspinatus part of the rotator cuff. In this type of pathology it is the pain caused by impingement of the torn part of cuff under the acromion and coracoacromial ligament which causes a painful arc and limits movements. Major tears, in which the rotator cuff is avulsed, are very uncommon, but com-

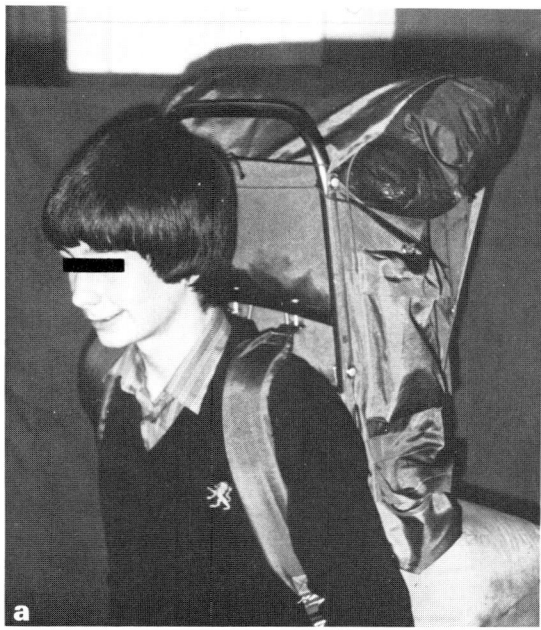

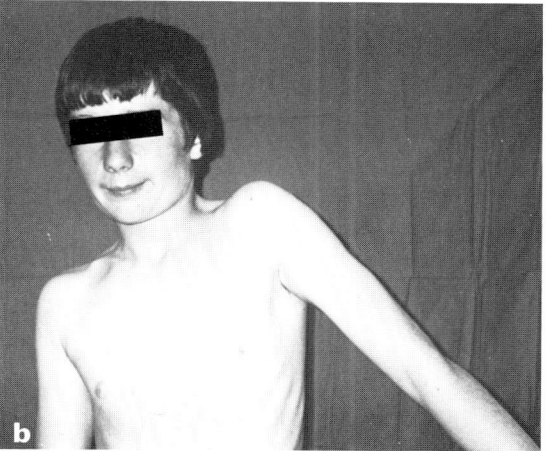

Fig. 11.10. (a) This boy developed paralysis of supraspinatus after carrying this heavy rucksack all day on a long walk. Observe how the strap presses on the top of his shoulder, compressing the suprascapular nerve.
(b) He cannot abduct the shoulder. He recovered within a few weeks. (Pictures kindly supplied by Professor W.A. Wallace.)

pletely prevent abduction. This may be because the deltoid rapidly becomes wasted.

Axillary nerve

This is one of the silliest examples of anatomical nomenclature. The axilla is full of nerves, and the first thing this nerve does is to leave the axilla, by passing through the quadrangular space below the glenohumeral joint. It then winds round the posterior aspect of the neck of the humerus, a course clearly described by its earlier and better name, the circumflex nerve. In this position, it lies beneath the deltoid, and its main function is to supply that muscle. It also innervates teres minor and finally supplies the skin overlying the deltoid.

The deltoid muscle, like supraspinatus, is active throughout the range of abduction, though it works at a better mechanical advantage in the upper part of the range.

Paralysis of the deltoid prevents active abduction of the glenohumeral joint. Supraspinatus cannot manage on its own. The patient, there-

fore, does the best he can with scapulothoracic movement, and the characteristic hunched shoulder results. In long-standing cases, wasting of the deltoid makes its abnormal condition very obvious and the humeral head can be felt and even seen through it.

The axillary nerve is important to the orthopaedic surgeon in two ways. Firstly, he must not cut it during a surgical approach to the shoulder. For this reason, the standard approach to the glenohumeral joint is from the front, freeing the anterior margin of the deltoid and retracting it posteriorly, which is safe because the nerve reaches the muscle from behind. In the transacromial approach to the top of the shoulder (Kessel 1982) the upper part of deltoid is split longitudinally down the middle, but care is taken not to split the muscle for more than 5 cms because if the separation was carried further down it would reach the level of the axillary nerve and thus risk denervating the anterior half of the deltoid.

Secondly, the axillary nerve may be damaged by injuries around the shoulder, especially inferior dislocation. It is important to examine the nerve before attempting to reduce the shoulder, to exclude this complication, and to carry out a gentle reduction to avoid damaging the nerve. Although this complication occurs in only a small proportion of dislocations, the latter are common, and this injury is seen from time to time. The nerve is stretched and the injury is usually an axonotmesis. Tulloch Brown (1952) reviewed 76 cases of nerve injury complicating dislocation of the shoulder, all seen at one hospital over six years and thought to constitute about 25% of all shoulder dislocations. There was no relationship to the type of injury, the method of reduction, or delay in reduction, but today the frequency of axillary nerve injury is less, possibly due to gentler methods of reduction. Six patients had only transient sensory loss in the distribution of the axillary nerve, but 53 had complete motor paralysis of this nerve, though most made a complete recovery. In 17 patients other nerves were affected or there were multiple nerve injuries. If electrical tests show no sign of recovery after three months, nerve grafting can give excellent results (Petrucci *et al.* 1982).

Musculocutaneous nerve

The muscular component of this nerve supplies the main elbow flexors; biceps and brachialis. It also supplies the coracobrachialis. The cutaneous branch continues to become the lateral cutaneous nerve of the forearm.

Injuries to this nerve are rare in civilian life, though Bristow (1947) reported 21 cases from the two World Wars, 19 being due to gunshot wounds, one to a fracture and one to a dislocation. It may, however, be damaged by retraction during the surgical approach to the front of the shoulder. Fortunately, the patients can still flex the elbow quite strongly, using brachioradialis and pronator teres (which are supplied by the radial nerve) though supination is weakened. In fact, excision of part of the musculocutaneous nerve has been recommended for severe spasticity of the elbow flexors in non-

functional arms (Garland *et al.* 1980).

Compression of the lateral cutaneous nerve of the forearm by the biceps tendon and aponeurosis has been described by Bassett and Nunley (1982) as causing aching on the anterolateral aspect of the elbow. Only the acute cases had burning dysaesthesiae, but most had impaired sensation on examination in the distribution of the nerve. The symptoms were made worse by pronation in extension which 'frequently occurs after an incorrectly executed forehand stroke at tennis'. This syndrome was difficult to distinguish from tennis elbow. Some cases were due to overuse of the arm and settled with rest; seven needed surgical decompression which apparently relieved the symptoms.

The lateral cutaneous nerve is also of interest to the surgeon as the source of a nerve graft (McFarlane & Mayer 1976). Only a short length is available, but it is very suitable to bridge a gap in a digital nerve, with the great advantage that it lies within the same sterile field and exsanguinated area as the recipient nerve. The bifurcation of the lateral cutaneous into its anterior and posterior branches can be used to reproduce the division of the common digital nerve into its branches to the adjoining sides of two fingers.

Radial nerve

The radial nerve supplies the muscles which prepare the hand for action (Beasley 1981); the extensors of the elbow and wrist, which place the hand where it is needed, and the extensors of the metacarpophalangeal joints of the fingers and all three joints of the thumb, which open the hand to surround an object to be held.* For this reason complete paralysis of the radial nerve greatly impedes the use of the hand. In fact, one of Dr William Littler's residents, who injected with local anaesthetic, on separate occasions, each of the three major nerves in his own arm, found that the radial nerve paralysis was the most dis-

---

* It also supplies supinator which is another muscle of placement, since the forearm spends most of its time pronated and is only supinated on demand.

abling of the three. Fortunately, however, the effects of radial paralysis are easier to overcome than those of median or ulnar paralysis.

In paralysis of the posterior interosseous branch of the radial nerve there is no wrist drop because extensor carpi radialis longus and usually brevis are still working. The patient may even be dismissed as hysterical because he can extend the wrist and also the interphalangeal joints of the fingers (which are extended by the intrinsic muscles of the hand, supplied by the ulnar nerve).

The examination of the muscles which are supplied by the radial nerve requires considerable care, as various trick movements may conceal paralysis. According to Sunderland (1978) 'Every movement normally controlled exclusively by the radial nerve may, with one exception, be preserved in complete lesions of this nerve. The exception is radial abduction of the thumb. . . . The most reliable test of radial nerve function is to ask the patient to extend the wrist and fingers and radially abduct the thumb simultaneously through a full range and against resistance.'

Pathology

General   Paralysis of the radial nerve may be a local manifestation of a general neurological disorder. This is seen most commonly in neuralgic amyotrophy, starting with severe pain around one scapula, radiating down the outer side of the arm to the elbow, and sometimes accompanied by paraesthesiae. After 2–14 days the pain subsides and muscle paralysis becomes apparent. This usually recovers in a few weeks or months (Sandifer 1967).

Radial nerve paralysis may also be the presenting feature of diabetes mellitus, polyarteritis nodosa, alcoholism or serum sickness. Lead poisoning may present with a wrist drop, though this is probably due to a muscle disorder rather than a nerve lesion; in this condition abductor pollicis longus is spared. Arsenic poisoning is similar.

In addition hysterical paralysis can occur.

External pressure   This may be due to pressure in the axilla from crutches or the back of a chair, or to a stuporous person sitting with his arms folded on a table in front of him and his head resting on the lateral side of the elbow. The latter is said to be the commonest cause of Saturday night palsy.

In the unconscious or anaesthetised patient, pressure may be caused by a tourniquet, or by the back of the arm resting on the edge of a bed or operating table. The effects upon the nerve of pressure of this sort depend on the amount of pressure and the period for which it is applied. The mildest is a *rapidly reversible physiological block* due to ischaemia. This can be seen when operating under local anaesthetic but using a tourniquet; after about 20 minutes, the patient develops weakness and sensory loss in the hand (and also complains of the pressure of the tourniquet). Nevertheless this remains a most useful and satisfactory technique for operations that can be done in 15 minutes, for example release of carpal tunnel syndrome or De Quervain's tenovaginitis.

More severe or prolonged pressure produces a *local demyelinating block,* which is not followed by Wallerian degeneration and which recovers in a few weeks.* Gilliatt (1975) has studied in detail the pathology of this type of lesion, using a pneumatic tourniquet, and shown that at each edge of the tourniquet excessive pressure squeezes the myelin sheath, like toothpaste in a tube, from the high to the low pressure area. This creates what amounts to an intussusception of the axon, with one myelinated segment being pushed into the next one, so that the node of Ranvier moves away from the high pressure, stretching the myelin sheath which eventually ruptures. Local demyelination follows, but remyelination occurs relatively quickly. In clinical practice this occurs when a nerve trunk is compressed by an outside object during a period of unnatural immobility (such as drunken stupor

---

* The term 'neurapraxia' thus embraces two different pathological processes: the rapidly reversible physiological block, and the local demyelinating block.

or an anaesthetic), when a nerve is retracted too vigorously during an operation, or when a tourniquet used for an operation is overinflated. It has been found that the pressure gauges on many hospital tourniquets are faulty, often seriously, and moreover in certain types of system the gauge measures the pressure in the box but not in the tourniquet. All surgeons using tourniquets should make sure that they are calibrated regularly, preferably every week. If the pressure is correct, a period of two hours is certainly safe (Klenerman 1980, Fletcher & Healy 1983). Experimental work in baboons has shown that similar changes are produced by compression of the nerve by a thin nylon cord, which is perhaps comparable to the sharp edge of a fracture sticking into a nerve.

If the pressure is very prolonged, as may occur after a barbiturate overdose, further changes take place. In the skin, lesions occur which are sometimes called 'barbiturate blisters', but which can develop in coma due to other drugs. In the muscle, swelling after the circulation is restored may cause a closed compartment syndrome requiring urgent decompression. The nerve itself undergoes *Wallerian degeneration* in at least some of its fibres, and an axonotmesis results.

Fractures   One in every ten fractures of the shaft of the humerus is complicated by immediate radial nerve paralysis. If the paralysis is only partial, it may be assumed that the nerve is in continuity and spontaneous recovery will occur. If the paralysis is complete, there is no way of telling whether the nerve is divided or not except by exploring it. Garcia and Maeck (1960) reported a series in which the policy was to operate on such patients immediately. In 23 explorations, the nerve was found to be divided in only one case. The other findings were two impaled, five bruised, two stretched, seven interposed, three normal and three not recorded. Recovery was complete in twenty patients and incomplete in three. Packer *et al.* (1972) in a follow-up study of the same patients, found 89% complete recovery in those explored after two weeks, but only 38% in those explored late or not at all and,

therefore, advised immediate operation in all cases with complete paralysis. They emphasised the technical difficulties of the operation if performed later, but on the other hand it should be remembered that many of the 89% would have had a similar result without operation. Shaw and Sakellarides (1967), found no recovery in 10 out of 25 patients with complete paralysis. In their series the initial treatment was conservative, but exploration was carried out if recovery was not taking place, at an average of 2½ months after injury. This was needed in 15 patients. In five the nerve was found to be contused and subsequently recovered. The nerve was completely divided in four, partly divided in two and involved in a neuroma in four; none of these recovered, though five of the operations were performed in the 1930s and with modern techniques better results should be possible. The onset of recovery in clinically complete lesions varied from one week to eight months, with an average of five weeks.

It appears that in at least 60% of cases and probably more, the nerve is in continuity and will recover spontaneously. Exploration may itself interfere with nerve function, as well as having other risks, and would not appear to be justifiable as a routine procedure. However, if the fracture is being operated on for any other reason the nerve should be examined. Most patients should be treated conservatively and watched closely. If there is no sign of recovery by eight weeks, exploration should be carried out. By this time the fracture is stable, and if the nerve is involved in callus it can be freed. In some cases the nerve will be found to be divided, in which case it can be repaired; in some it will be contused, in which case the operation was unnecessary, but many needless operations will have been avoided. It may seem logical to delay exploration until enough time has passed for regeneration of an axonotmesis to the most proximally innervated of the paralysed muscles (brachioradialis), but this takes 13–16 weeks, by which time the nerve may be deeply embedded in bone, and in any case nerve suture after so long a delay is less likely to give useful recovery.

Paralysis may develop after manipulation of humeral fractures, especially spiral fractures at the junction of the middle and lower thirds with lateral displacement of the distal fragment, where manipulative reduction may trap the nerve between the fracture surfaces. Nerve function must be tested before manipulating these or any other fractures, and this type of fracture should be manipulated with particular care. If paralysis does develop, the fracture should be exposed and the nerve freed from between the bone ends (Holstein & Lewis 1963).

Supracondylar fractures of the humerus are notorious for causing arterial damage but may also cause nerve injury. According to Watson-Jones (1930), the radial nerve is the most commonly affected in this fracture, although many surgeons find that the median nerve is more often injured.

Fractures of the upper third of the radius and dislocation of the radial head may cause posterior interosseous paralysis. Stein *et al.* (1971) reported seven cases complicating Monteggia fracture-dislocations. Three of these also had ulnar nerve paralysis. Paralysis of the radial or posterior interosseous nerve may follow operative treatment of fractures. This is considered below.

Wounds   The deep situation of the important part of the nerve, compared to the median and ulnar nerves, means that it is seldom divided in lacerations. When it is, the results of repair are good in 50% and fair in 25% (Seddon 1972). In normal civilian life the incidence of nerve involvement in open and closed fractures is similar, indicating that the injury is due to the fractured bone ends and not to external agents, but in fractures of the humerus due to gunshot wounds the radial nerve is severed in 50% of cases, and is often irreparable (Sunderland 1978).

Injections in the upper arm may damage the radial nerve, and it (or its branches) may inadvertently be divided during surgical operations, especially if there is much scar tissue present. Fortunately radial nerve paralysis appearing after surgery is usually a neurapraxia caused by a retractor. To some extent this is unavoidable, but the incidence of postoperative paralysis can be greatly reduced by familiarity with the anatomy and gentle retraction. Garcia and Maeck reported nearly 25% incidence of paralysis after internal fixation of the humerus between 1929 and 1949 but none between 1950 and 1959. Strachan and Ellis (1971) have shown that in pronation the proximal part of the posterior interosseous nerve moves medially; when exposing the head of the radius the forearm should therefore be kept pronated. Similar care is necessary when using Boyd's posterolateral approach to the proximal part of the shaft of the radius, though the AO (Arbeitsgemeinschaft für Osteosynthesefragen) group of surgeons (who use this approach for plating the radius) make a point of exposing the nerve to protect it.

The superficial radial branch is at risk in the operation for de Quervain's stenosing tenosynovitis and if a transverse incision is used it must be through skin only. According to Dellon and Mackinnon (1984), this nerve has a particular propensity to form a painful neuroma. They attribute this to the fact that it is normally tethered proximally beneath the deep fascia, and if it also becomes tethered distally after an injury, it is repeatedly stretched during the normal movements of the wrist.

Tumours   Compression by tumours can occur where the mobility of the nerve is restricted so that it cannot retreat before the tumour.

Most of the reported cases have been in the supinator region, causing posterior interosseous paralysis. The supinator muscle itself may be spared, presumably because the nerve gives off some branches of supply to the muscle before entering it. The diagnosis of tumour may not be obvious, as the onset of symptoms is often sudden and the tumour may not be palpable externally. The commonest tumour is a lipoma (Capener 1966) which may be detectable on X-ray as an area of translucency. Pain may be due to a benign lipoma and does not necessarily indicate a malignant or inflammatory condition. Posterior interosseous paralysis may also be caused by other benign tumours, by a ganglion (Bowen & Stone 1966) or by massive synovial swelling with dislocation of the superior radio-ulnar joint due to rheumatoid arthritis (Marmor *et al.* 1967).

Compression of the superficial radial nerve, producing a sensory deficit, has been recorded due to a lipoma (Leffert 1972) and a haemangioma (Spinner 1972).

Compression syndromes, not due to tumours, have been described at two sites where the nerve passes through narrow tunnels.

Lotem *et al.* (1971) reported three cases of complete paralysis in the muscles supplied by the radial nerve below its branches to the triceps. Each case followed vigorous muscular activity. Clinically and electrically the lesions were neurapraxias and complete recovery took place within a few days. Dissections in cadavers revealed that although the lateral head of the triceps arose mainly from the superolateral lip of the spiral groove, there was frequently an accessory origin from the distal end of the infero-medial lip of the groove, the two origins being connected by a fibrous arch. These authors postulated this as the site of compression, but surgical decompressions were not carried out as they were not necessary.

Sharrard (1966) described four patients with posterior interosseous palsy due to 'traumatic neuritis', three associated with minor hyperextension injuries of the elbow and one with long-standing cubitus varus. All recovered, though not immediately, after decompression and mobilization of the posterior interosseous nerve. Spinner (1968) similarly decompressed the nerve in six patients with posterior interosseous paralysis showing no sign of recovery after eight weeks, and considered that the fibrous arch of Frohse was the compressing factor.

However, Burns and Lister (1984) who explored three patients with radial nerve lesions of unknown cause, found well localized hour-glass constrictions of the radial nerve that could not be attributed to extrinsic compression. The cause of this remains unknown, though the nerves showed some recovery; it was concluded that all were probably due to medical disorders such as polyarteritis and allergic angio-neuropathy. In the light of this, some of the earlier papers describing 'compression' of various nerves on the basis of the operative findings may need to be re-assessed.

Roles and Maudsley (1972) believe that tennis elbow can be due to compression of the radial nerve and its branches, usually at the arcade of Frohse but also, in some cases, by the medial edge of the extensor carpi radialis brevis and by adhesions binding down the nerve to the capsule of the radiohumeral joint. They treated 38 resistant tennis elbows by division of these structures to release the nerve, with improvement in all. Van Rossum *et al.* (1978) could find no clinical or electrical evidence of nerve compression in ten of their patients with resistant tennis elbow. Heyse-Moore (1984) offered an explanation as to how exploration of the radial nerve relieved the symptoms in such cases.

Treatment

Treatment of the causative condition This has already been discussed, but it is worth emphasising that in posterior interosseous paralysis of unknown case, a surgical exploration is advisable, since the nerve may be compressed by a tumour which is not detectable by external examination.

Supportive treatment while awaiting recovery This is specially important in radial nerve lesions, since most recover spontaneously. The aim is to prevent the development of joint contractures. The simplest method is a passive splint (usually an anterior plaster slab) holding the wrist and metacarpophalangeal joints in extension, but prolonged immobilization of the metacarpophalangeal joints in extension leads to stiffness. This may be avoided by using a dynamic or lively splint, which permits active flexion of the joints but automatically returns them to the extended position. In practice, these are rather cumbersome and the patient often finds it easier to use a wrist splint and leave the hand free. Flexion contractures at the metacarpophalangeal joint are not a problem, and ordinary use probably provides enough passive extension, though this can be reinforced.

Electrical stimulation of the denervated muscles to prevent atrophy is a traditional method, but there is no real evidence that it is effective. It is certainly of no value unless carried out at least five times a week. Wynn Parry (1981) did not employ it as a routine measure but considered it may be useful in the later stages when recovery was beginning.

Treatment of the residual disability
Sunderland (1978) gave full details of recovery times. If there is no sign of recovery within a year, it should be assumed that there will be permanent loss and reconstructive surgery carried out in the form of tendon transfers.

Tendon transfers for radial nerve paralysis were developed by Robert Jones (1916) in the First World War. He used the following transfers:

1   Pronator teres to the radial extensors of the wrist;
2   Flexor carpi ulnaris to the extensors of middle, ring and little fingers;
3   Flexor carpi radialis to the extensors of the index finger and pollicis longus.

The pronator teres transfer is still the best procedure for providing wrist extension. It is convenient and easy to carry out and fulfils the basic requirements for tendon transfer; moreover the transferred muscle continues to act as a pronator as well as becoming a wrist extensor. The pronator teres tendon is usually sutured to extensor carpi radialis longus because its tendon extends more proximally than that of the brevis, but Brand (1966) advised detaching a strip of periosteum with the insertion of pronator teres and making the transfer to extensor carpi radialis brevis whose insertion is more central on the back of the wrist. This gives dorsiflexion with less radial deviation.

The transfer of the wrist flexors, however, has been changed, since Zachary (1946) showed that leaving one wrist flexor in place gave better results. Transfer of both wrist flexors causes loss of active wrist flexion and also inability to stabilize the wrist when the fingers are extended, so that even the finger-extending action of the transferred muscles is impaired. Palmaris longus is not good enough on its own as a wrist flexor (and may be absent anyway), so it is now agreed that one of the main wrist flexors should be left *in situ*. Boyes and Brand prefer to retain flexor carpi ulnaris on the grounds that this is the direct antagonist of the re-activated radial wrist extensors. Brand transferred flexor carpi radialis to the finger extensors. Boyes (1970) transferred the flexor digitorum superficialis tendons of the middle and ring fingers through the interosseous membrane to the long extensors of the fingers and thumb, since their range of excursion is greater than that of the wrist flexors. However, most surgeons, especially in Britain, prefer to retain flexor carpi radialis *in situ,* because it is more centrally placed on the wrist, and also not to disturb the finger flexors. Therefore, they transfer flexor carpi ulnaris around the ulnar border of the wrist to extensor digitorum communis, and this gives very satisfactory results.

The line of this transfer is such that it can be very easily continued into extensor pollicis longus; this is the simplest method of restoring thumb extension and, in the author's experience, is usually all that is needed.

If lack of radial abduction remains a problem, it can be provided by transfer of palmaris longus, if present, to abductor pollicis longus and extensor pollicis brevis. (Boyes, having used flexor digitorum superficialis to extend the fingers, still has flexor carpi radialis available to transfer to abductor pollicis longus and extensor pollicis brevis). Alternatively, palmaris longus can be transferred to the rerouted extensor pollicis longus, which gives an excellent combined extension and abduction of the thumb, almost impossible to distinguish from normal thumb function (Scuderi 1949).

If palmaris longus is absent, then, if necessary,

the thumb can be stabilized in abduction by arthrodesis of the carpometacarpal joint.

In posterior interosseous paralysis the problem is easier because the radial wrist extensors
do not need to be replaced and in addition one of
them can be transferred for other purposes. The
procedure is modified accordingly.

One point about these transfers is worth noting, since it does not apply in other sites. Owing
to the greater power of the flexors, the tendons
should be sutured with the muscles in almost
maximum tension. However if extensor digiti
minimi is included in the operation (which it
need not be) it should be sutured in less tension
than extensor digitorum communis or the little
finger will hyperextend (White 1960).

The arm should be immobilized with the
wrist, fingers and thumb in extension, not just in
the neutral position, for five weeks, followed by
a week or two in a dynamic splint.

Tendon transfers are so satisfactory that arthrodesis of the wrist is hardly ever needed. Elton
and Omer (1972) observed that patients with
radial nerve palsy, whether treated by tendon
transfer or experiencing nerve recovery, often
developed tightness in the extensors preventing
simultaneous flexion of the wrist and fingers, but
this is a rather unnatural movement, seldom
needed in ordinary life. In fact, in an irrecoverable radial nerve lesion, it is possible by tendon
transfers to restore function to something
approaching normal, unlike the median and
ulnar nerves where the sensory component is
more important.

Median nerve lesions

The median nerve has no branches above the
elbow; its proximal half is simply a cable carrying nerve fibres from one point to another.
Below the elbow, it supplies all the muscles in the
flexor compartment of the forearm, except for
flexor carpi ulnaris and the ulnar half of flexor
digitorum profundus. The deep group of muscles
(profundus, flexor pollicis longus, and pronator
teres) are supplied through the anterior
interosseous branch of the median.

In the hand, this is the nerve which makes
possible the precision handling of small objects.
Such objects are held and manipulated between
the thumb, index and middle fingers. It is the
thenar muscles, supplied by the median nerve,
which oppose the thumb to the other fingers, but
still more important it is the median nerve which
provides sensation for those three digits, without
which these fine manipulations are almost
impossible. Thus it is the most important nerve
in the arm.

Pathology

As this is a long nerve, it is worth considering in
sections the different types of pathology which
may affect it.

In the upper arm it is deeply placed and seldom divided in lacerations, but may be pressed
upon or damaged by fractures of the humerus,
by an aneurysm of the brachial artery, or by a
careless surgeon operating in this region. An
overinflated tourniquet may also cause a median
nerve lesion, though usually all three major
nerves in the arm will be affected.

Just above the elbow, it may be compressed by
a supracondylar fracture or beneath a ligament
of Struthers. Posterior dislocation of the elbow
itself, or anterior dislocation of the radial head
may also cause median nerve paralysis.

Just below the elbow, the median nerve (like
each of the three major nerves of the arm) passes
under a fibrous arch of muscle origin to enter the
plane between the superficial and deep muscles.
In this case the arch is that from which flexor
digitorum superficialis arises and it is said that
an entrapment neuropathy may occur here. It is
also claimed that the median nerve may be compressed slightly more proximal, where it passes
between the two heads of pronator teres, or
more proximal still, under the lacertus fibrosus.
Hartz *et al.* (1981) reported 39 patients whom
they considered to have median nerve compression in this region, causing aching and easy
tiring in the flexor muscles in the forearm. Sometimes there was numbness in the median nerve

distribution, brought on by repeated pronation, but not waking the patient at night; despite this, seven patients had undergone carpal tunnel decompression which, of course, had not helped them. Others were diagnosed as neurotic or hysterical. The key physical sign, which almost always was present, was tenderness over the proximal part of the pronator teres muscle. In many cases, paraesthesiae could be produced by getting the patient to pronate the extended forearm against resistance, which tightens the pronator and reproduces the symptoms. In others, symptoms were produced by flexing the middle finger against resistance. This paper, like others on these less well established nerve compression syndromes, leaves the reader with a sense of unease. Here is an alleged compression syndrome, in which nerve conduction studies are usually normal, the operative findings are variable (if they want to, surgeons can always convince themselves at operation that *something* is compressing a nerve), and a fair proportion of patients had evidence at the time or later of another nerve compression syndrome in the arm. The possibility of 'double-crush' further confuses the issue. The author has not knowingly seen either of these conditions, but they must be borne in mind, especially in the case of 'carpal tunnel syndrome' which is atypical or fails to respond to treatment.

The same may be said about compression of the anterior interosseous branch of the median nerve, which runs down the front of the interosseus membrane. Since flexor pollicis longus and profundus are both paralysed, the patient cannot form an O with the fingers, a gesture which in most parts of Europe means good or OK, though in Belgium and France it may mean zero, and in Malta, Greece and Turkey it is used as an insult or comment (Morris *et al.* 1979). However, it is convenient to regard the ability to make this ring sign as OK, and inability (with the distal joints being pushed into extension so that their distal phalanges are parallel) as demonstrating paralysis of the anterior interosseous nerve. This nerve is at risk during arteriography in this area, and may be affected by fractures of the radius

and ulna (Warren 1963). However, the reported compression syndromes are again not completely convincing, with descriptions of 'adhesions' around the nerve. Spinner (1970) stressed that many patients with anterior interosseous paralysis will recover spontaneously; the commonest cause is neuralgic amyotrophy (though it must be admitted that even this is not an entirely satisfactory diagnosis, since it is a disease without a pathology). One cannot help wondering whether 'pronator teres syndrome' and 'superior thoracic aperture syndrome' are not also often due to a self-limiting local neuropathy and would have recovered without surgical intervention.

Much the commonest site of median nerve pathology is *around the wrist,* and, of course, the commonest of all is the *carpal tunnel syndrome.* It is hard to realize that this was not understood forty years ago. There are plenty of doctors still working who had never heard of carpal tunnel syndrome in their medical training. What will the next forty years reveal?

Doctors were familiar with the syndrome of nocturnal acroparaesthesiae in middle-aged women, but they did not understand what caused it, nor how easily it could be relieved until they read the paper by Brain *et al. (*1947). This is one of the few old papers which is still worth reading, as its description of the condition is so clear; it is also entertaining to read the spirited, sometimes heated, correspondence which it evoked in the next few issues of *The Lancet.*

The only respect in which one might take issue with Brain's description is that it is of late cases. In early cases, there are no physical signs, and one should not wait until they appear, as there is evidence that after six months complete recovery is less likely (Semple & Cargill 1969). The diagnosis should be made on the history. Readers of this book will have treated many patients with carpal tunnel syndrome, and it would be insulting to describe it here. The key feature is painful pins-and-needles waking the patient during the night. If this does not occur a diagnosis of carpal tunnel is doubtful, and other conditions such as a cervical disc lesion or one of those in-between compression syndromes at the superior thoracic aperture or upper forearm must be considered. A digital neuritis is easily confused with carpal tunnel syndrome, an error the author has made on at least one occasion. The symptoms are very similar and may even wake the patient at night, but affect only *part* of the median nerve distribution. Nerve conduction studies can make the distinction. The possibility of the median nerve being compressed at the level of the carpal tunnel but by outside factors, such as the handle of a walking stick on which the patient leans heavily, must also be considered. The author develops median nerve paraesthesiae after wearing double surgical gloves for about half an hour.

Obviously physical signs must be looked for, and of these the most subtle is weakness of abductor pollicis brevis. Opponens may be supplied by the ulnar nerve and is thus of no diagnostic value. If full flexion of the wrist reproduces the symptoms within one minute (Phalen's test), the pathology is probably at wrist level, though unfortunately this test is quite often negative in carpal tunnel syndrome and can be positive in 'pronator teres syndrome' (Hartz *et al.* 1981).

Although surgeons are familiar with the clinical effects of nerve compression, many are surprisingly ignorant of the changes which take place in the nerve itself. The pathology of chronic nerve compression (as opposed to acute compression, which has been discussed in the radial nerve section of this chapter) can be divided into different stages of severity:

1 *Intermittent compression,* such as that which causes the nocturnal acroparaesthesiae. Since these symptoms can usually be made to disappear within 5 or 10 minutes by shaking or moving the hand, or altering its posture, they must be produced by a rapidly reversible physiological block; similar, in fact, to the effect of a tourniquet. The actual cause of the symptoms is probably ischaemia (Gilliatt & Wilson 1954, Lundborg *et al.* 1982b). It is thought that the ischaemia is produced by oedema of the nerve causing slowing or stasis of the capillary blood flow.

2 *Slight but longstanding compression* of nerves may be present but insufficient to produce symptoms: it is sometimes revealed by nerve conduction studies on the supposedly normal opposite limb tested for comparison with the symptomatic one.

Careful examination of lengths of the median and ulnar nerves from cadavers (not known to have complained of neurological symptoms previously) have sometimes shown changes in the median nerve in the carpal tunnel or ulnar nerve in the cubital tunnel which are thought to indicate mild compression. The reason they are considered pathological is that the nerves above and below the tunnels do not show these changes, and the reason they are thought to indicate mild compression is that they appear to be the early stages of changes seen more severely in patients known to have severe nerve compression.

There are two types of pathological change due to mild compression. First, there is thickening of the epineurium and perineurium in the compressed area. Secondly there are changes in the actual nerve fibres, though these are too subtle to be obvious on cross-sections and can only be demonstrated if individual axons are teased out (Neary *et al.* 1975). It is then seen that the myelinated segments between the nodes of Ranvier are not of equal thickness throughout their length, but are swollen and bulbous at the end furthest from the centre of compression (Fig. 11.11a).

3 *Moderate chronic compression.* In patients with clinical evidence of nerve compression more extensive structural changes have been seen. The segments of myelin sheath are not only swollen at the end furthest from the centre of compression, but are also thinned and tapered at the other end, i.e. nearest to the centre of compression (Fig. 11.11b). It seems that the ends of the lamellae which form the myelin sheath have become detached from the axon 'and have retracted along the fibre away from the node, so that the tapering is, in fact, a stepwise rather than a continuous process' (Gilliatt 1975). It is not

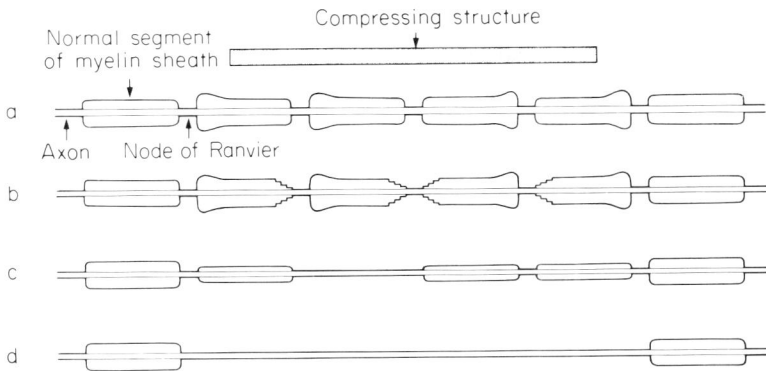

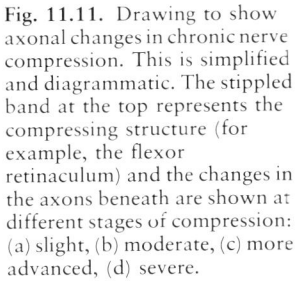

Fig. 11.11. Drawing to show axonal changes in chronic nerve compression. This is simplified and diagrammatic. The stippled band at the top represents the compressing structure (for example, the flexor retinaculum) and the changes in the axons beneath are shown at different stages of compression: (a) slight, (b) moderate, (c) more advanced, (d) severe.

surprising that this damage to the sheath may lead to complete loss of the myelin sheath in that segment. It often reappears, but thinner than before (Fig. 11.11c). Thus the nerve contains a mixture of fibres: some with normal myelin sheaths, others which are demyelinated, and still others showing evidence of remyelination (Neary & Eames 1975).

4 *Severe compression.* In these, a greater proportion of axons, especially the larger fibres, have lost their myelin sheaths, not only in the compressed area but distal to it (Fig. 11.11d). There is thus a detectable reduction in the diameter of myelinated nerve fibres when the nerve is examined in cross-section. Similar changes in nerve fibre size have been observed in a patient with minimal weakness and wasting of abductor pollicis, and normal sensory testing and nerve conduction studies (Thomas & Fullerton 1963). It therefore seems that, as in other systems in the body, there is a great deal of reserve capacity or planned redundancy: very considerable pathological changes are present by the time symptoms appear. It will be recalled that the situation in polio is similar (*see* above). This makes it easy to understand why operative decompression at an early stage is more likely to be followed by complete recovery than if delayed until clinical signs are present.

5 *Very late cases.* In extreme degrees of severity or chronicity, the changes in the nerve become visible to the naked eye. This takes the form of swelling or 'neuroma' of the nerve proximal to the compressed area (Fig. 11.12). This

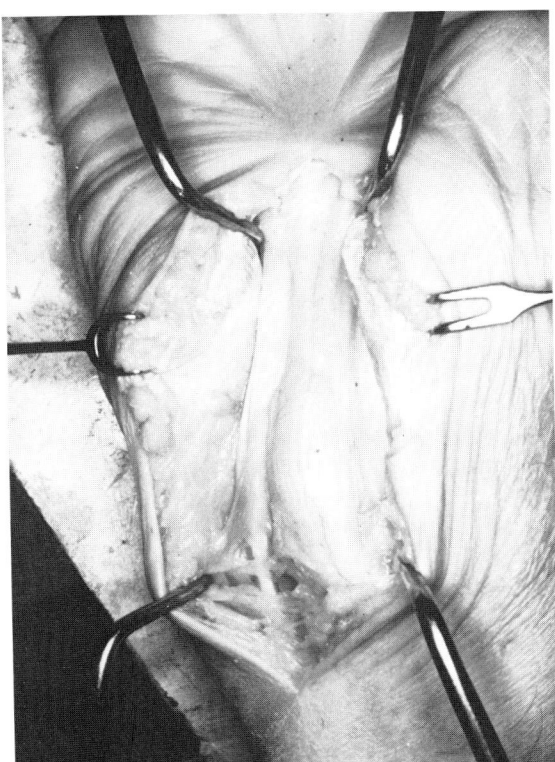

Fig. 11.12. Operative photograph showing proximal 'neuroma' on the median nerve in an extremely longstanding and severe case of carpal tunnel syndrome. The upper half of the wound shows the flexor retinaculum incised to reveal the median nerve in the carpal tunnel; below this (i.e. just proximal to the wrist) is the swollen section of nerve.

may be due to obstruction of the normal distal flow of endoneural fluid, obstruction to the normal flow of blood down the nerve, or both. A cut nerve bleeds from its proximal end. In addi-

tion, the 'neuroma' contains considerable proliferation of the supporting connective tissue in
and around the nerve.

Treatment

It is not necessary to obtain electrical studies in
the typical case, but they are useful in cases of
doubt: not so much doubt as to whether there is
or is not compression (cases which are clinically
equivocal may be electrically equivocal) but
doubt as to the level of the nerve pathology.

In bilateral cases one must be especially careful to exclude a cervical disc lesion as the cause of
the trouble, but carpal tunnel syndrome is quite
often bilateral and the surgeon must then decide
whether to operate on both together or separately with an interval between. This depends
upon the patient's circumstances and in particular who she has at home to look after her: if
both hands are operated on simultaneously, the
patient will be very handicapped for a week or
two and will need much care and attention. If
first one hand is operated on and later the other,
the patient can maintain some independence but
the whole process is more drawn out.

If only one hand is to be operated on, this can
be done perfectly well under local anaesthetic:
one simply infiltrates the area of the operation. A
tourniquet must be used, but most patients can
tolerate this for 15 or 20 minutes, which is all
that is needed.

The incision should be planned with care,
because the commonest complication is tenderness of the scar. The palmar cutaneous
branch leaves the main trunk of the median
nerve about 10 cm above the wrist and runs
parallel to it on the radial side, close to the tendon of flexor carpi radialis, in 98.3% of cases
(Das & Brown 1976). The incision should be in
the midline of the hand or slightly to the ulnar
side: certainly not to the radial side, as damage to
the palmar cutaneous branch may cause very
troublesome hyperaesthesia in the proximal part
of the palm. At the proximal end of the carpal
tunnel, the palmar cutaneous branch divides and

some of its fine terminal branches run across or
even within the flexor retinaculum. One can
hardly avoid dividing these, which is probably
the cause of that tenderness in the proximal part
of the scar which is the most common complication of this operation: fortunately it usually
settles in a month or two. The author has found
that the least troublesome incision is a straight
one, from the centre of the distal flexor crease of
the wrist and running for about 5 cms towards
the web between the middle and ring fingers
(Fig. 11.12).

One must remember that, so far as surface
anatomy is concerned, the flexor retinaculum is
a structure in the *hand*. The incision should not
only cross the col between the bases of the thenar
and hypothenar eminences, but continue down-
hill on the distal side until the flat plain of the
palm is reached, because the commonest cause of
failure of the operation is incomplete division of
the flexor retinaculum (MacDonald *et al.* 1978).
Here caution must be used, as it is easy to hook
up one of the digital branches of the median
nerve or the superficial palmar arterial arch, and
division of these structures does not improve the
result. The surgeon must know exactly where all
these structures lie.

The thenar branch of the median nerve is also
divided occasionally and the surgeon should be
aware that it may arise within the carpal tunnel
and pierce the flexor retinaculum, instead of arising in the more usual way just beyond the flexor
retinaculum (Das & Brown 1976). In patients
with severe wasting of the thenar eminence, the
writer exposes the little motor branch and
decompresses it separately where it passes
through the fascia over the thenar eminence.
This must be done carefully, as to divide the
branch only makes matters worse, and it must be
admitted that there is no evidence that separate
decompression of the motor nerve is of benefit.

Colles' fractures cause mild compression of
the median nerve more often than is generally
realized. Fortunately, reduction of the fracture is
usually all that is needed to decompress the
nerve. In some cases, however, symptoms of
carpal tunnel syndrome develop a few weeks or

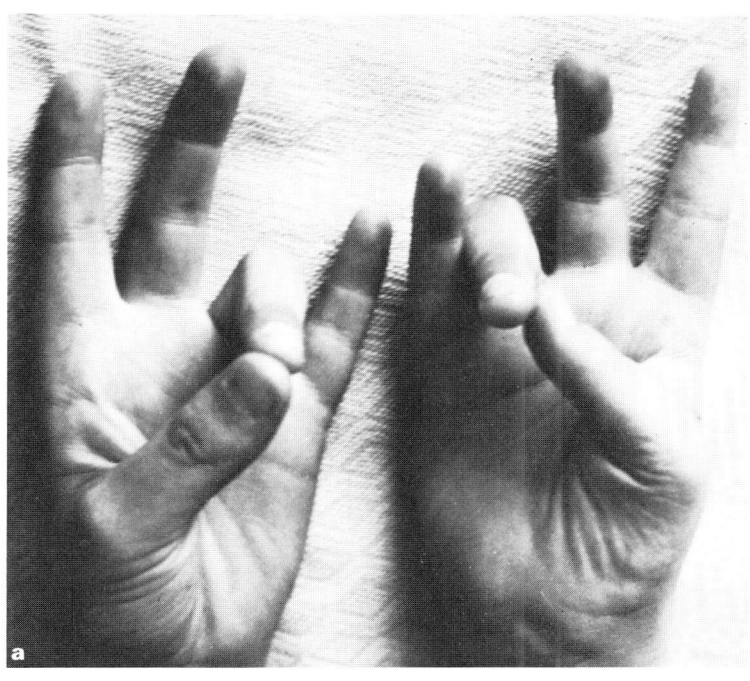

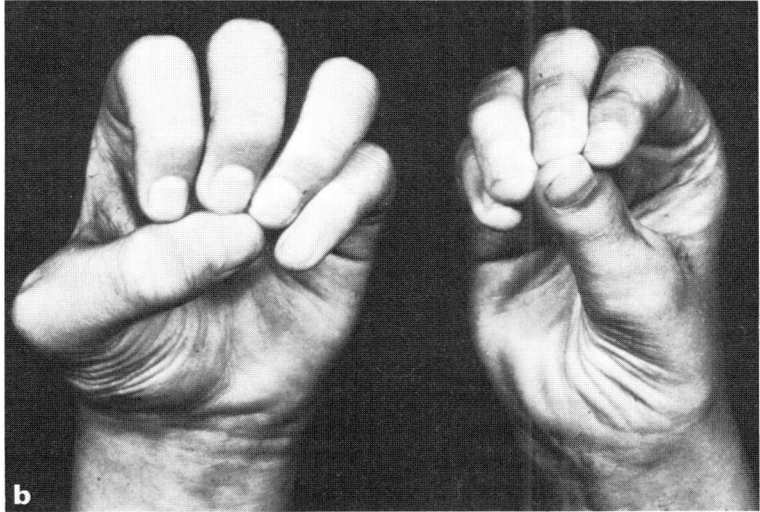

Fig. 11.13. Opponens transfer. (a) The patient had a median nerve injury with poor motor recovery. He can adduct his right thumb but not rotate it to face the pulps of the fingers. (b) After opponens transfer, using flexor digitorum sublimis of the ring finger, he can rotate the right thumb much better and can achieve satisfactory opposition.

months after the fracture, and are presumably caused by the deformity. In operating on such patients, the incision should be extended more proximally, with an ulnar step, so that it reaches at least to the level of the fracture and preferably slightly proximal to that. The same applies when the compression is due to rheumatoid tenosynovitis.

The median nerve is not far beneath the skin at the wrist and it is often cut in *lacerations*. At that level, the motor fibres are the most superficial, and the nerve may be only partly divided. However, the diagnosis of a partial injury is often due to inadequate examination, particularly of sensation. A pin and cotton wool must be used.

Whether total or partial, a cut nerve should be repaired within 24 hours if the cut is a clean one by a sharp instrument. If there is an element of crushing, or any infection, or an experienced surgeon is not available, secondary suture will be wiser, but this inevitably involves resecting a scarred area so that the ends will no longer match exactly. The use of an operating microscope enables both this matching and the actual suturing to be done more accurately, and there is evidence to suggest that the use of magnification gives better results. However, there is no evidence that any particular method of repair (for example, perineural as opposed to epineural) is superior.

Probably the commonest nerves to be injured are the digital nerves, especially those which are branches of the median nerve. Honner *et al.* (1970) have shown that primary repair gives satisfactory recovery of sensation, especially in younger patients. It was also noticed that the results were better in those with skilled or dexterous occupations: perhaps because their work involved an element of sensory re-education. A particularly interesting finding was that blocking the *uninjured* digital nerve with local anaesthetic usually produced considerable loss of sensation on the injured side. This did not happen in control patients, and suggests that sensory recovery is at least partly by the development of 'overlap' from the other digital nerve. The mechanism of this remains a fascinating puzzle. More recent work suggests that the strongest reason for primary repair of a digital nerve is to prevent the development of a painful neuroma, which is rare after repair but common if nothing is done to the injured nerve.

Management of residual disability

If a median nerve lesion, from whatever cause, proves irrecoverable, it is usually impossible to improve sensation, though one can improve the patient's awareness of the problem so that he avoids inadvertent injury. Bedeschi *et al.* (1984) have reported sensory nerve transfers in five cases of irrecoverable injury to the median nerve or its roots. The dorsal cutaneous branches of the ulnar nerve, or the terminal branches of the radial nerve (except that to the thumb) were divided distally, mobilized around to the front of the hand, and sutured to the digital branches of the median nerve. Only a few patients have been so treated and the quality of the results is not described in detail (in particular, whether the patient learned the new source of the sensory impulses) but the idea is an interesting one.

In contrast, the motor function of opposition can be restored fairly easily, provided that no contracture has been allowed to develop (Fig. 11.13). The types of tendon transfers used to restore opposition have already been described in connection with poliomyelitis (p. 210–214).

Ulnar nerve

The ulnar nerve is the main nerve for power grip, such as that used in holding a hammer. The handle is held on the radial side between the thumb and index finger (by the adductor pollicis and first dorsal interosseous) and on the ulnar border of the hand by the flexed little and ring fingers (whose profundus is ulnar-innervated). The importance of the little finger to power grip is often not appreciated, but loss of the little finger causes more disability than loss of the index finger, almost all of whose functions can readily be taken over by the middle finger.

Pathology

The ulnar nerve is particularly subject to external pressure because it lies close beneath the surface for much of its course. Thus it may be compressed by crutches in the axilla, by hanging the arm over the back or side of a chair, by the end of an above-elbow plaster, or by the edge of an unskilfully applied roller towel to elevate a hand after surgery. It is similarly at risk in lacerations, especially around the elbow and wrist where it is subcutaneous. It can also be compressed by tumours or by the displaced fragments in almost any fracture or dislocation in the arm, from a dislocated shoulder to a fractured 4th or 5th metacarpal.

Its superficial position, and consequent slightly lower temperature, is also thought to be the reason why the ulnar nerve is particularly liable to be affected by leprosy.

down the back of the ulnar side of the wrist and hand: thus it will be spared if the pathology is in the front of the wrist or palm, but affected if the lesion is at the elbow.

At the wrist or hand The pathology is usually a ganglion, but deep-seated so that it cannot be felt from the outside though it compresses part or all of the ulnar nerve against other structures. Compression of the nerve by a rheumatoid synovial cyst has also been reported (Dell 1979).

If the lesion is in Guyon's canal in front of the wrist, all the branches of the ulnar nerve in the hand will be compressed. If it is distal to the division into superficial and deep branches, the latter will be compressed where it passes beneath the fibrous arch of origin of the hypothenar muscles (Fig. 11.14), causing weakness of the small muscles of the hand supplied by the deep branch of the ulnar nerve, but sparing sensation which is

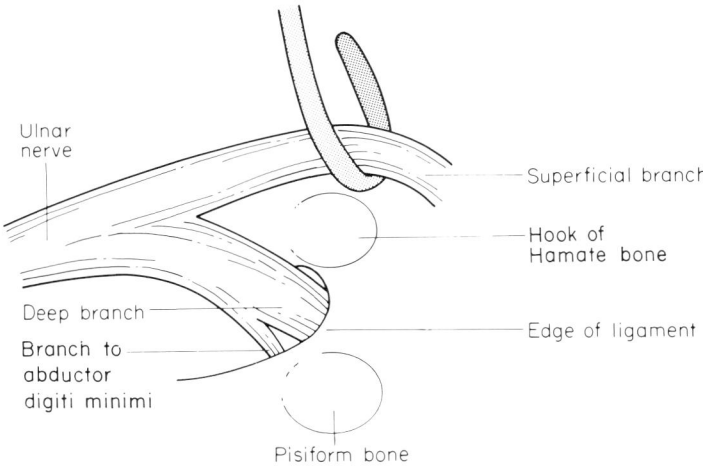

Fig. 11.14. Drawing of the branching of the ulnar nerve in the proximal part of the palm, from which it can be seen how some branches may be compressed and others spared, depending upon the precise site of the pathological lesion. (Reproduced with permission from Hayes *et al.* 1969.)

Ulnar nerve

Superficial branch

Hook of Hamate bone

Deep branch

Edge of ligament

Branch to abductor digiti minimi

Pisiform bone

In Western countries, nontraumatic ulnar nerve lesions are usually either at the elbow or in the proximal part of the hand; at both of these levels the nerve passes through a tunnel beneath the fibrous arch of origin of a muscle.

It is often possible to localize the level of the lesion by clinical examination, and electrical tests are seldom necessary. Involvement of the dorsal cutaneous branch is useful in this respect. It arises about 10 cms above the wrist and runs

mediated by the superficial branches. If the lesion is just a little further distal, the most proximal motor branch (to abductor digiti minimi) may be spared while the rest of the nerve (supplying the intrinsics, including the fourth palmar interosseous which adducts the little finger) are compressed, so that muscle imbalance causes abduction of the little finger (Hayes *et al.* 1969).

At the elbow The great majority of closed

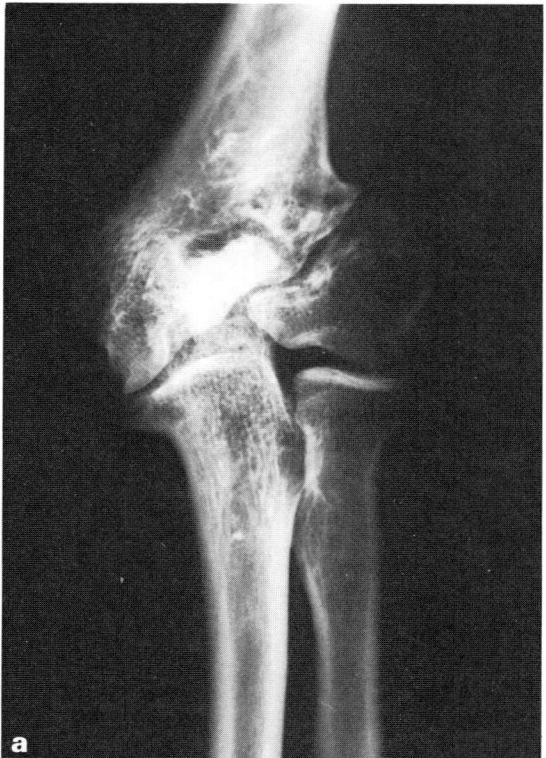

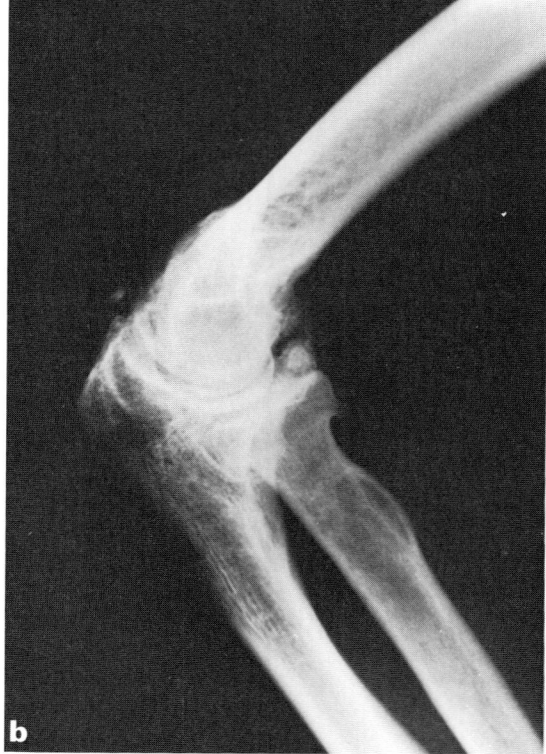

Fig. 11.15. X-rays of the elbows of two patients who presented with recent ulnar nerve lesions.
(a) Old ununited fracture of the lateral condyle sustained forty years previously.
(b) Primary osteoarthritis of the elbow.

ulnar nerve lesions are at the level of the elbow, where the nerve passes under the fibrous arch of origin of flexor carpi ulnaris. The elbow joint should be examined clinically and X-rayed, as some cases are secondary to abnormalities in that joint, the classic example being an old ununited or malunited fracture of the lateral condyle (Fig. 11.15a). The term 'old' is used advisedly, as the neurological signs and symptoms may not appear for very many years after the accident: the longest interval in one of the author's patients has been sixty years, and eighty years has been recorded! The mechanism of this tardy ulnar palsy is far from clear. Sunderland (1978) gave a full account of the different theories and concluded that 'the evidence suggests that the

basic cause of most of the cases of delayed palsy is arthritis of the elbow', that is osteoarthritis secondary to the altered anatomy caused by the old injury. 'Limitation of movement brings in its train fibrosis of the synovial structures, and fibrous change in the margins of the articular cartilage'. This is supported by the fact that ulnar neuropathy may also occur in primary osteoarthritis of the elbow (Fig. 11.15b).

However, in 50% of ulnar nerve lesions at elbow level, the elbow joint appears normal. Osborne (1959) argued strongly that the nerve is simply compressed in its tunnel and showed that the fibrous arch of origin of flexor carpi ulnaris tightens as the elbow is flexed: 'any pathological condition developing in the joint beneath may cause bony, cartilaginous or soft tissue thickening and encroachment on the space necessary for free passage of the ulnar nerve beneath the fibrous band. Compression of the nerve against the band is then inevitable in the flexed position and a conduction block or neuritis develops' (Osborne 1959). Pathological changes, similar to those described above as resulting from chronic compression of the median nerve in the carpal tunnel, have been demonstrated in the ulnar nerve at the elbow, and were most strongly marked precisely beneath the fibrous arch now sometimes called Osborne's band (Neary & Eames 1975).

Wadsworth (1982) went further and suggested that the medial collateral ligament bulged out in flexion and further compressed the nerve from its deep side. This sounds a little like having it both ways: if a structure becomes tight, one blames it for compressing the nerve, and if it becomes loose, one still blames it.

The difficulty with the simple compression theory, making the condition analogous to carpal tunnel syndrome, is that the symptoms are quite different. The complaint is not of painful pins-and-needles but of diminished sensation, weakness and wasting of the small muscles of the hand (because of this, these patients are often referred to neurological clinics in the first instance). However, this can be countered by the argument that, whereas the median nerve contains over 90% of sensory fibres, the ulnar nerve is about half sensory and half motor, so the effects of compression would be different. The present writer does not find this wholly convincing: the sensory fibres surely would be affected in the same way, be they few or many.

Whatever the exact pathology, there are many patients with a well-localized impairment of conduction in the ulnar nerve at the level of the elbow, and this is often amenable to relief by surgical treatment.

Treatment

What is the best operation? The simplest is just to decompress the nerve by dividing the fibrous arch across it, sometimes called Osborne's band in deference to the surgeon who recommended this procedure. He now advises that it should not only be divided, but should be resutured

deep to the nerve to prevent recurrence of the compression (Osborne 1970).

However, one may go further and remove the nerve from that area altogether by transposing it anteriorly. MacNicol (1979) reviewed 110 operations for ulnar neuritis and concluded that simple release should be restricted to patients with a short history (the presence of physical signs means that there is a long history) in whom at operation there is an obvious constriction without adhesions. Anterior transposition is recommended where no abnormality is seen or where the nerve is dislocated, compressed or tethered proximal to the aponeurosis of flexor carpi ulnaris. If there is any radiographic abnormality, the bed of the nerve must be assumed to be abnormal and transposition seems wise.

If the surgeon decides to transpose the nerve, where should it be put? MacNicol (1979) cited nine different papers and concluded that deep transposition was less prone to postoperative complications than superficial placement. Leffert (1982) also favoured the deep position beneath the common flexor origin, which has to be detached and resutured. There must be some risk of weakening the flexor muscles by this method and, presumably for this reason, Leffert did not do it in professional athletes, but in his review of the results of deep transposition, he did not mention flexor strength after operation, let alone give figures for it. This problem can be avoided by detaching and later reattaching the bony origin of the flexor muscles (i.e. the medial epicondyle) but this introduces a new set of possible complications. Moreover, the deep position itself may lead to scarring which constricts the nerve (King & Morgan 1970, Froimson & Zahrawi 1980) and the present writer has had to remove a nerve from the deep position into which it had earlier been transposed and place it superficially, a procedure which relieved the patient's symptoms.

In fact, it is not necessary to choose between a subcutaneous and a submuscular placement of the nerve. The author makes a shallow cut across the front of the common flexor mass, taking particular care to divide any strong aponeurotic fibres within it. The muscle fibres pull the cut edges apart to form a trough or groove, and the nerve is placed in that, so that the superficial surface of the nerve does not project above the surface of the muscle and is not liable to minor trauma. Neither the muscle nor the fascia should be sutured over the nerve, because this might compress it again as scar forms, but a small flap may be raised from the fascia over the muscle and sutured to the subcutaneous fat to prevent the nerve from slipping back into its original position (Eaton *et al.* 1980).

Broudy *et al.* (1978) reported ten patients needing re-operation after transposition of the ulnar nerve. In nine of these, the medial intermuscular septum was intact and was kinking the transposed nerve. Various other problems were found, and it is stated that in four cases 'the nerve was located in a channel cut into muscle which subsequently had become densely scarred.' However, the arithmetic suggests at least three of these four patients also had the nerve kinked at the septum, so the scarring in the muscular trough was not necessarily causing any symptoms.

The author has reviewed 20 consecutive cases of ulnar neuritis operated on under his own care. Their ages ranged from 15 to 67, with an average of 46 years. One woman and one man had bilateral involvement; in six other women and ten other men only one elbow was affected. There were equal numbers of right and left elbows. X-rays showed old fractures in three patients, and primary osteoarthritis in three; three other patients had rheumatoid disease. Eleven patients showed no radiographic abnormality. Three of this last group, all of whom had mild symptoms and signs, were treated by decompression of the nerve: at review one was cured and two improved. Fourteen had transposition into a groove in the muscle, as described above: four were cured, five improved, and five remained the same. One was worse: the nerve was re-explored and found to be kinked by an undivided medial intermuscular septum: this was excised and the nerve transposed deeply, after which the

symptoms were improved. Two patients had the nerve transposed to a deep position in the first instance; one was improved and one cured. It was noted that relief of symptoms was seldom as rapid as in carpal tunnel syndrome, and often took place just when one was beginning to give up hope, usually about 8 weeks after operation.

The problem of where to put the nerve can be avoided altogether by leaving the nerve where it is and removing the underlying bone: medial epicondylectomy, an operation seldom done in Britain, but from which good results have been reported in other countries (King & Morgan 1959, Craven & Green 1980, Froimson & Zahrawi 1980). It perhaps deserves more consideration here. The advantage is that it involves much less dissection and handling of the ulnar nerve than does transposition, and it is claimed that, in consequence, relief of symptoms occurs more quickly. The medial collateral ligament must not be damaged, and the flexor origin is reattached: it is said that no weakness of wrist or finger flexion or forearm pronation results since the muscle origin always heals firmly to the humerus and, in any case, the medial epicondyle is only part of its origin.

The ulnar nerve, uniquely, is subject to spontaneous recurrent dislocation: that is to say it is transposed anteriorly when the elbow is flexed but returns to its normal position on extension (Fig. 11.16). This was found to occur in 16.2% of apparently normal individuals examined specifically for this condition (Childress 1956). Childress found that in 75% the nerve only moved onto the tip of the medial epicondyle, which may perhaps be regarded as a subluxation, but in 25% it passed 'completely across and anterior to the epicondyle when the elbow is flexed to more than 90°'.

None of these subjects was aware that he had such an abnormality, and plainly no treatment was required. Sometimes, however, patients present with ulnar nerve symptoms and careful examination reveals the dislocation of the nerve. Those whose nerves sublux onto the epicondyle are subject to direct trauma or repeated pressure, such as a 48-year-old orthopaedic surgeon described by Childress who used to develop pain in the elbow and tingling on the ulnar side of his hand when driving his car with the inner side of his elbow supported on an elbow rest. Similar pressure may occur during a general anaesthetic or from a plaster shoulder spica. Surgical treatment is seldom needed in this type.

Patients whose nerves dislocate fully may develop a friction neuritis with progressive sensory and motor loss. In such cases surgery is indicated to keep the nerve permanently in the anterior position. Childress recommended deep transposition.

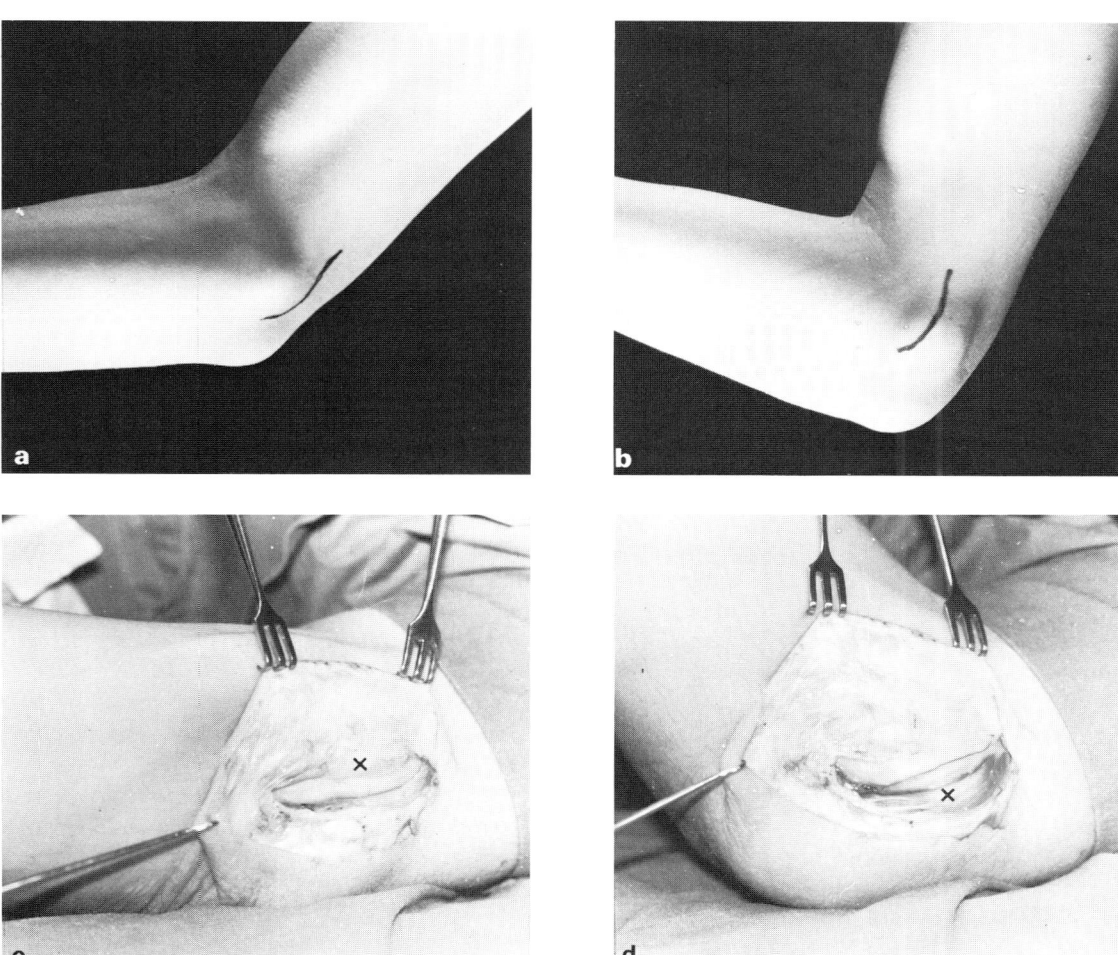

Fig. 11.16. Dislocating ulnar nerve in a medical student who had recently developed symptoms in the ulnar nerve distribution in the hand.
(a) With the elbow in extension, the ulnar nerve lies in the normal place. (The position of the nerve has been drawn on the skin.)
(b) In flexion, the nerve slips forwards to lie anterior to the medial epicondyle.
(c) Operative photograph of same patient, with elbow extended. The cross marks the medial epicondyle.
(d) In flexion, the ulnar nerve has moved to the front of the medial epicondyle, now covered by the medial edge of triceps, which also has slipped forwards.

Management of permanent or residual disability

Can anything be done to alleviate the effects of paralysis of the ulnar nerve whose cause cannot be cured?

Firstly, one must be sure that the nerve has been given sufficient time to recover. If it is completely divided at the elbow, recovery in the ulnar forearm muscles will not begin until 3–7 months have passed, and one must wait 6–11 months for the onset of recovery of sensation in the hand and 10–20 months for recovery in the hypothenar muscles. (There is never likely to be much recovery in the interossei or adductor pollicis in an adult.) Even if the nerve is cut more distally, at the wrist, sensory return does not start for 4–10 months.

Secondly, one must decide whether anything *need* be done. It has been said that the ulnar nerve is a luxury in a working man. This is not true since it plays an important part in grip; nevertheless, it must be admitted that many patients can manage without it, especially if the damage is at the wrist level so that the flexor carpi ulnaris and flexor digitorum profundus are unaffected. Sensation in the ulnar distribution is not as important as in the median nerve. Although the disability is less the ulnar nerve is largely motor and in theory it should be possible to improve the motor function.

Solonen and Bakalim (1976) have reported useful results following tendon transfers to replace the actions of the paralysed adductor pollicis and first dorsal interosseous muscles, thus strengthening pinch grip and the use of the thumb in power grip.

This leaves the clawing of the fingers. In the relatively stiff Caucasian hand, this is seldom more than a minor nuisance and cosmetic blemish, but in the more flexible Oriental hand it may alter the pattern of flexion to such an extent as to cause real disability, especially in grasping large objects. This is especially the case if the median nerve is also affected and all the lumbricals are paralysed, as is often the case in leprosy.

Many ingenious operations have been devised in the attempt to overcome this problem. This is not the place to describe them all, and in any case some are of historical interest only; a full account is given by Omer (1982). These operations may be divided into two main types.

The simplest procedures aim only to *prevent the hyperextension at the metacarpophalangeal joint.* It is easy to show, in almost all cases of intrinsic paralysis, that if metacarpophalangeal hyperextension is prevented (for example, by the examiner blocking it with his own fingers) the patient can actively extend the interphalangeal joints very much better and sometimes fully. This is because in the uncontrolled situation the long extensors (supplied by the radial nerve and therefore working) waste their limited excursion in the unwanted movement of hyperextension of the metacarpophalangeal joints. If this is prevented, their action is transferred to the more distal joints and these are extended instead.

The metacarpophalangeal hyperextension can be prevented by a lively splint but this is cumbersome and does not improve the function or appearance of the hand. Surgically, it can be achieved by a bone block on the dorsum, or by shortening the soft tissues on the front of the joint as described by Zancolli. The latter is generally preferred, and its efficacy can be increased by incising the fibrous flexor sheath so that the long flexor tendons bowstring across the metacarpophalangeal joint and thus can help flex it (Leddy *et al.* 1972). The disadvantage of this purely passive procedure is that the soft tissues may stretch, with recurrence of the clawing.

A more dynamic approach can be used, and the most successful of these methods in leprosy patients appears to be the *tendon transfers* evolved by Brand (1977) in which thin tendon grafts (plantaris split into two) are sutured proximally to the tendon of extensor carpi radialis brevis and tunnelled first through the interosseous spaces to pass in front of the deep transverse metacarpal ligament and then back into the dorsum of the fingers where they are sutured to the lateral band of the extensor tendons. This distal half of the graft thus follows the same line as the intrinsic muscles and can perform the same function: flexion of the metacarpophalangeal joints and extension of the interphalangeal joints.

Parkes (1973), whose paper included a useful review of earlier procedures, simplified this procedure by omitting the proximal part; the tendon grafts do not pass between the interossei but are sutured to the flexor retinaculum. They are still made to work by extension of the wrist, but indirectly by a *tenodesis* effect.

Conclusion

The orthopaedic surgeon needs to be a good neurologist, as far as the peripheral nervous system is concerned. He can neither diagnose nor treat patients without knowing the branching pattern of such nerves, the nerve supply of each muscle, and the method of testing them. In addition, he should know, as part of his instinctive background knowledge (like the multiplication tables), the nerve root supply of the main muscle groups and the areas of the sensory dermatomes. He must appreciate the key role of sensation, know how to test it appropriately, and understand what it is that he is really testing and why.

He must never forget that he may be dealing with a local manifestation of a systemic disorder, and will need to work with a neurologist in such cases, and in those with peripheral nerve lesions in whom electrical tests are needed. In particular, it is important to know whether the neurological condition is likely to be progressive or not.

In considering treatment, a realistic goal should be defined and this should be in terms of functional activities, not just achieving an anatomical movement.

The actual operations may be the easiest part of the management, but can improve life for many patients and transform it for a few. The orthopaedic surgeon is privileged to be able to help.

Acknowledgments

I should like to thank my colleagues Dr A. M. Whiteley, Mr C. L. Colton and Professor W. A. Wallace for their advice on different parts of this chapter, and Mrs D. Beesley for typing the manuscript. The section on radial nerve lesions incorporates material from my paper on that subject published in *The Hand* (1973) 5, 200–8.

References

ASHER R. (1972) *Talking Sense*, pp. 145–55. Pitman Books Ltd., London.

ASSIN J.L.T. (1983) Paralysies obstétricales du plexus brachial, evolution spontanée, resultats des interventions reparatrices precoces. Thesis, University of Paris, St-Louis.

BARR J.S., FREIBERG J.A., COLONNA P.C. & PEMBERTON P.A. (1942) A survey of end results on stabilization of the paralytic shoulder. *Journal of Bone and Joint Surgery*, **24**, 699–707.

BASSETT F.H. & NUNLEY J.A. (1982) Compression of the musculocutaneous nerve at the elbow. *Journal of Bone and Joint Surgery*, **64A**, 1050–2.

BEASLEY R.W. (1981) *Hand Injuries*. W.B. Saunders Co., Philadelphia, London and Toronto.

BEDESCHI P., CELLI L. & BALLI A. (1984) Transfer of sensory nerves in hand surgery. *Journal of Hand Surgery*, **9B**, 46–9.

BOWEN T.L. & STONE K.H. (1966) Posterior interosseous nerve paralysis caused by a ganglion at the elbow. *Journal of Bone and Joint Surgery*, **48B**, 774–6.

BOOME R.S. (1982) Brachial plexus palsies following traumatic false aneurysms. *Journal of Bone and Joint Surgery*, **64B**, 143.

BOYES J.H. (1970) *Bunnell's Surgery of the Hand*, 5th ed. J.B. Lippincott Co., Philadelphia and Toronto.

BRAIN W.R., DICKSON WRIGHT A.D. & WILKINSON M. (1947) Spontaneous compression of both median nerves in the carpal tunnel; 6 cases treated surgically. *Lancet*, ii, 277–82.

BRAND P.W. (1966) Tendon transfers in the forearm. In *Hand Surgery* (ed. J.E. Flynn), pp. 331–42. Williams & Wilkins, Baltimore.

BRAND P.W. (1977) Paralysis of the intrinsic muscles of the hand. In *Operative Surgery – The Hand* (ed. R.G. Pulvertaft) pp. 238–57. Butterworth & Co., London & Boston.

BRAND P.W. (1980) In *Management of Peripheral Nerve Problems* (eds. G.C. Omer & M. Spinner) pp. 862–72. W.B. Saunders Co., London & Toronto.

BRAND P.W., BEACH R.B. & THOMPSON D.E. (1981) Relative tension and potential excursion of muscles in the forearm and hand. *Journal of Hand Surgery*, **6**, 209–19.

BRISTOW W.R. (1947) Injuries of peripheral nerves in two World Wars. *British Journal of Surgery*, **34**, 333–48.

BROUDY A.S., LEFFERT R.D. & SMITH R.J. (1978) Technical problems with ulnar nerve transposition at the elbow: findings and results of re-operation. *Journal of Hand Surgery*, **3**, 85–9.

BUNNELL S. (1964) In *Surgery of the Hand* (ed. J.H. Boyes) 4th ed. revised pp. 438–59. J.P. Lippincott Co., Philadelphia and Montreal.

BURNS J. & LISTER G.D. (1984) Localized constrictive radial neuropathy in the absence of extrinsic compression: three cases. *Journal of Hand Surgery*, **9A**, 99–103.

BURKHALTER W., CHRISTENSEN R.C. & BROWN P. (1973) Extensor indicis proprius opponensplasty. *Journal of Bone and Joint Surgery*, **55A**, 725–32.

CALDWELL C.B., WILSON D.J. & BOURN R.M. (1969) Evaluation and treatment of the upper extremity in the hemiplegic stroke patient. *Clinical Orthopaedics and Related Research*, **63**, 69–93.

CAPENER N. (1966) The vulnerability of the posterior interosseous nerve of the forearm: a case report and an anatomical study. *Journal of Bone and Joint Surgery*, **48B**, 770–3.

CHILDRESS H.M. (1956) Recurrent ulnar nerve dislocation at the elbow. *Journal of Bone and Joint Surgery*, **38A**, 978–84.

COCHRANE R.G. (1964) Neuritis in leprosy. In *Leprosy in Theory and Practice* (eds. R.G. Cochrane and T.F. Davey) 2nd ed. pp. 410–17. John Wright & Sons Ltd., Bristol.

CRAVEN P.R. & GREEN D.P. (1980) Cubital tunnel syndrome: treatment by medial epicondylectomy. *Journal of Bone and Joint Surgery*, **62A**, 986–9.

DAS S.K. & BROWN H.G. (1976) In search of complications in carpal tunnel decompression. *The Hand*, **8**, 243–9.

DAWSON D.M., HALLETT M. & MILLENDER L.H. (1983) *Entrapment Neuropathies*. Little Brown and Co., Boston and Toronto.

DELL P.C. (1979) Compression of the ulnar nerve at the wrist secondary to a rheumatoid synovial cyst. Case report and review of the literature. *Journal of Hand Surgery*, **4**, 468–73.

DELLON A.L. (1981) *Evaluation of Sensibility and Re-education of Sensation in the Hand*. William and Wilkins, Baltimore and London.

DELLON A.L. & MACKINNON S.E. (1984) Susceptibility of the superficial sensory branch of the radial nerve to form painful neuromas. *Journal of Hand Surgery*, **9B**, 42–5.

EATON R.G., CROWE J.F. & PARKES J.C. (1980) Anterior transposition of the ulnar nerve using a noncompressing fasciodermal sling. *Journal of Bone and Joint Surgery*, **62A**, 820–5.

ELTON R.C. & OMER G.E. (1972) Tendon transfers for the nerve-injured upper limb. *Journal of Bone and Joint Surgery*, **54A**, 1561.

FLETCHER I.R. & HEALY T.E.J. (1983) The arterial tourniquet. *Annals of the Royal College of Surgeons of England*, **65**, 409–17.

FOO C.L. & SWANN M. (1983) Isolated paralysis of the serratus anterior. A report of 20 cases. *Journal of Bone and Joint Surgery*, **65B**, 552–6.

FROIMSON A.I. & ZAHRAWI F. (1980) Treatment of compression neuropathy of the ulnar nerve at the elbow by epicondylectomy and neurolysis. *Journal of Hand Surgery*, **5**, 391–5.

GARCIA A. & MAECK B.H. (1960) Radial nerve injuries in fractures of the shaft of the humerus. *American Journal of Surgery*, **99**, 625–7.

GARLAND D.E., THOMPSON R. & WATERS R.L. (1980) Musculo-cutaneous neurectomy for spastic elbow flexion in non-functional upper extremities in adults. *Journal of Bone and Joint Surgery*, **62A**, 108–12.

GILLIATT R.W. (1975) Peripheral nerve compression and entrapment. In *Eleventh Symposium on Advanced Medicine* (ed. A.W. Lant) Pitman Medical Books, London.

GILLIATT R.W. (1979) The classical neurological syndrome associated with a cervical rib and band. In *Pain in the Shoulder and Arm: an Integrated View* (eds. J.M. Greep, H.A.J. Lemmens, D.B. Roos & H.C. Urschel) Martinus Nijhoff Publishers, The Hague, Boston and London.

GILLIATT R.W. & WILSON T.G. (1953) A pneumatic tourniquet test in the carpal tunnel syndrome. *Lancet*, **ii**, 595–7.

GOLDNER J.L. (1974) Upper extremity tendon transfers in cerebral palsy. *Orthopedic Clinics of North America*, **5**, 389–414.

GREEN W.T. & BANKS H.H. (1962) Flexor carpi ulnaris transplant and its use in cerebral palsy. *Journal of Bone and Joint Surgery*, **44A**, 1343–52.

GUTTMAN SIR L. (1973) *Spinal Cord Injuries*. Blackwell Scientific Publications Ltd., Oxford.

HANSON R.W. & FRANKLIN M.R. (1976) Sexual loss in relation to other functional losses for spinal cord injured males. *Archives of Physical Medicine and Rehabilitation*, **57**, 291–3.

HARDY A.E. (1981) Birth injuries of the brachial plexus. *Journal of Bone and Joint Surgery*, **64B**, 98–101.

HARTZ C.R., LINSCHEID R.L., REED GRAMSE R. & DAUBE J.R. (1981) The pronator teres syndrome: compressive neuropathy of the median nerve. *Journal of Bone and Joint Surgery*, **63A**, 885–90.

HAYES J.R., MULHOLLAND R.C. & O'CONNOR B.T. (1969) Compression of the deep palmar branch of the ulnar nerve. *Journal of Bone and Joint Surgery*, **51B**, 469–72.

HELLER C.A., STANLEY P., LEWIS-JONES B. & HELLER R.F. (1983) Value of X-ray examinations of the cervical spine. *British Medical Journal*, **287**, 1276–8.

HEYSE-MOORE G.H. (1984) Resistant tennis elbow. *Journal of Hand Surgery*, **9B**, 64–6.

HEYWOOD A.W.B. (1979) The pathogenesis of the rheumatoid swan-neck deformity. *The Hand*, **11**, 176–83.

HOLSTEIN A. & LEWIS G.B. (1963) Fractures of the humerus with radial nerve paralysis. *Journal of Bone and Joint Surgery*, **45A**, 1382–8.

HONNER R., FRAGIADAKIS E.G., & LAMB D.W. (1970) An investigation of the factors affecting the results of digital nerve division. *The Hand*, **2**, 21–30.

INGLIS A.E. & COOPER W. (1966) Release of the flexor-pronator origin for flexion deformities of the hand and wrist in spastic paralysis. *Journal of Bone and Joint Surgery*, **48A**, 847–57.

INMAN V.T., SAUNDERS M. & ABBOTT L.C. (1944) Observations on the function of the shoulder joint. *Journal of Bone and Joint Surgery*, **26**, 1–30.

JAMES J.I.P. (1969) The relationship of Dupuytren's contracture and epilepsy. *The Hand*, **1**, 47–9.

JEFFREYS T.E. (1980) *Disorders of the Cervical Spine*. Butterworth & Co., London.

JONES R. (1916) On suture of nerves, and alternative methods of treatment by transplantation of tendon. *British Medical Journal*, 1, 641–3, 679–82.

KESSEL L. (1982) *Clinical Disorders of the Shoulder*, pp. 68–71. Churchill Livingstone, Edinburgh, London, Melbourne and New York.

KING R.J. (1984) Personal communication.

KING R.J. & BONNEY G. (1983) Analysis of 82 thoracic outlet explorations. *Journal of Bone and Joint Surgery*, 65B, 218.

KING R.J. & MOTTA G. (1983) Iatrogenic spinal accessory nerve palsy. *Annals of the Royal College of Surgeons of England*, 65, 35–7.

KING T. & MORGAN F.P. (1959) Late results of removing the medial humeral epicondyle for traumatic ulnar neuritis. *Journal of Bone and Joint Surgery*, 41B, 51–5.

KLENERMAN L. (1980) Tourniquet time — how long? *The Hand*, 12, 231–4.

LAMB D.W. & CHAN K.M. (1983) Surgical reconstruction of the upper limb in traumatic tetraplegia. A review of 41 patients. *Journal of Bone and Joint Surgery*, 65B, 291–8.

LEDDY J.P., STARK H.H., ASHWORTH C.R. & BOYES J.H. (1972) Capsulodesis and pulley advancement for the correction of claw-finger deformity. *Journal of Bone and Joint Surgery*, 54A, 1465–71.

LEFFERT R.D. (1972) Lipomas of the upper extremity. *Journal of Bone and Joint Surgery*, 54A, 1262–6.

LEFFERT R.D. (1982) Anterior submuscular transposition of the ulnar nerves by the Learmonth technique. *Journal of Hand Surgery*, 7, 147–55.

LINGE B. VAN & MULDER J.D. (1963) Function of the supraspinatus muscle and its relation to the supraspinatus syndrome. *Journal of Bone and Joint Surgery*, 45, 750–4.

LOTEM M., FRIED A., LEVY M., SOLZI P., NAJENSON T. & NATHAN H. (1971) Radial palsy following muscular effort. A nerve compression syndrome possibly related to a fibrous arch of the lateral head of the triceps. *Journal of Bone and Joint Surgery*, 53B, 500–6.

LOUIS D.S., LAMP M.K. & GREENE T.K. (1985) The upper extremities and psychiatric illnesses. *Journal of Bone and Joint Surgery*, 10A, 687–93.

LUNDBORG G., DAHLIN L-B., DANIELSEN N., HANSSON H-A., JOHANNESSON A., LONGO F.M. & VARON S. (1982a) Nerve regeneration across an extended gap: a neurobiological view of nerve repair and the possible involvement of neurotrophic factors. *Journal of Hand Surgery*, 7, 580–7.

LUNDBORG G., GELBERMAN R.H., MINTEER-CONVERY M., LEE Y.F. & HARGENS A.R. (1982b) Median nerve compression in the carpal tunnel — functional response to experimentally induced controlled pressure. *Journal of Hand Surgery*, 7, 252–9.

MCCUE F.C., HONNER R. & CHAPMAN W.C. (1970) Transfer of the brachioradialis for hands deformed by cerebral palsy. *Journal of Bone and Joint Surgery*, 52A, 1171–80.

MACDONALD R.I., LICHTMAN D.M., HANLON J.J. & WILSON J.N. (1978) Complications of surgical release for carpal tunnel syndrome. *Journal of Hand Surgery*, 3, 70–6.

MCFARLANE R.M. & MAYER J.R. (1976) Digital nerve grafts with the lateral antebrachial cutaneous nerve. *Journal of Hand Surgery*, 1, 169–73.

MACNICOL M.F. (1979) The results of operations for ulnar neuritis. *Journal of Bone and Joint Surgery*, 61B, 159–64.

MARMOR L., LAWRENCE J.F. & DUBOIS E.L. (1967) Posterior interosseous nerve palsy due to rheumatoid arthritis. *Journal of Bone and Joint Surgery*, 49A, 381–3.

MATEV I. (1963) Surgical treatment of spastic 'thumb-in-palm' deformity. *Journal of Bone and Joint Surgery*, 45B, 703–8.

MOBERG E. (1976) Reconstructive hand surgery in tetraplegia, stroke and cerebral palsy: some basic concepts in physiology and neurology. *Journal of Hand Surgery*, 1, 29–34.

MOBERG E. (1978) *The Upper Limb in Tetraplegia: a New Approach to Surgical Rehabilitation*. George Thieme, Stuttgart.

MORRIS D., COLLETT P., MARSH P. & O'SHAUGHNESSY M. (1979) *Gestures: Their Origins and Distributions*, pp. 99–118. Jonathan Cape, London.

NARAKAS A.O. (1981) The effects on pain of reconstructive neurosurgery in 160 patients with traction for crush injury to the brachial plexus. In *Phantom and Stump Pain* (eds. J. Siegfried and M. Zimmerman) Springer Verlag, Berlin, Heidelberg and New York.

NARAKAS A.O. (1985) The treatment of brachial plexus injuries. *International Orthopaedics*, 9, 29–36.

NEARY D. & EAMES R.A. (1975) The pathology of ulnar nerve compression in man. *Neuropathology and Applied Neurobiology*, 1, 69–88.

NEARY D., OCHOA J. & GILLIATT R.W. (1975) Sub-clinical entrapment neuropathy in man. *Journal of the Neurological Sciences*, 24, 283–98.

NICKEL V.L., PERRY J. & GARRETT A.L. (1963) Development of useful function in the severely paralysed hand. *Journal of Bone and Joint Surgery*, 45A, 933–52.

OMER G.E. (1980) In *Management of Peripheral Nerve Problems* (eds. G.E. Omer & M. Spinner) pp. 779–89. W.B. Saunders Co., Philadelphia, London and Toronto.

OMER G.E. (1982) Ulnar nerve palsy. In *Operative Hand Surgery* (ed. D.P. Green) pp. 1061–80. Churchill Livingstone, Edinburgh, London and Melbourne.

OMER G.E. & SPINNER M. (1980) *Management of Peripheral Nerve Problems*. W.B. Saunders Co., Philadelphia, London and Toronto.

OSBORNE G.V. (1959) Ulnar neuritis. *Postgraduate Medical Journal*, 35, 392–6.

OSBORNE G.V. (1970) Compression neuritis of the ulnar nerve at the elbow. *The Hand*, 2, 10–13.

OSBORNE G.V. (1983) The hysterical hand. Paper read to British Society for Surgery of the Hand at Buxton on 14th May 1983.

PACKER J.W., FOSTER R.R., GARCIA A. & GRANTHAM S.A. (1972) The humeral fracture with radial nerve palsy: is exploration warranted? *Clinical Orthopaedics and Related Research*, 88, 34–8.

PARKES A. (1973) Paralytic claw fingers — a graft tenodesis operation. *The Hand*, 5, 192–9.

PETRUCCI F.S., MORELLI A. & RAIMONDI P.L. (1982) Axillary nerve injuries — 21 cases treated by nerve graft and neurolysis. *Journal of Hand Surgery*, 7, 271–8.

POLLOCK G.A. (1962) Surgical treatment of cerebral palsy. *Journal of Bone and Joint Surgery*, 44B, 68–81.

RANNEY D.A. (1976) The superficialis minus deformity and its operative treatment. *The Hand*, 8, 209–14.

RANSFORD A.O. & HUGHES S.P.F. (1977) Complete brachial plexus lesions. A ten-year follow-up of twenty cases. *Journal of Bone and Joint Surgery*, 59B, 417–20.

ROLES N.C. & MAUDSLEY R.H. (1972) Radial tunnel syndrome. Resistant tennis elbow as a nerve entrapment. *Journal of Bone and Joint Surgery*, 54B, 499–508.

RORABECK C.H. & HARRIS W.R. (1981) Factors affecting the prognosis of brachial plexus injuries. *Journal of Bone and Joint Surgery*, 63B, 404–7.

SAMILSON R.L. & MORRIS J.M. (1964) Surgical improvement of the cerebral palsied upper limb. *Journal of Bone and Joint Surgery*, 46A, 1203–16.

SANDIFER P.H. (1967) *Neurology in Orthopaedics*, Butterworth & Co., London.

SCUDERI C. (1949) Tendon transplants for irreparable radial nerve paralysis. *Surgery, Gynaecology and Obstetrics*, 88, 643–51.

SCHNEIDER L.H. (1969) Opponensplasty using the extensor digiti minimi. *Journal of Bone and Joint Surgery*, 51A, 1297–302.

SEDDON H.J. (1972) *Surgical Disorders of Peripheral Nerves*. Churchill Livingstone, Edinburgh and London.

SEDEL L. (1982) The results of surgical repair of brachial plexus injuries. *Journal of Bone and Joint Surgery*, 64B, 54–66.

SEGAL A., SEDDON H.J. & BROOKS D.M. (1959) Treatment of paralysis of the flexors of the elbow. *Journal of Bone and Joint Surgery*, 41B, 44–50.

SEMPLE J.C. & CARGILL A.O. (1969) Carpal tunnel syndrome. Results of surgical decompression. *The Lancet*, i, 918–9.

SHARRARD W.J.W. (1957) Muscle paralysis in poliomyelitis. *British Journal of Surgery*, 44, 471–80.

SHARRARD W.J.W. (1966) Posterior interosseous neuritis. *Journal of Bone and Joint Surgery*, 48B, 777–80.

SHARRARD W.J.W. (1971) *Paediatric Orthopaedics and Fractures*. Blackwell Scientific Publications Ltd., Oxford.

SHAW J.L. & SAKELLARIDES H. (1967) Radial nerve paralysis associated with fractures of the humerus. A review of 45 cases. *Journal of Bone and Joint Surgery*, 49A, 899–902.

SIMMONS B.P. & VASILE R.G. (1980) The clenched fist syndrome. *Journal of Hand Surgery*, 5, 420–7.

SMITH R.J. (1975) Factitious lymphedema of the hand. *Journal of Bone and Joint Surgery*, 57A, 89–94.

SPIEGEL D. & CHASE R.A. (1980) The treatment of contractures of the hand using self-hypnosis. *Journal of Hand Surgery*, 5, 428–32.

SPINNER M. (1968) The arcade of Frohse and its relationship to posterior interosseous nerve paralysis. *Journal of Bone and Joint Surgery*, 50B, 809–12.

SPINNER M. (1970) The anterior interosseous nerve syndrome with special attention to its variations. *Journal of Bone and Joint Surgery*, 52A, 84–94.

SPINNER M. (1972) *Injuries to the Major Branches of Peripheral Nerves of the Forearm*. W.B. Saunders Company, Philadelphia, London and Toronto.

SOLONEN K.A. & BAKALIM G.E. (1976) Restoration of pinch grip in traumatic ulnar palsy. *The Hand*, 8, 39–44.

STEIN F., GRABIA S.L. & DEFFER P.A. (1971) Nerve injuries complicating Monteggia lesions. *Journal of Bone and Joint Surgery*, 53A, 1432–6.

STRACHAN J.C.H. & ELLIS B.W. (1971) Vulnerability of the posterior interosseous nerve during radial head resection. *Journal of Bone and Joint Surgery*, 53B, 320–3.

SUNDERLAND S. (1978) *Nerves and Nerve Injuries*, 2nd ed. Churchill Livingstone, Edinburgh and London.

SWAFFORD A.R. & LICHTMAN D.H. (1982) Suprascapular nerve entrapment — case report. *Journal of Hand Surgery*, 7, 57–60.

SWANSON A.B. (1960) Surgery of the hand in cerebral palsy and the swan-neck deformity. *Journal of Bone and Joint Surgery*, 42A, 951–64.

TAKAMI H., TAKASHI S. & ANDO M. (1984) Latissimus dorsi transplantation to restore elbow flexion to the paralysed limb. *Journal of Hand Surgery*, 9B, 61–3.

THOMAS P.K. & FULLERTON P.M. (1963) Nerve fibre size in the carpal tunnel syndrome. *Journal of Neurology, Neurosurgery and Psychiatry*, 26, 520–27.

TULLOCH BROWN J. (1952) Nerve injuries complicating dislocation of the shoulder. *Journal of Bone and Joint Surgery*, 34B, 526.

UPTON A.R.M. & McCOMAS A.J. (1973) The double crush in nerve-entrapment syndrome. *The Lancet*, 2, 359–62.

VAN BEEK A.L., EDER M.A. & ZOOK E.G. (1982) Nerve regeneration — evidence for early sprout formation. *Journal of Hand Surgery*, 7, 79–83.

VAN ROSSUM J., BURUMA O.J.S., KAMPHUISEN H.A.C. & ONVLEE G.J. (1978) Tennis elbow — a radial tunnel syndrome? *Journal of Bone and Joint Surgery*, 60B, 197–8.

WADSWORTH T.G. (1982) *The Elbow*, Churchill Livingstone, Edinburgh, London and New York.

WARREN J.D. (1963) Anterior interosseous nerve palsy as a complication of forearm fractures. *Journal of Bone and Joint Surgery*, 45B, 511–2.

WATSON-JONES R. (1930) Primary nerve lesions in injuries of the elbow and wrist. *Journal of Bone and Joint Surgery*, 12, 121–40.

WHITE W.L. (1960) Restoration of function and balance of the wrist and hand by tendon transfers. *Surgical Clinics of North America*, 40, 427–59.

WYNN PARRY C.B. (1981) *Rehabilitation of the Hand*, 4th ed. Butterworth & Co., London.

ZACHARY R.B. (1946) Tendon transplantation for radial paralysis. *British Journal of Surgery*, 33, 358–64.

ZANCOLLI E. (1979) *Structural and Dynamic Bases of Hand Surgery*, 2nd ed., J.P. Lippincott Co., Philadelphia and Toronto.

Chapter 12
The Orthopaedic Management of the Stroke Patient

B. A. ROPER

Introduction

Stroke is a colloquialism for the upper motor neuron lesion consequent upon a cerebrovascular accident. The frequent sequel of a cerebrovascular accident is a hemiplegia; quadriplegia is relatively uncommon. The incidence of hemiplegia following a cerebrovascular accident in the United Kingdom is 2 per 1000 of the population each year (Acheson & Fairbairn 1970). This means that there are half a million people in the United Kingdom suffering from hemiplegia.

There are four main types of cerebrovascular accident: cerebral thrombosis, intracerebral haemorrhage, subarachnoid haemorrhage and cerebral embolism. The prognosis varies with each condition. For instance, with cerebral embolism, one in three are dead within three months and a further one third die within three years. With cerebral infarction, one in four die within three months and a further one quarter are dead within three years. It is not easy to make a differential diagnosis but this is improving with advances in radiological diagnostic techniques, radio-isotope scanning, ultrasound techniques and the development of magnetic resonance imaging. Life expectancy varies inversely with age, with the severity of any pre-existing hypertension and of any accompanying cardiac dysfunction, with the existence of diabetes mellitus, and with the duration and depth of the initial period of unconsciousness.

The severity of the resulting hemiplegia depends on the density of the initial ischaemia, the adequacy of any collateral circulation and the severity of the residual brain damage. The response to rehabilitation depends upon associated illnesses such as arteriosclerosis, hypertension, diabetes, cardiac insufficiency, osteoarthritis and defects in vision and hearing. Age is of considerable importance. Seventy-five per cent of patients with strokes are over the age of 60 and of those patients referred for rehabilitation, 70% are over 50 years of age (Nichols 1980). Rehabilitation should commence as soon as possible but this obviously depends upon the prognosis.

A gradually extending paralysis and prolonged deepening unconsciousness are bad prognostic signs as are persistent flaccidity and intense hypertonicity. The normal sequence of events is a period of initial flaccidity and then hypertonicity with brisk reflexes. Recovery is optimal in the first few months with a crest at two months.

Neurophysiology

After a cerebrovascular accident, the sensory and motor cortices are damaged. The dysfunction experienced by a patient is due to disruption of the selective control and the consequent exposure of primitive reflexes, together with sensory disturbances. The disturbance of the central nervous system results in increased muscle excitation arising from alteration of the Sherringtonian 'central excitatory state'. This response depends on an intact reflex arc. The increased muscle excitation is diminished by sleep, sedation and coma, increased by anxiety and motor activity (Calne 1975) and manifest as spasticity and rigidity. These terms describe the phenomenon of resistance to passive movement, thought to be typical of a pyramidal tract lesion. Sustained resistance is thought to be more typical for corticospinal lesions (Dimitrijević & Nathan 1967). 'Lead pipe' or 'cog-wheel' rigidity is thought to be typical of extrapyramidal lesions. Spasticity and rigidity have been attributed to increased alpha and fusi-motor (gamma neuron) activity but the evidence for this is controversial (Dietrichson 1971, McLellan 1973).

Presumably large lesions in the central nervous system lead to complex changes in the neurotransmitter function. These could either be defective synthesis or inactivation of storage release mechanism. At the present time, these mechanisms are not understood, but this is a field for intensive research. There is some optimism because it is now clearly understood that Parkinson's disease is due to a striatal depletion of dopamine and this discovery has allowed a rational therapeutic regimen to be developed. The evaluation of medical treatment is exceedingly difficult. It is possible to reduce spasticity by the use of drugs, but there is a very narrow borderline between an effective therapeutic dose and that producing sleep. Matthews (1966) developed a technique for using electromyograms comparing the H reflex response to maximum excitation of the motor nerve. This proved to be a difficult technique.

There are different types of disturbed motor control in hemiparetic patients and this has been particularly demonstrated by studies of the characteristics of the movement patterns of gait in hemiparesis (Drillis 1958, Liberson et al. 1962, Brunnstrom 1964, Finley & Karpovich 1964, Murray & Clarkson 1966, Perry 1969a). A few have been more directly concerned with the disturbed control of muscle activation. Surface electromyograms taken from different leg muscles during walking have suggested a low degree of activity, in general both in the paretic and in the nonparetic limb. Hirschberg and Nathanson (1952), Marks and Hirschberg (1958) and Peat et al. (1976) determined the

average electromyographic activity in full muscle groups of the paretic leg in different phases of gait and found more complex changes. Thus in the gastrocnemius muscle low average levels of activity were found in all the different phases of the gait cycle, but in the other muscles examined average levels of activity were decreased in some phases and increased in others.

The dispersion of levels of activity in the different phases of gait were considerable in all muscles examined and signified a marked individual variation. Such variation was also apparent from electromyography of lower limb muscles in the stance phase of hemiparetic gait (Carlsöo et al. 1974) and was noticed in a study using this method to evaluate the effects of gait training (Bogardh & Richards 1974). Knutsson and Richards (1979), in a study of this problem of the pattern of muscle activation in walking, compared 26 hemiparetic patients with 10 normal patients. In nine hemiparetic patients the calf muscles were prematurely activated in the stance phase probably due to enhanced stretch reflexes: this was called Type 1. In another nine patients (Type 2) the electromyographic activity was reduced to an extremely low level in two or more of the muscles examined. In four patients there was a pathological coactivation of several or all of the muscles during part of the gait cycle thus disrupting the normal sequential shift of activity in antagonistic muscles: this was called Type 3. In four patients the muscle activation pattern was much more complex and no common pattern was discernible.

Perry et al. (1978) identified three features pertinent to walking during a series of experiments involving the hemiparetic lower limb. Extension of the hip and knee sharply increased the quick stretch response of the ankle plantar flexors compared to that elicited with these joints flexed (limb synergy); and the upright posture doubled the tone of the extensor muscles compared to that found with the patient supine (vestibular reflex). During walking, these two effects were further enhanced by the overlay of the primitive locomotor patterns in patients dependent on this method of limb control.

Extension of the knee in preparation for stance simultaneously activated the plantar flexors of the ankle. This premature activity exposed the patient's spastic state to stretch at a time when the muscles normally would be relaxed.

Motor deficits alone are seldom the bar to functional recovery. Sensory defects, especially of proprioception and two-point discrimination, are of vital importance and can have a profound bearing on rehabilitation. The most profound sensory loss is anosognosia. This is a denial of the true self-image and occurs when the patient is totally unaware of the hemiplegic side. This is usually associated with a lesion of a right non-dominant hemisphere and has a very poor prognosis for functional recovery. Disturbance of the body image also gives a sensation of falling which is unrelated to involvement of the vestibulocerebral tract and impairment of the visiospatial perception. Defects of position sense, stereognosis and spacial orientation may markedly restrict the redevelopment of functional activities. Apraxia is the inability to perform previously learned skilled tasks and is frequently linked with ataxia which is a loss of muscular coordination. Agnosia is the loss of the ability to recognize sensory stimuli and, in addition, there may well be impairment of intellectual function and changes in personality which often are demonstrated by marked emotional lability. A right-sided hemiplegia is frequently accompanied by aphasia or dysphasia.

Nonsurgical treatment

Rehabilitation is an organized therapeutic programme directed towards recovering maximal function in patients with permanent or severely protracted physical disability. Early mobilization either actively or passively is of paramount importance (Matthews 1975). The longer a patient is idle the more profound the loss of function becomes. There are two aspects to this. The first is physical, but, probably more importantly, there is the mental attitude of the patient. The sooner the patient is persuaded that there

will be some degree of recovery, the greater will be the functional recovery. Many treatments for patients with strokes have been proposed and one of the few constant findings is that any treatment designed to increase the sensory input and facilitate motor output of the brain will be beneficial. The increase of the sensory input is possibly the most important factor.

Sensation

It is very easy to forget that a substantial amount of the cerebral cortex is concerned with sensation and that after a cerebrovascular accident considerable damage to these areas can result. It is not uncommon to find patients who are tripping over things and bumping into things and it is assumed that this is a disturbance of balance, but in fact the reason why they are exhibiting this phenomenon is because they have an homonymous hemianopia and just cannot see anything to one side of the body. By far the most serious sensory loss in terms of possible recovery of function is loss of proprioception. There can be very extensive loss of an awareness of the position of the body or part of the body in space. Obviously if this does not recover the potential for function in that person is markedly reduced. The most satisfactory method of assessing this is to get the patient to make a line drawing of their body image. In severe cases of hemiplegia with a loss of body image they will totally ignore one side of the body. Where merely the distal part of a limb is concerned then they may draw a limb with totally disassociated hand. There is no doubt that recovery of sensation does occur, but how much is merely a result of resolution of oedema and whether there is any genuine restoration of function is almost impossible to know. Most of the evidence in support of recovery of sensation is anecdotal; this is largely because there are no simple and consistent techniques available for measuring sensation. It certainly seems that if a person is exposed to repeated sensory stimulation associated with an educational programme recovery of function can occur.

Motor

The motor effects as a result of a cerebrovascular accident are usually manifest. The flexed upper limb and the dragging lower limb held fairly stiffly, are well recognized by lay people as being due to stroke. As a result of it being more obvious, possibly more attention has been focused on

progressive spasticity and deformity (Fig. 12.1) and very limited return of function. Travis and Woolsey (1956) questioned how much of the dysfunction was related to the neurological lesion and how much was the result of associated deformities. They and other workers (Bucy *et al.* 1966, Beck & Chambers 1970) found that in monkeys after pyramidal tract lesions good

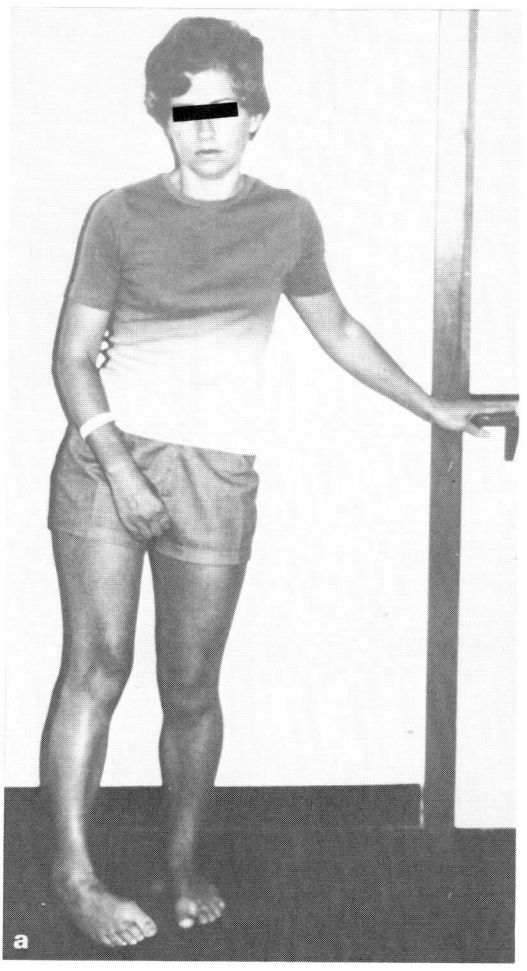 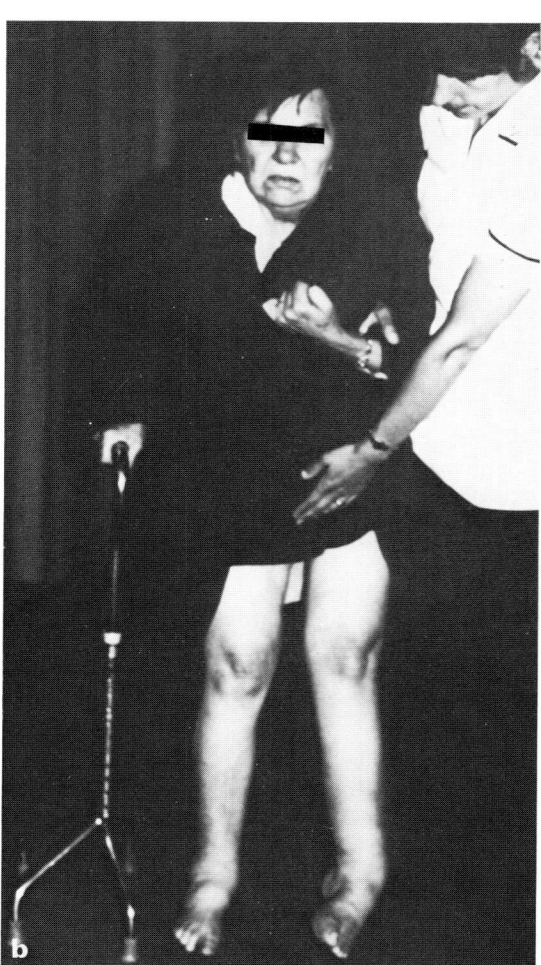

Fig. 12.1. (a) and (b) Typical pattern of deformity due to hemiplegia.

the motor side of strokes than the sensory deficit although, of course, the two cannot really be separated.

In 1951 Twitchell described the natural course of patients with hemiplegia. This was of

results were obtained provided that early mobilization and functional assistance were carried out. This approach has been confirmed in the treatment of patients with strokes (Matthews 1975) who nowadays have markedly less loss of function and are less spastic than those described by Twitchell. The fundamentals of the rehabilitation programme are early mobilization and the direction of the resultant neurocontrol into effective function. As a result contractures are minimized and erroneous use of the patient's available control is avoided. The prime concern is the avoidance of contractures since a true shortening of the muscle tendon unit, if allowed to persist, will produce a secondary shortening of the capsule and ligamentous structures of the associated joints.

Contracture has to be differentiated from spasticity which is an exaggerated stretch reflex. Stretch receptors are activated when the applied force exceeds a certain threshold (Granit 1970). The forces accompanying movement will be transmitted more completely if the tissues are stiff rather than flexible. Contractures stiffen tissues, immobility creates contractures. Spasticity preserves the contracture by excluding the intramuscular fibrous tissues from the stretching force. Muscles are more sensitive to contractures than the joint capsules. If the tissues have normal flexibility the range of movement needed for function may be passed before a spastic response is elicited. Clinical experience suggests that passive tissue flexibility decreases progressively as the period of inactivity lengthens and, therefore, early and frequent movement of the limbs are required to prevent contractures. Personal experience has shown that passive movement of a limb for only half an hour a day is adequate. Active mobilization is obviously the best since as the muscles change their length they also alter the alignment of their sheaths and therefore, physiologically, stimulate the ground substance and mobilize the collagenous interfibrous junction. Conversely, stimulation of the antagonists leads to contralateral relaxation thereby exposing the contractures to stretching forces.

To stimulate muscle activity in patients who lack direct control of their muscles, physiotherapists use various reflex patterns. Various techniques are available and the exercise systems of Brunnstrom, Knott, Bobath and Rood are currently used. Most therapists employ a mix-

ture of these systems and seem to get the best results when treatment is provided during the patient's period of spontaneous recovery, preventing or correcting contractures before the collagenous tissues have undergone permanent change. However, very few satisfactory attempts have been made to evaluate the effects of physiotherapy on recovery; this is largely because it is difficult to standardize the actual technique and treatment. Furthermore, it is even more difficult to standardize stroke patients; even with a gross clinical picture each stroke patient is different from the next one and the complexities of electomyographic attempts at classification are such that the problem becomes even greater. Therefore it is almost impossible to set up a true scientific controlled trial of different treatment regimens. As a consequence, most papers discussing physiotherapy treatment tend to rely on anecdotal information.

A more direct means of inducing muscle activity is through functional electrical stimulation which has always been an extremely attractive approach since it is a direct attempt to replace the central control mechanism and manipulate what is, to all intents and purposes, a reasonably normal peripheral nervous system. The problem with functional electrical stimulation has always been the transmission across the skin interface of an electrical stimulus of sufficient intensity to generate effective muscle activity. Recent research on the size and material of the electrode and the quality of the stimulating current (Nelson et al. 1980) has given hope that in the future a universally acceptable therapeutic mechanism will be come available. The group from Ljubljana (Dimitrijević et al. 1968, Vodovnik et al. 1978) are also carrying out extensive clinical trials. With the developments of technology multimuscle stimulation of key lower extremity muscles will be feasible. A second experimental therapeutic programme combining postural feedback by goniometer with electrical stimulation and voluntary effort is giving encouraging results (Bowman et al. 1979). This aspect of research is developing very rapidly and offers the greatest hope for the future.

It may not be possible to institute active stretching and therefore, passive stretching has to be substituted. Manual stretching techniques are not terribly satisfactory because the stretch period is too brief. The objective of passive stretching is to fatigue the spastic muscle, thereby exposing the fibrous tissue element to the stretching force. Serial plaster casting has proved very acceptable. By keeping the joint at rest the stretch response is not elicited so the

does is to stimulate the exaggerated stretch response and can only increase the deformity (Fig. 12.3). Orthotic restraint is particularly useful in two areas, the wrist and the ankle. Both of these joints have a single posture that is an acceptable functional compromise. In the hemiplegic lower limb with foot drop due to spastic equinovarus and diminished proprioception, a short leg orthotic device is needed. Provided that it has an absolutely rigid ankle then not only is

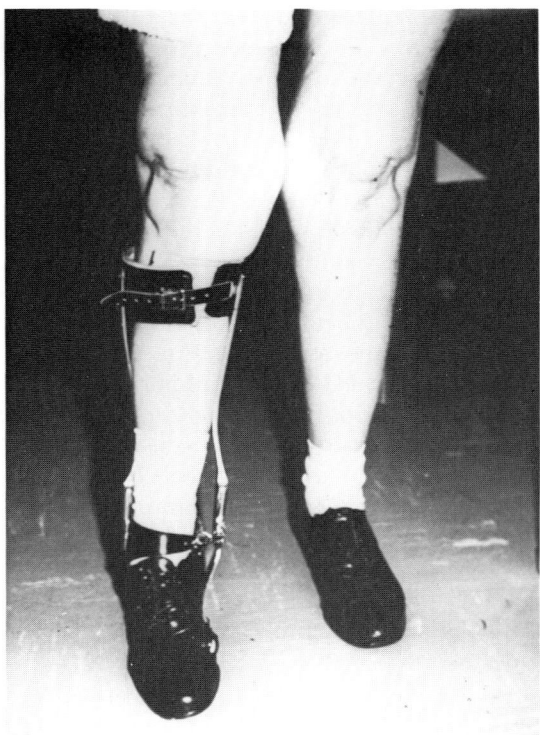

Fig. 12.2. Fixed ankle–below knee orthosis with wide calf cuff.

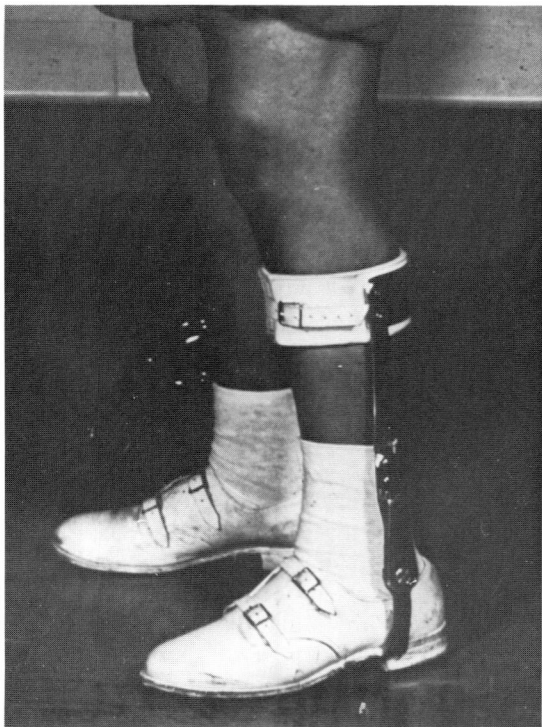

Fig. 12.3. Spring loaded below knee orthosis increasing spasticity.

collagenous tissues are exposed to the corrective force. Another means of reducing spasticity and deformity is by orthotic restraint (Fig. 12.2). By locking a joint in neutral functional position the stretch stimulus is avoided and hence a spastic response does not occur (Perry 1969b). Obviously any orthotic device incorporating a spring system is totally contraindicated because all this

the deformity of the ankle controlled but the instability of the knee is also controlled. The hyperextended knee is caused by weak quadriceps muscles, impaired proprioception and severe spasticity or contracture in the plantar flexor muscles of the calf and foot. Persistence of the flexor pattern throughout the swing phase increases the spasticity of the knee flexors and prevents the patient from reaching forward for a full step. A short leg brace locked in slight dorsiflexion will prevent the knee from going into hyperextension, it will correct the plantar flexion deformity and produce proprioception through contact between the brace and the skin. During forward progression the force of the posterior cuff of the brace against the calf will hold the knee in the neutral position by preventing the tibia from angling backward. The unstable knee in flexion will similarly be controlled provided that the brace is locked at 90° or in slight plantar flexion. The locked ankle joint preventing dorsiflexion causes cuff pressure against the anterior part of the tibia and this stimulus causes the patient to contract the quadriceps and the hip extensors to pull away from the brace, thereby gaining the desired stability of the knee. There is no indication for a long leg brace. The patient with hemiplegia needs strength in the extensor of the hip to use either a long or a short leg brace. To walk with a long leg brace he needs enough control of extension to counteract spasticity or tightness of the hip flexors, that is to stabilize the trunk over the weight-bearing extremity. When there is this much control there is adequate stability of the thigh for a short leg brace to be worn to stabilize the knee.

When confronted with obstructive spasticity that has failed to respond adequately to the previously described techniques, controlled chemolysis or operative intervention may be indicated. Temporary chemolysis is used in patients who have an overwhelming spasticity in one group of muscles and yet function in the antagonist muscles is present but weak, the principle being that if the stronger muscle is weakened then the strength of the weaker muscle can be increased. When the nerve regenerates and power is returned to the stronger muscle, the strength of the antagonist muscle may well be sufficient to allow reasonably normal function. It is also of use when trying to evaluate the longterm effects of surgery. Three per cent aqueous phenol was first used by Khalili et al. (1964) and reported again in 1967 (Khalili & Betts 1967). Their method was percutaneous identification of the peripheral nerve using a needle electrode. This technique has not had universal acceptance because phenol infusion of a mixed nerve is apt to cause troublesome hyperaesthesia or causalgia. However, Copp and Keenan (1972) described their extensive experience without a significant incidence of complications. The alternative is to use three per cent phenol in glycerine injected directly into the motor branches which have been exposed at open operation (Mooney et al. 1969) to create a partial peripheral nerve lesion which has the potential for 75% recovery over a period of six months. The positive advantage of this technique is that there is a direct attack on specifically spastic and overactive muscles whilst not damaging other muscles which may be considerably less troublesome or may even have normal function. The side-effect of sensory disturbance is avoided but, of course, the disadvantage is that it demands an open operation. An alternative technique is to inject 45% alcohol into the motor points of muscles, which is particularly useful in those muscles whose nerve supply is either mixed or not easily approached. It is a very simple technique which can be used on outpatients. Fortuitously the motor end-plates are usually in the region of the centre of the muscle belly and, if this can be identified, direct injection of about 10 millilitres of 45% double-distilled alcohol into this region will produce marked alleviation of spasticity. This technique is particularly useful in dealing with spastic quadriceps.

Surgical treatment

Once the patient has reached a stable neurological state, permanent correction of an obstructive spasticity may well be desirable. It can be accomplished by surgical release of the appropriate tendons, by selected neurectomies, or by transferring tendons to produce the antagonistic action. The choice of which technique is to be used depends entirely on whether one wishes to remove the offending muscle action totally, to weaken it or to reverse it. With increasing experience, the indication for surgical intervention is becoming quite clearcut.

Following damage to the motor cortex several levels of activity result. The most severe situation is where the motor cortex is virtually destroyed and the patient is left totally flail. The next most severe lesion is where the residual is primitive reflex activity, of which the most common example is the mass flexor withdrawal response. If this is the the only activity that is left there is very little to be gained by active rehabilitation and the only indication for intervention is to improve the nursing care. The next most severe lesion leaves usable reflex activity, that is an extensor thrust response which will allow standing or phased flexion response which will allow walking. These reflex actions may be too strong to allow their proper use and this is the main group where surgery is indicated. The next level of severity is where there is voluntary control but demonstrable spasticity. By reducing this level of spasticity almost normal function may be achieved and this is the other indication for operation. Where there is voluntary control without any demonstrable spasticity, there in no indication for any surgical intervention.

Over the years, the surgical approach has been viewed with a certain amount of displeasure. This has largely been due to the unpredictability of the results because of the difficulty in accurately identifying which muscle was the offending force. The complex interaction of normal muscle action, abnormal muscle action, reflex action, stretch reflexes and phasing that occurs during use creates a total pattern of muscle action which differs greatly from that which is capable of being elicited by a standard diagnostic test. A greater understanding of the common variations after a stroke by clinical examination and by trial and error has produced a greater predictability. Very careful clinical examination must be carried out. This clinical examination must be carried out in the particular posture in which the function being assessed is normally performed, thus if one is looking at the lower limb then the clinical examination and assessment must be carried out with the patient in an upright functional position and preferably during walking. Examination with the patient supine on the examination couch has no part to play. Examination during walking also implies that the treatment programme for each patient has to be designed and adapted to the particular disturbance in each individual case.

With regard to the upper limbs if the function being analysed is normally carried out in the sitting position then the examination should be with the patient sitting, if it is with the patient standing then the examination should be with the patient standing. There are very substantial variations from day to day because of alterations in temperature, humidity and, more particularly, in the temperament of the patient. If the patient is tense the spasticity will be more marked, if the patient is temperamentally relaxed the spasticity will be decreased. This means that before embarking on any surgical treatment the patient should be examined on several occasions by different people and an overall evaluation made.

The use of local nerve blocks to obliterate spastic obstruction, particularly in the upper limb, has most certainly produced a very distinct advance allowing an accurate assessment of whether there is any underlying activity in the antagonist group of muscles and the strength of this activity. This allows a decision to be made whether merely a total release or a specific elongation be done where there is antagonistic activity, or whether a transfer of an overacting muscle to perform an absent antagonist function should be carried out. Perhaps, more importantly, it shows the patient exactly what the operation can achieve. It is important to remember that these people have had an absolutely shattering experience and may be totally alien to any form of intervention no matter how carefully it is explained; actually to see an improvement may well be the turning point.

The greatest benefit from using local nerve blocks has been the ability to differentiate between a deformity due to spasticity and deformity due to a contracture, that is a true muscle tendon or joint capsule shortening. The results of surgery for spastic deformity are infinitely better than in those cases where there is a true contracture. Provided that after careful assessment a true muscle balance is achieved after surgery for spasticity, it is extremely rare for a further deformity to appear. However, in cases where there is a contracture there is a very marked tendency for contractures to recur even after extensive treatment either be stretching or by surgical intervention. The tendency, therefore, is not to hope for improvement in function where there is a contracture but to be very hopeful for an increase in function where one is dealing with a spastic deformity. The other great advance is the analysis of dynamic electromyography using wire electrodes introduced into muscles and telemetric transmission. Muscle activity can be recorded and, more importantly, the phasing of muscle activity can be timed. This technique has been developed extensively by Perry (Perry *et al.* 1974, Perry & Hoffer 1977) and surely represents one of the greatest advances that there has been in this particular problem. The use of dynamic electromyography certainly increases the predictability of any operative intervention.

Surgical treatment of the upper limb

The painful shoulder

The painful shoulder is a major impairment to the entire rehabilitation programme because the patient with an adducted, medially rotated, painful shoulder makes no attempt to use the affected arm and often fails to participate in walking training. The pain often persists in spite of early onset of positioning and active assisted exercises. Caldwell *et al.* (1969) found that of 100 hemiplegic patients no less that 70 had painful shoulders; the pain subsided in 30 of these patients after treatment to improve the range of movement; 15 patients were found to have common orthopaedic causes for their pain, such as tendinitis or bursitis, but 25 patients were left with remarkably painful contractures. On careful examination it was found that most of the

spasticity was in the subscapularis muscle and to a lesser extent in the pectoralis major. Therefore an operation was devised to divide both these muscles. The subscapularis tendon was dissected from the anterior capsule and then resected leaving the capsule intact. The tendon of pectoralis major was transected at its insertion. This operation has proved to be very beneficial in terms of relief of pain and also in producing an increase in abduction and lateral rotation of the shoulder (Braun *et al.* 1971).

The subluxating shoulder has frequently been considered a major problem. The author has found that downward subluxation of the shoulder was only a feature immediately after the stroke when there was considerable muscle flaccidity. If a programme of assisted active movement is embarked upon then, as the muscle tone returns, the incidence of subluxation gets progressively less and the condition becomes extremely rare when the patients are reviewed after neurological stabilization has occurred.

The flexed spastic elbow

The habitual posture of the hemiplegic arm usually includes considerable flexion of the elbow which is particularly marked during walking. Severe spasticity of the flexors does not respond to remedial exercises. The deformity is unsightly and prevents the patients from positioning the hand appropriately while attempting purposeful grasp. If the problem is purely one of spasticity musculocutaneous neurectomy will decrease the deformity (Garland *et al.* 1980). The technique of musculocutaneous neurectomy is that an incision is made over the deltopectoral groove which is opened up, the coracobrachialis tendon arising from the tip of the coracoid is identified and the musculocutaneous nerve is found as it approaches the medial side of this muscle during the course of its first 5cm, the exact point of entry is very variable. The nerve is then transected.

Where the deformity is partly due to spasticity and partly to true flexion contracture the deformity can be reduced by division of the brachialis with or without lengthening the biceps tendon. The brachialis is exposed with an incision lateral to the biceps tendon above the elbow, the brachialis muscle lies immediately behind the tendon, the muscle belly is transected horizontally about two inches above the elbow joint. The biceps tendon is lengthened in a routine 'Z' plasty fashion if this is necessary.

In the author's experience, where there is a true contracture of the anterior capsule of the elbow, capsulectomy has not proved to be very satisfactory. Almost invariably there is a recurrence of the deformity because very frequently in these patients there is no activity in the triceps and extension of the elbow is merely gravity assisted. This does not seem to be strong enough to counteract the overactivity of the elbow flexors.

extremely difficult to clean and it can have a very unpleasant odour. This is a clear indication for surgical correction. Some patients would rather have a somewhat floppy hand than the fairly easily recognized deformity of the flexed wrist and fingers and this may also be an indication for surgical intervention. The operation of choice is a flexor slide which involves elevation of all the forearm muscles from the bones and interosseous membrane, an extensive procedure.

In some patients, after careful evaluation and particularly after assessment using local anaesthetic nerve blocks, it may be felt that there is potential for improving function by selected tendon elongations and tendon transfers. One common situation is where there is flexion of the wrist and fingers but no action of the extensors. Some of this flexion control may be reflex and some voluntary. In these circumstances it is poss-

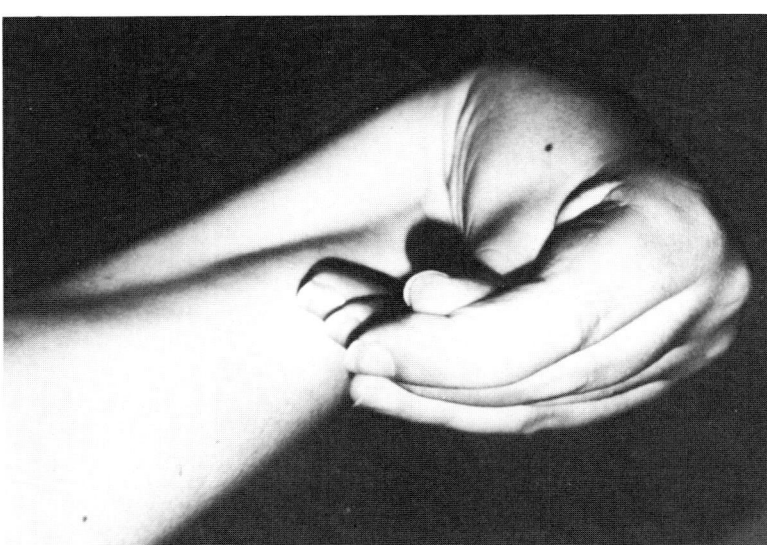

Fig. 12.4. Severe spastic hand deformity (pre-operative).

Flexion of the wrist and fingers (Fig. 12.4)

There are two main indications for surgical intervention for flexion of the wrist and fingers. One is to improve cosmesis and hygiene and the second is to try and improve function (Chapter 11). When the deformity is severe the fingers become firmly embedded in the palm and as the palm sweats the hand becomes macerated. It is

ible to lengthen the flexor tendons to the fingers and the thumb individually, and to place the hand into the position of rest transfer the wrist flexors into the extensors. Flexor tendon lengthening is carried out through a longitudinal midline incision on the volar aspect of the forearm, the muscle tendon junction of the muscle to be lengthened is exposed and identified; the tendon is then separated from the muscle belly. It is normally a long attachment of about two inches, and if the muscle fibres are detached from the tendon it is then possible to slide the tendon distally down the muscle belly and then resuture it in place at the appropriate length with the fingers in the desired position (Fig. 12.5). When the wrist flexors are required to be transferred into the wrist extensors the incision is made on the radial side of the volar aspect of the wrist joint and flexor carpi radialis is identified and detached from its insertion. An incision is made on the radial side of the dorsal aspect of the wrist and extensor carpi radialis longus and brevis are identified, a subcutaneous tunnel is then fashioned between the volar and the dorsal aspect of the forearm and the flexor carpi radialis is rerouted through the tunnel and brought out on to the dorsum of the wrist. The end of this tendon is then tunnelled through the side of extensor carpi radialis longus and brevis and is sutured *in situ* with the wrist held maximally dorsiflexed.

lent functional result, especially in the rare cases with almost normal sensation.

Surgical treatment of the lower limb

Operations on the lower limb fall into two main groups. The first involves purely destructive surgery. These are the cases where there is a very severe motor cortical lesion which has left purely primitive reflex arcs. The indication here is to facilitate nursing care. Where there is a mass withdrawal response with very severe spasticity, secondary joint contractures very frequently develop and the care of the perineum and the prevention of bedsores become a great problem. To get rid of the hip flexion, iliopsoas release, adductor release and obturator neurectomy are indicated. These operations are all carried out through an incision parallel to and just below the flexor crease in the groin. In an adductor release, adductor longus and gracilis are usually divided,

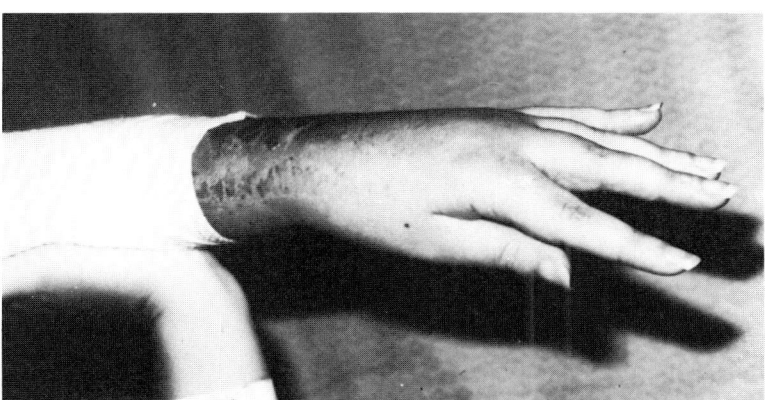

Fig. 12.5. Same hand as shown in Fig. 12.4 after flexor slide procedure.

Some patients do obtain some voluntary movement after this operation but the usual useful recovery results from a tenodesis effect: as the wrist is allowed to drop into flexion the fingers extend and as the wrist comes up into extension so the fingers flex. This gives a useful grasp and release. In the fairly rare circumstance where the finger flexors are spastic but there is an underlying extension activity for the wrist and fingers, it is possible merely to do flexor tendon lengthening procedures. This will produce an excel-

the other adductor muscles are only divided if they are manifestly tight. The division is made at the level of their origin from the pubic bone. Iliopsoas is identified at its insertion to the lesser trochanter and the tendon is divided immediately adjacent to its insertion. The obturator nerve is found three inches distal to the origin of adductor longus running between adductor longus and magnus. In order to make sure that an adequate neurectomy is carried out normally an inch of the nerve is resected.

For pronounced knee flexion contracture hamstring tenotomies are used. Hamstring tenotomies and lengthening are usually performed distally at the muscle tendon junction just proximal to the popliteal fossa and the posterior aspect of the femur through longitudinal incisions.

The other indication for operation is in patients who have usable reflex activity or in whom muscles which are under voluntary control are sufficiently spastic as to interfere with the normal function of the hip. Commonly, as the patient tries to walk, there is overriding spasticity in the adductors which overpower the abductors producing a scissoring gait. This is treated by releasing those adductors which are overacting, at their origin from the pubic bone. If the spasticity is very marked then anterior obturator neurectomy may well be beneficial.

The most common problem which arises at the knee is persistent extension due to spasticity in the quadriceps muscle. This can be alleviated by distal division of one of the heads of the quadriceps muscle as described by Waters *et al.* (1979). Knee flexion is very rarely a problem but when it does arise, a hamstring elongation seems to be a more appropriate operation than the Eggers transfer of the hamstrings into the femur.

The ankle and foot

One of the most common deformities after a stroke is equinovarus of the involved foot. This deformity is produced by hypertonicity in the plantar flexors and invertors, and paresis of the dorsiflexors and evertors of the foot. If otherwise unimpaired, patients with this deformity can walk although the gait is laborious and unsafe. There is an 8% incidence of fracture around the hip in hemiplegics due to falling (Treanor & Reifenstein 1961). The objectives of the operation are to allow enough dorsiflexion of the foot to give adequate toe clearance during the swing phase of gait and to produce the correct angle at the ankle so that if possible heel strike is achieved, or failing this, a flatfooted gait

is produced. By balancing the dorsiflexion in the neutral position a stable platform for acceptance of weight can be obtained.

In order to produce surgical correction two elements have to be tackled. The first is the spastic equinus which may be caused by two muscles, the soleus and gastrocnemius. In order to try to decide which of these two muscles is the predominant deforming force, most clinicians use the Silfverskiöld technique (Silfverskiöld 1923–4). Because only the gastrocnemius crosses the knee, spastic equinus that occurs with extension but not with flexion is attributed to this muscle. If the position of the knee makes no difference the soleus is credited. Anyone who has any experience in the problem and who has attempted specific release of individual muscles rapidly realizes the use of this test will give thoroughly inconsistent results. This is one situation in which a walking electromyograph allows the surgeon to come to a precise differential diagnosis. An appropriate operation based on this analysis of the obstructive spastic equinus gives excellent results (Perry *et al.* 1974). Where such an electromyograph is not available most surgeons now would elect for elongation of the Achilles tendon. In the author's experience the most satisfactory method is a percutaneous triple-cut lengthening as described by Mooney and Goodman (1969). Only where there is a muscle tendon shortness (that is, a true contracture) has he found it necessary to use an open slide technique as described by White (1943), and Banks and Green (1958). In a triple-cut operation, the most distal incision is on the medial aspect of the tendon just above its insertion into the os calcis. A second incision is made on the lateral aspect in the middle of the palpable mass and a third incision on the medial aspect of the muscle tendon junction. The foot is then forcibly dorsiflexed to provide new length. Any varus of the heel is almost certainly due to spasticity in tibialis posterior and this is best treated by simple division of the tendon immediately behind the medial malleolus.

As a result of the EMG studies it has become clear that the forefoot varus is due to overactivity of the tibialis anterior muscle (Fig. 12.6). The most satisfactory operation to correct this deformity has been found to be a split tibialis anterior transfer (Fig. 12.7, 12.8). The rationale for a split transfer is to avoid overcorrection and yet to supply appropriate dynamic corrective tension. Merely transferring the tibialis anterior tendon to the middle of the dorsum of the foot or to the lateral aspect of the foot has proven to be unsatisfactory because the exact placing of the transfer has to be very precise with very little margin for error and one frequently finishes up with either the original deformity or, even worse, the opposite deformity. Patients appropriate for this operation are those in whom the equinovarus posture cannot be corrected by bracing but who have minimal deformity due to spasticity and could become free of the brace and revert to a fairly normal gait as a result of the operation. The patient with selective motor control sufficient to override his postural patterns is able to plantarflex and dorsiflex his foot to some degree with the knee extended even though the foot is in varus. He should be able to discard the

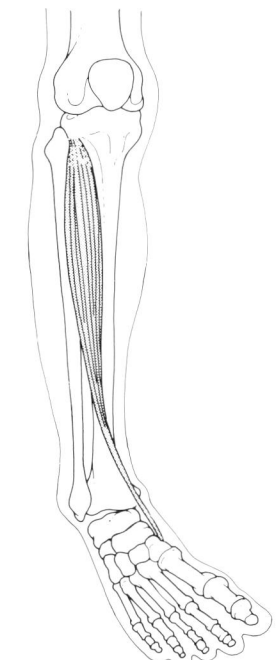

Fig. 12.6. Diagram of varus foot caused by isolated anterior tibialis pull.

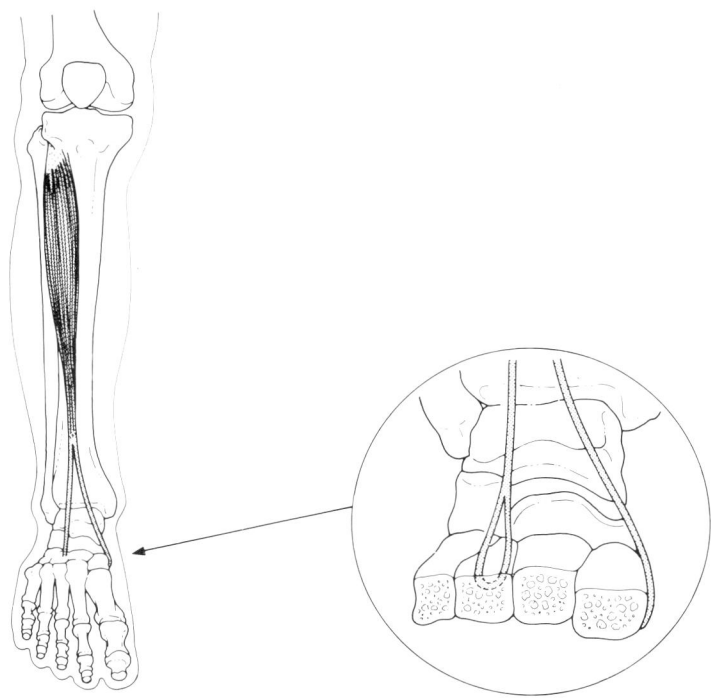

Fig. 12.7. Diagram of rerouting split anterior tibialis tendon to balance dorsiflexion.

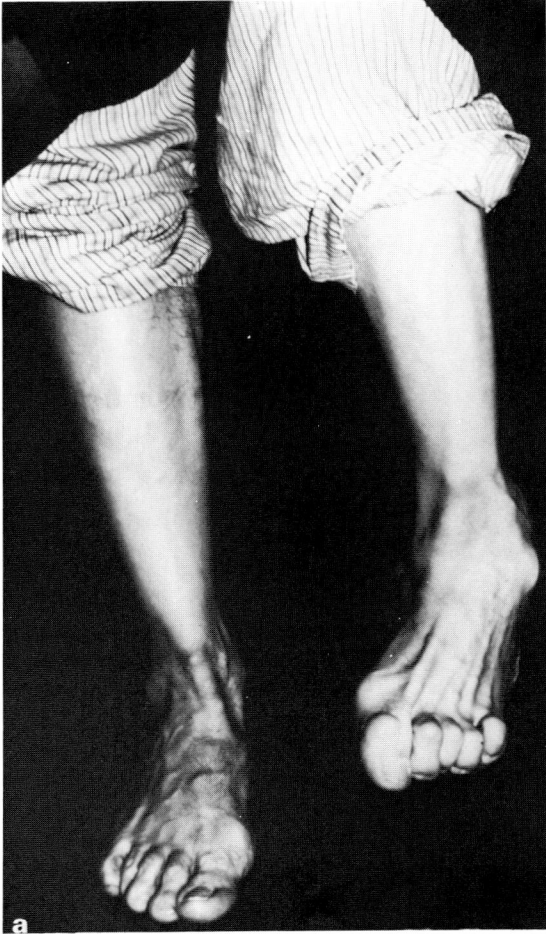
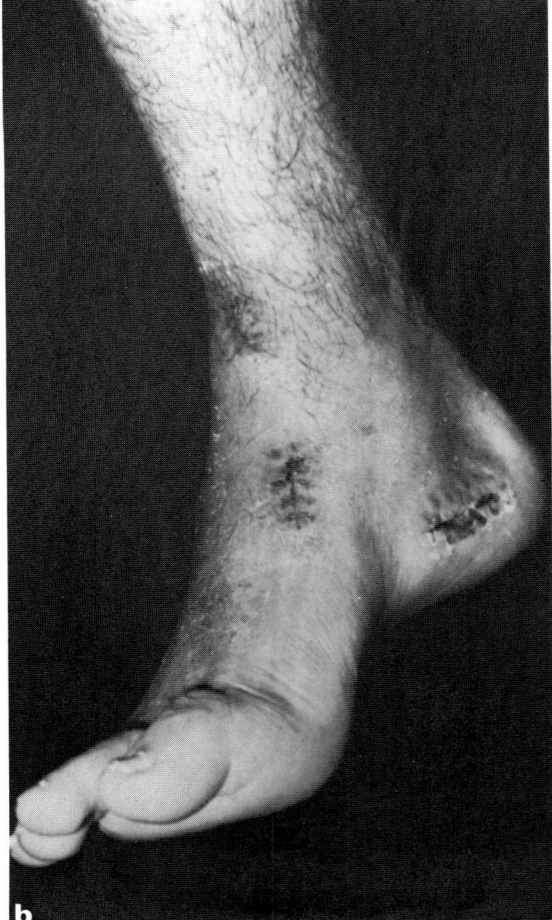

Fig. 12.8. (a) Equinovarus deformity with claw toes and adducted heel.
(b) Postoperative photograph showing the scars of split anterior tendon transfer and tibialis posterior release.

brace after the operation. Those patients who have insufficient selective control to overwhelm their primitive postural patterns may also avoid a brace provided that their reflex can be initiated at the appropriate point in the gait cycle. In those patients where the action of tibialis anterior in the flexor pattern is insufficient to allow clearance of the forefoot in the swing phase of gait, bracing will still be required.

For the transfer, an incision is made over the insertion of the tibialis anterior*. The lateral half of the tendon is separated and divided at its insertion. An incision is then made over the tibialis anterior tendon five centimetres above the ankle and the divided lateral part of the tendon withdrawn through the more proximal wound. An incision is made over the third cuneiform and the tendon is passed distally subcutaneously into this third incision. Two drill holes are made in the cuneiform angled towards each other and joined in the depth of the bone. The bony bridge must be maintained between these two drill holes. The tendon is passed through this bony tunnel, the foot is maximally

---

* The technique is slightly different to that described on page 176.

dorsiflexed and the tendon is pulled as tightly as possible and sutured to itself. A below-knee walking plaster is maintained for six weeks after which a protective plastic orthosis is worn for a further six weeks, We have reviewed our own series of patients all of whom had reached a neurologically stable state and had had intensive physiotherapy before operation. Out of a group of 60 patients there were six who could not walk before this operation, and were able to do so afterwards. All the patients achieved dorsiflexion during walking, We used a classification of the degree of spasticity according to a scale, 0 = none, 1 = increased stretch reflex, 2 = moderate clonus, 3 = severe clonus, to compare the degree of spasticity before operation with that found after operation. We found that overall the spasticity in the calf muscles was reduced by 60% by elongation of the Achilles tendon.

All the patients were able to walk significantly faster after the operation. We found that the best results were achieved if operation was carried out four to six months after their stroke, and that the younger the patient, the better the result. As a result of longterm review we have found that if improvement is achieved then it is maintained. Any deterioration implies that there has been a further episode of cerebrovascular damage. On a more recent review we have found that after elongation of the Achilles tendon and a split tibialis anterior transfer 10% of patients were able to discard walking aids, 24% were able to discard all aids.

Perhaps the most painful deformity after a stroke is clawing of the toes, usually of the lateral four toes, but occasionally there is a significant deformity of the great toe which frequently gives rise to blisters and callosities and quite often to infected paronychia. This deformity is easily corrected by the Girdlestone flexor to extensor transfer. Girdlestone flexor to extensor transfers are carried out through dorsolateral incisions over the base of the proximal phalanges of the appropriate toes. The flexor sheath is incised, the flexor sublimus tendon is identified and divided at the insertion of the two slips into the middle

phalanx. The longus tendon is identified, is divided at the level of the proximal interphalangeal joint, and a black silk suture is introduced through the end of the tendon. The extensor tendon is then identified distal to the proximal interphalangeal joint and an end to side suture of the flexor longus tendon to the extensor tendon is carried out. The toes are immobilized for six weeks.

Conclusions

Rehabilitation of the patient after a stroke is now accepted practice. It is clear that the best results are obtained if the rehabilitation process, which should consist of early positioning, early physiotherapy and bracing as necessary, is started immediately after the stroke. Surgery does have a part to play once a stable neurological state has been reached. By using careful clinical assessment, local nerve blocks and dynamic EMG studies, the indications for surgery are becoming more clear-cut and the results more predictable. The advances in the future will undoubtedly come from a clearer understanding of the neurophysiology of strokes and in the use of functional electrical stimulation for more precise diagnosis.

References

ACHESON R.M. & FAIRBAIRN A.S. (1970) Burden of cerebrovascular disease in the Oxford area in 1963 and 1964. *British Medical Journal,* 11, 621–6.

BANKS H.H. & GREEN W.T. (1985) The correction of equinus deformity in cerebral palsy. *Journal of Bone and Joint Surgery,* 40A, 1359–79.

BECK C.H. & CHAMBERS W.W. (1970) Speed, accuracy and strength of forelimb movement after unilateral pyramidotomy in Rhesus monkeys. *Journal of Comparative and Physiological Psychology,* 70, 1–22.

BOGARDH E. & RICHARDS C. (1974) Gait analysis and relearning of gait control in hemiplegic patients. In *Seventh International Congress of the World Confederation for Physical Therapy,* Montreal, 443.

BOWMAN B.R., BAKER L.L. & WATERS R.L. (1979) Positional feedback and electrical stimulation: an automated treatment for the hemiplegic wrist. *Archives of Physical Medicine and Rehabilitation,* 60, 497–502.

BRAUN R.M., WEST F., MOONEY V., NICKEL V.L., ROPER B. & CALDWELL C. (1971) Surgical treatment of the painful shoulder contracture in the stroke patient. *Journal of Bone and Joint Surgery*, **53A**, 1307–12.

BRUNNSTROM S. (1964) Recording gait patterns of adult hemiplegic patients. *Journal of the American Physical Therapy Association*, **44**, 11–8.

BUCY P.C., LADPLI R. & EHRLICH A. (1966) Destruction of the pyramidal tract in the monkey: the effects of bilateral section of the cerebral peduncles. *Journal of Neurosurgery*, **25**, 1–23.

CALDWELL C.B., WILSON D.J. & BRAUN R.M. (1969) Evaluation and treatment of the upper extremity in the hemiplegic stroke patient. *Clinical Orthopaedics and Related Research*, **63**, 69–93.

CALNE D.B. (1975) Drug treatment of spasticity and rigidity. In *Modern Trends in Neurology*, 6 (ed. D. Williams) pp. 205–21. Butterworth & Co., London.

CARLSÖÖ S., DAHLÖFF A.-G. & HOLM J. (1974) Kinetic analysis of the gait in patients with hemiparesis and in patients with intermittent claudication. *Scandinavian Journal of Rehabilitation Medicine*, **6**, 166–79.

COPP E.P., KEENAN J. (1972) Phenol nerve and motor point block in spasticity. *Rheumatology and Physical Medicine*, **11**, 287–92.

DIETRICHSON P. (1971) Phasic ankle reflex in spasticity and Parkinsonian rigidity. The role of the fusimotor system. *Acta Neurologica Scandinavica*, **47**, 22–51.

DIMITRIJEVIĆ M.R. & NATHAN P.W. (1967) Studies of spasticity in man. Some features of spasticity. *Brain*, 90, 1–30.

DIMITRIJEVIĆ M.R., GRAĆANIN F., PREVEC T. & TRONTELI J. (1968) Electronic control of paralysed extremities. *Biomedical Engineering*, **3**, 8–14.

DRILLIS R. (1958) Objective recording and biomechanics of pathological gait. *Annals of the New York Academy of Science*, **74**, 86–109.

FINLEY F.R. & KARPOVICH P.V. (1964) Electromagnetic analysis of normal and pathological gaits. *Research Quarterly of the American Association for Health, Physical Education and Recreation*, **35**, 379–84.

GARLAND D.E., THOMPSON R. & WATERS R.L. (1980) Musculocutaneous neurectomy for spastic elbow flexion in nonfunctional upper extremities in adults. *Journal of Bone and Joint Surgery*, **62A**, 108–12.

GRANIT R.A. (1970) *The Basis of Motor Control*. Academic Press, London.

HIRSCHBERG G.G. & NATHANSON M. (1952) Electromyographic recording of muscular activity in normal and spastic gaits. *Archives of Physical Medicine*, **33**, 217–25.

KHALILI A.A. & BETTS H.B. (1967) Peripheral nerve block with phenol in the management of spasticity. *Journal of the American Medical Association*, **200**, 1155–7.

KHALILI A.A., HARMEL M.H., FORSTER S. & BENTON J.G. (1964) Management of spasticity by selective peripheral nerve block with dilute phenol solutions in clinical rehabilitation. *Archives of Physical Medicine*, **45**, 513–9.

KNUTSSON E. & RICHARDS C. (1979) Different types of disturbed motor control in gait of hemiparetic patients. *Brain*, **102**, 405–30.

LIBERSON W.T., HOLMQUEST H.J. & HALLS A. (1962) Accelerographic study of gait. *Archives of Physical Medicine and Rehabilitation*, **43**, 547–51.

MARKS M. & HIRSCHBERG G.G. (1958) Analysis of the hemiplegic gait. *Annals of the New York Academy of Science*, **74**, 59–77.

MATTHEWS W.B. (1975) *Practical Neurology*, 3rd ed. Blackwell Scientific Publications, London.

MATTHEWS W.B. (1966) Ratio of maximum H reflex to maximum H response as a measure of spasticity. *Journal of Neurology, Neurosurgery and Psychiatry*, **29**, 201–4.

McLELLAN D.L. (1973) Dynamic spindle reflexes and the rigidity of Parkinsonism. *Journal of Neurology, Neurosurgery and Psychiatry*, **36**, 342–49.

MOONEY V. & GOODMAN F. (1969) Surgical approaches to lower extremity disability secondary to strokes. *Clinical Orthopaedics and Related Research*, **63**, 142–52.

MOONEY V., FRYKMAN G. & McLAMB J. (1969) Current status of intraneural phenol injections. *Clinical Orthopaedics and Related Research*, **63**, 122–31.

MURRAY M.P. & CLARKSON B.H. (1966) The vertical pathways of the foot during level walking. II Clinical examples of distorted pathways. *Journal of American Physical Therapy Associations*, **46**, 590–9.

NELSON H.E. JR., SMITH M.B., BOWMAN B.R. & WATERS R.L. (1980) Electrode effectiveness during transcutaneous motor stimulation. *Archives of Physical Medicine and Rehabilitation*, **61**, 73–7.

NICHOLS P.J.R. (1980) Strokes. In *Rehabilitation Medicine*, 2nd ed. pp. 159–81. Butterworth & Co., London.

PEAT M., DUBO H.I.C., WINTER D.A., QUANBURY A.O., STEINKE T. & GRAHAME R. (1976) Electromyographic temporal analysis of gait: hemiplegic locomotion. *Archives of Physical Medicine and Rehabilitation*, **57**, 421–5.

PERRY J. (1969a) The mechanics of walking in hemiplegia. *Clinical Orthopaedics and Related Research*, **62**, 23–31.

PERRY J. (1969b) Lower extremity bracing in hemiplegia. *Clinical Orthopaedics and Related Research*, **63**, 32–8.

PERRY J., GIOVAN P., HARRIS L.J., MONTGOMERY J. & AZARIA M. (1978) The determinants of muscle action in the hemiparetic lower extremity and their effect on the examination procedure. *Clinical Orthopaedics and Related Research*, **131**, 71–89.

PERRY J. & HOFFER M.M. (1977) Preoperative and post-operative dynamic electromyography as an aid in planning tendon transfers in children with cerebral palsy. *Journal of Bone and Joint Surgery*, **59A**, 531–7.

PERRY J., HOFFER M.M., GIOVAN P., ARTONELLI D. & GREENBERG R. (1974) Gait analysis of the triceps surae in cerebral palsy. A preoperative and postoperative clinical and electromyographic study. *Journal of Bone and Joint Surgery*, **56A**, 511–20.

SILFVERSKIÖLD N. (1923–1924) Reduction of the uncrossed two-joints muscles of the leg to one-joint muscles in spastic conditions. *Acta Chirurgica Scandinavica*, **56**, 315–30.

TRAVIS A.M. & WOOLSEY C.N. (1956) Motor performance of monkeys after bilateral partial and total cerebral decortications. *American Journal of Physical Medicine*, **35**, 273–310.

TREANOR W.J. & REIFENSTEIN G.H. (1961) Potential reversibility of the hemiplegic posture. *American Journal of Cardiology*, **7**, 370–8.

TWITCHELL T.E. (1951) The restoration of motor function following hemiplegia in man. *Brain,* **74,** 443–80.

VODOVNIK L., KRALJ A., STANIC U., ACIMOVIC R. & GROS N. (1978) Recent applications of functional electrical stimulation to stroke patients in Ljubljana. *Clinical Orthopaedics and Related Research,* **131,** 64–70.

WATERS R.L., GARLAND D.E., PERRY J., HABIG T. & SLABAUGH P. (1979) Stiff-leg gait in hemiplegia: surgical correction. *Journal of Bone and Joint Surgery,* **61A,** 927–33.

WHITE J.W. (1943) Torsion of the Achilles tendon: its surgical significance. *Archives of Surgery,* **46,** 784–7.

Index